£12.9

OCCUPATIONAL THERAPY WITH THE ELDERLY

OCCUPATIONAL THERAPY WITH THE ELDERLY

Edited by

MARJORIE HELM DipCOT SROT

Head Occupational Therapist,
Astley Ainslie Hospital, Edinburgh

Churchill Livingstone 🏛️

EDINBURGH LONDON MELBOURNE AND NEW YORK 1987

599/93809

CHURCHILL LIVINGSTONE
Medical Division of Longman Group Limited

Distributed in the United States of America by Churchill
Livingstone Inc., 1560 Broadway, New York, N.Y. 10036,
and by associated companies, branches and
representatives throughout the world.

First published 1987

ISBN 0-443-03469-9

British Library Cataloguing in Publication Data
Occupational therapy with the elderly.
  1. Occupational therapy 2. Aged
  I. Helm, Marjorie
  615.8′5152   RM735

Library of Congress Cataloging in Publication Data
Occupational therapy with the elderly.
  Includes index.
  1. Occupational therapy for the aged. 2. Aged —
Rehabilitation. I. Helm, Marjorie. [DNLM: 1. Occupa-
tional Therapy — in old age. WB 555 0158]
RC953.8.022025 1987   615.8′515′0880565 86–32741

Produced by Longman Singapore Publishers (Pte) Ltd.
Printed in Singapore

Preface

The occupational therapy profession views the treatment of a large ageing population in a progressive, positive and optimistic manner which, it is hoped, will be reflected in the following chapters.

Fifteen years ago my introduction to elderly patients came as a visiting occupational therapy student to a ward for old people of mixed abilities. Some would return home, but others were destined for long-term care. I noticed that nothing but the most rudimentary occupational therapy treatment was given — purses to be thonged were handed out to a group of elderly ladies, and the thonging was removed again by the therapist and her student back in the occupational therapy department. This stimulating hour's activity took place once a week!

At that time I thought there has to be something better than this: and happily it can now be said that there is. In *Occupational Therapy with the Elderly* modern, dynamic approaches will be described, advice given and solutions suggested.

There seems to be no better way to illustrate the need for this book, with its descriptions of services for elderly people, than to quote verbatim the story of Miss Reed, which happened as recently as 1982, to remind us that even now mistakes can be made and the elderly and their carers can suffer quite needlessly. In the population of over-65-year olds in the United Kingdom, females exceed males by two thirds; therefore the patient/client will be referred to as 'she' throughout the book.

Miss Reed's story
(related in August 1984)

Although it is now some nineteen months since my mother died at the age of 94, I still keep wondering whether there was anything more my sister (67) and I (70) could have done to have made her more comfortable. She was very fit and active until she was 89 but then she fell during one night and broke her femur or pelvis. (We were never told which — and neither was my mother!) Up till then she had done most of the housework and all the cooking, and it was very difficult for her after the fall to watch us trying to cope. But she still did as much as she could — including dressmaking.

Unfortunately, though, she was not able to walk without a zimmer after she came out of hospital as her leg never healed properly, and later on she required a walking trolley. During the operation I understand the pin had not been inserted correctly and she had to go back from the convalescent hospital to the general hospital to have it removed. She was then sent back to convalesce again but had to remain in hospital much longer than should have been necessary.

Overall, my mother suffered from the following complaints: myxoedema since 1948, severe anaemia, diverticulitis, arthritis of the hands and knees, osteoarthritis of the spine, incontinence, partial deafness, cataract operation on one eye two or three years before her death. (She had a haemorrhage in the other eye which was inoperable.)

Looking back I feel that we were not given very much support from the authorities. We were loaned a commode from the hospital and an orthopaedic chair from the social work department, after I had approached our doctor. I had previously done voluntary work for about two years with Age Concern after doing 20 weeks' training, so had it not been for that I do not know what we would have done, as our doctor at that time knew very little. Actually he was not very well himself and subsequently retired.

My mother also received a day attendance allowance which I applied for on her behalf, but again, had it not been for Age Concern, we would never have known about it. I also applied later for a night attendance allowance but my mother died before arrangements could be made for a doctor to examine her.

From the beginning of October 1982, when we knew that my mother had osteoarthritis of the spine, she was confined to her bed most of the time. I kept worrying because she was never comfortable either in or out of bed, and asked the doctor whether we could have a nurse to help her wash and perhaps to make her more comfortable. At the beginning of December we managed to get a nurse once a fortnight to wash my mother. Previous to this, she had twice fallen out of bed and our new doctor did arrange for bars to be fixed to the floor in front of the bed to prevent her falling out.

But as the bed was a double one and against the wall, this made it very awkward for my mother to get up to the commode, as she then had to get out at the foot of the bed where there were no bars. In turn this made it difficult for my sister and me to get her back to bed, as we had to start at the foot of the bed and push and pull her up — not very comfortable for her with a sore back!

I have practically no power in my left hand and arm (the result of radiotherapy) and my sister broke her pelvis and arm in a road accident, so neither of us was really very able; and as my mother got weaker, it became more and more difficult for us to manage — especially as by this time my mother was becoming incontinent and much less able to help herself.

During this time the nurse never assisted in making my mother's bed. Perhaps this was beyond her duties — I do not know! Now I keep wondering why I did not phone the health visitor and I am sorry this idea did not occur to me at the time. It would also have been very nice for my mother to have had an outside visitor. The doctor did say that we should think about getting a private nurse, but both my mother and I could not see how this would work as she would sleep for periods during the day and did not need any attention. The nurse would probably not have been there when she was needed.

I thought it would help my mother if she got through to the living-room and sat in different surroundings, so I arranged to hire a wheelchair from the Red Cross so that we could wheel her through. Our hall was ten yards long so she could not possibly have managed to walk. This was just before Christmas but unfortunately the chair was never used as by then my mother was too weak. We also bought an orthopaedic chair in the previous October for £170 because she was never comfortable in the chair from the social work department. Unfortunately this new chair was never used either.

Before hiring the wheelchair from the Red Cross, I was in touch with the orthopaedic clinic who were very helpful. It was from them I discovered that physiotherapists visited patients in their own homes when necessary, and I was most upset to think that my mother had been unable to avail herself of this service when she came home from hospital. She had great spirit and practised walking up and down the three steps to our back garden. I used to wish that we had someone capable of helping her and to this day it makes me extremely angry to think I did not have the sense to think of finding out about a physiotherapist myself. My mother so wanted to help herself and it is disgraceful to think that there were facilities available and we were unable to take advantage of them. It may be that we had too much to do to think clearly!

I might just add that a few years before my mother's back got so bad, I made arrangements for her to have some teeth out. After various phone calls trying to find the right person to contact, a dentist and a nurse came at my request. We paid for this to be done and then our own dentist came to the house to make new dentures for her. The same thing happened when she required new glasses. Our own optician agreed to come to the house. In addition, I arranged for a hairdresser to do my mother's hair until she was too ill to have it done, and I also arranged for a chiropodist to visit her.

For some reason, it was always the doctor's assistant who came to see her, and although I often mentioned that my mother would like to see her own doctor, it was still the assistant who came. Now, too late, I think that I should have insisted on her seeing the doctor with whom she was registered.

You will gather from the above that not a lot of help was offered to us and it was a continual struggle to get the necessary help. Our feeling towards the end was one of helplessness and aloneness, and my mother felt the same way.

Conclusion

This story shows that sometimes, in spite of availability of back-up services, it is possible for elderly people to slip through the 'care agencies' net. It is the aim of this book to alert all health care workers so that such a tale or one of similar mismanagement need never again be told.

Edinburgh, 1987   M. H.

Dedication of this book comes in three parts:

Firstly to Miss Reed and all other unsung heroines and (some heroes) who strive to care for elderly relatives.

Secondly to one of the founder members of the Edinburgh occupational therapists' interest in the elderly group, Miek Duncan, who died in 1984. She would have been an enthusiastic contributor, and I hope that the publication reflects her optimistic and original view of the subject.

Thirdly to my friend M. F. for the encouragement, advice, faith and patience shown during the past two years.

Acknowledgements

I would like to thank all occupational therapists at the local interest in the elderly group for suggesting topics for inclusion in *Occupational Therapy with the Elderly*.

Professor James Williamson was of great help in commenting on information to be included in the introduction and in the geriatric medical assessment unit chapter.

Medical ethics is a significant subject when working with elderly people and Dr Ian Thompson's approach was essential to clarify the subject simply and logically.

Dr Brian Pentland's expertise was of great value in advising on chapters with a neurological content.

I am also grateful to Mrs Evelyn McPake and to Mr B. Hunter, both of whom act as legal advisors to the Alzheimer Societies of Scotland and England. They explain patients' legal rights in the introduction. My infinite gratitude goes to Mrs Catherine Verth for typing most of the (at times indecipherable) manuscript cheerfully and uncomplainingly.

Contributors

Sheena E. E. Blair DipCOT SROT
Occupational Therapy Tutor, Royal Edinburgh Hospital

Jeanette Caspers BSOTR
Ex-Head Occupational Therapist, Princess Margaret Rose Hospital, Edinburgh, now practising in Copenhagen

Gillian Crosby DipCOT SROT
Divisional Assistant (Rehabilitation), Lothian Regional Council

Fiona G. M. Docherty DipCOT SROT
Head Occupational Therapist, Royal Victoria Hospital, Edinburgh

Isabel Duncan BA(Hons) CertSocSci CQSW
Regional Development Officer, Lothian Supported Accommodation Team; Vice-Chairman, Kirk Care Housing Association, Edinburgh

Elspet M. R. Ewing RGN LCST
Senior Speech Therapist, Astley Ainslie Hospital, Edinburgh

Anne K. G. Fraser DipCOT SROT
Head Occupational Therapist, St Columba's Hospice, Edinburgh

Roseann Gerber MChS SRCh
Edinburgh Foot Clinic & School of Chiropody, Edinburgh

Alison Glen DipCOT SROT
Senior Occupational Therapist, Royal Edinburgh Hospital

Susan Grindley DipCOT SROT
Senior Occupational Therapist, Liberton Hospital, Edinburgh

Isobel Harley DipCOT SROT
Area Occupational Therapist, Lothian Health Board, Edinburgh

Linda E. Harris DipCOT SROT
Senior Occupational Therapist, Bangour Village Hospital, West Lothian

Marjorie Helm DipCOT SROT
Head Occupational Therapist, Astley Ainslie Hospital, Edinburgh

Enid C. Henery HEC SRD
Senior Dietitian, City Hospital, Edinburgh

Norman Hood MBChB FRCPE
Consultant Physician in Geriatric Medicine, Longmore Hospital, Edinburgh

Brian K. Hunter MA(Cantab)
Solicitor

Kay Kennedy DipOTNZ SROT
Tutor, Glasgow School of Occupational Therapy

Jean J. Maclean DipCOT SROT
Lecturer in Occupational Therapy, Queen Margaret College, Edinburgh

Evelyn R. McPake MA(Hons)
Solicitor

Catriona J. C. Mason DipCOT
Regional Occupational Therapist, Lothian Region

Finola R. Meikle DipCOT SROT
Head Occupational Therapist, City Hospital, Edinburgh

Nancy Munro DipCOT SROT
Senior Occupational Therapist, Astley Ainslie Hospital, Edinburgh

Elizabeth L. Ostle DipCOT SROT
Occupational Therapist, Princess Margaret Rose Orthopaedic Hospital, Edinburgh

Carol Peterson DipCOT SROT
Senior Occupational Therapist, Astley Ainslie Hospital, Edinburgh

Margaret E. Rainey DipCOT SROT
Senior Occupational Therapist, Lothian Disabled Living Centre, Astley Ainslie Hospital, Edinburgh

Roz Reynolds DipCOT SROT
Senior Occupational Therapist, Royal Edinburgh Hospital, Edinburgh

Kathleen M. Rumney SRCN DipCOT SROT
Senior Occupational Therapist, Queensberry House Hospital, Edinburgh

Roger G. Smith MB ChB FRCPE
Senior Lecturer, Department of Geriatric Medicine, University of Edinburgh, and Honorary Consultant, Lothian Health Board

J. Rachael Trevan DipCOT SROT
Head Occupational Therapist, Acute and Elderly Services, Harrow, Middlesex

Contents

The right to know
The right to privacy
The right to treatment

Hospital patients and the law

Introduction
M. Helm

The need for this book has arisen because of the increasing life-expectancy of the population, and the simultaneous reduction of statutory or voluntary resources available to help the elderly. Those who care for the elderly often apply the adjective 'geriatric' to patients of 65 and over: but, as we know, some people are old at 60 while others remain active into their 90s. 'Being old' therefore depends as much on the life-style, personality and attitude of individuals as on their actual physical condition.

In 1900 the average lifespan was 47 years; in 1985 it was over 70 years. The following statistics illustrate the predicted growth of the ageing population in the United Kingdom:

By 2001 the number of pensioners 60–74 will decrease by 10% compared to the 1981 figure. In the same year the number aged over 75 years will increase by 14.8% and the number over 85 years by 36.2% In 2001 'old' pensioners (i.e. over 75 years) will represent half of the retired population.

In 1975 2% of the retired population were living in institutional care; by 1985 this figure had increased to 6%. This is the context in which we will have to operate over the next two decades and it is precisely here that our profession has a distinctive and vital contribution to make. The Occupational Therapy Diploma Course of 1981 defined occupational therapy as 'the treatment of physical and psychiatric conditions through specific and selected activities in order to help people

The elderly population — future dimension UK (1980)
(Source:- Office of Population Consensus and Surveys)

In thousands	1981			1991			2001		
	65+	75+	85+	65+	75+	85+	65+	75+	85+
Total	8137	3127	559	8339	3547	736	7992	3620	847
Living alone	2839	1450	266	2954	1633	349	2856	1660	400

reach their maximum level of function and independence in all aspects of daily life'. This definition most aptly describes our role in the care of the elderly. The elderly are confronted with a number of difficult problems which can so easily make them a misery to themselves and a burden to others. There is retirement, the death or incapacity of a partner, boredom, loneliness, social isolation or even, paradoxically, over-solicitude by well-meaning relatives. All these, on top of failing sight and/or hearing, unreliable memory and a general slowing down of the system, not to mention acute illness or chronic disability, can lead many to give up on life and to become totally dependent on family, the social services or the medical profession for everyday support. The last choice is often reinforced by an attitude that the doctor and his pills are the answer to all human afflictions, so one might as well hand over all responsibility and effort for one's well-being to them.

Those of us involved in producing this book submit that this attitude must be fundamentally modified, that we must encourage old people to come to terms with their disabilities. We must explain to them the need to pay much greater attention to diet (reducing fats and sweets consumption), the importance of exercise, simple self-disciplines like cutting down on alcohol and cigarettes, and any other self-help remedies appropriate to each individual case.

The purpose of this book, therefore, is to outline ways and to contribute ideas by which occupational therapists can help the elderly to help themselves, so that as many as possible can live independent and satisfying lives without relying on already over-stretched professional services.

But before describing the detail of day-to-day work, it is vital that we consider essential aspects of caring, namely, the ethical dilemmas involved.

The subject of medical ethics is huge, complex and controversial. It is not our intention to go into great detail but simply to remind readers of those ethics which especially relate to the elderly, whether in or out of hospital. *Dorland's Medical Dictionary* defines medical ethics as 'the rules or principles governing the professional conduct of physicians'. (For more detail read the 'Hippocratic oath' in the *Dictionary of Medical Ethics* 1977 by A. A. Duncan, G. R. Dunstan & R. M. Welbourn.)

In society, our ethical and moral values are governed by the 'spirit of the community', that is by a set of generally acceptable and commonly agreed rules by which we run our affairs. Ethics, besides being a guide for how we should behave towards our patients, also provides a description of patients' expectations of the medical profession and those allied to it.

The principles: Respect for persons, Justice and Beneficience has been covered in depth in *The Belmont Report* (US DHEW 1978). The Commission which prepared this report comprised health professionals, lawyers, theologians and specialists in bio-ethics. They agreed that on both general cultural grounds and in the traditions of health care, specifically health care research, the principles of Respect for persons, Justice and Beneficience are basic and fundamental. Thompson (1983) describes these principles as follows:

Respect for persons means treating people as persons with rights. In general, this means that professionals and those in a caring role have a responsibility to give people the right kind of information to enable them to make responsible choices for themselves. It means adopting an enabling rather than a controlling role, so as to facilitate individual autonomy and elicit people's full potential to help themselves. It means not turning people into dependants medically or educationally. With respect to patients in particular, it involves recognising that they have a right to know, a right to privacy (i.e. a right to the protection of their personal dignity and confidential disclosures), and a right to adequate care or treatment.

Justice or non-discrimination, means both equality of opportunity for individuals and equality of outcome for groups. For individuals justice primarily means fairness, in particular non-discrimination on the basis of sex, race, class or religion, and not taking advantage of or neglecting those who are vulnerable by virtue of extreme youth, old age, handicap or mental disorder. However, the opportunities for self-fulfilment and self-determination of individuals might have to be restricted where the common good demands this, to facilitate more equal distribution of resources, or where others may be put at risk. The political dimensions of justice in terms of equality of outcome for groups has particular relevance to health care, not only in making services acceptable and accessible to all groups in the population, but also by the exercise of political control and reverse discrimination to provide for the needs of the most vulnerable and needy groups. Justice at this level is not only concerned with rational planning of public health and the provision, for example, of a National Health Service, but demands adequate public consultation, consumer feedback and participation in the planning of services. In protecting the public from harm there may be a need for public health legislation or legal controls to sanc-tion the compulsory hospitalisation and treatment of those who are dangerous to themselves or others by virtue of serious mental disorder. It also means providing adequate facilities for their rehabilitation and taking measures to ensure professional accountability.

Beneficence relates most obviously to the duty of professionals or others to care for vulnerable individuals entrusted into their care — children, the elderly, incompetents or the mentally disordered — but it also relates to the responsibility of the professional to act as an advocate in the best interests of his clients: the role of advocacy and fiduciary responsibility go together. Secondly, it refers to the responsibility of the professional to share his knowledge and expertise for the benefit of the patient or client. Knowledge is power, and being kept in a state of ignorance may mean being kept in a state of powerlessness. Sharing knowledge is not just a matter of obtaining informed consent to treatment, but using the disclosure of relevant information as an aid to therapy and the progressive restoration of autonomy to the patient.

In the light of the foregoing, it is important to examine how we are managing in practice. In an analysis of the development of British Social and Health Care Policy for the Elderly between 1834 and 1976, Sally MacIntyre (1977) notes that policies reflect differing balances between two opposing concerns: the humanitarian view of the 'problem' of ageing, which emphasises the need for public policy to create the conditions for minimising the personal pain of growing old, and the organisational view which emphasises the need to minimise the cost to the productive sector of society of the 'burden' of the elderly as a social group.

An open-ended commitment to providing institutional care for a rising number of elderly, sick and dependent people inevitably implies an open-ended drain on our economic resources. Nevertheless, the humanitarian need to give long-term care to patients who cannot be discharged from hospital is a clear embarrassment to the organisational objectives of social and health care policy.

We have learnt from studies by Kayser Jones (1981) and Townsend (1962) that 'institutionalisation causes mental and physical deterioration', so we must consider the value of home care over hospital, and the problems involved in home care, such as:

— How can elderly people be sustained at home?
— Is it a family obligation to look after frail elderly relatives?
— Who is responsible for whom?
— Are offspring responsible solely for their parents?
— Who looks after maiden aunts?
— At what stage may the family realistically relinquish their responsiblity of an elder to professional carers?
— What are the physical, emotional, social and economic consequences of home care as opposed to hospital care, and who ought to bear the cost?

There is general agreement that it is preferable to keep elderly people functioning independently at home for as long as possible. Those who cope on their own receive much more esteem from the community than those who are dependent; and, more importantly, dependency leads to a loss of self-esteem and a reduction in the sense of personal dignity and worth. It should be remembered that, despite the prevalent attitude that 'the State' should provide for the elderly, it is still the continuing common practice for the family (mainly daughters and daughters-in-law) to look after frail and ageing parents.

Then there is the question of the ethical use of resources. In the Age Concern publication *Challenge of Ageing*, Professor Brocklehurst (1978) suggests, in his chapter 'Ageing and Health', that the health visitor trained in health education would be the best person to identify an elderly patient's problems and refer them to the appropriate professional for action. Using the age/sex register which

general practitioners are advised to keep, the health visitor trained to give health education could test special senses, assess mental state, and obtain samples of blood and urine, so that reversible and treatable conditions could be speedily identified and treated.

All too often, many straightforward complaints go unreported by the elderly population, and unnoticed by general practitioners.

In Williamson's survey, 'Old People at Home' (1964), he found, on examining patients at home, that general practitioners were aware of 60% of conditions affecting the following systems: cardiovascular, respiratory, gastrointestinal, and central nervous; however they were unaware of 60% to 80% of problems such as: impaired vision, deafness, foot troubles, urinary tract abnormalities, anaemia, depression, dementia, diabetes, and myxoedema.

Equally, the well-intentioned but somewhat fatalistic 'you've got to expect this at your age' approach of some general practitioners can undermine natural fortitude and discourage old people from revealing the symptoms they are experiencing. The elderly must be made to see that they need not expect ill health just because they are getting old, that they themselves can take steps to prevent ill health and that there is available a professional team whose purpose is to help them remain fit and independent for as long as possible.

This suggests that money spent on health education, particularly in relation to preventive measures, to assist old people to enjoy good health in old age, could reduce the amount of money needed to provide hospital care for the elderly in the future.

But probably the most difficult dilemma faced by the medical profession is that of ethics and research. Geriatricians know that it is not necessarily in an elderly patient's best interests to continue administering tests and treatments for the sake of prolonging life: for instance, radiotherapy or cytotoxic drugs may cause more suffering than the actual disease. Doctors are trained to treat patients to make them better, so to withdraw treatment and allow 'nature to take its course' goes against the ethic of that training. This dichotomy begs the following questions:

— If a patient is too ill to make her own decisions should her family be asked for their opinion?
— Should the doctor alone take the responsibility for prolonging life?
— At what point should clinical treatment be withheld to allow a patient to die in relative peace and comfort, and with dignity?

In a 1983 lecture, Dr Ian Thompson (1983a: Senior Educationist, Scottish Health Education Group) suggested that if there is no cure, the original contract between patient and doctor should be renegotiated. A covenant should be offered to provide care, friendship and palliative treatment designed to minimise the patient's pain and suffering: this care should be provided at home or in a hospice (see Ch. 21).

The object of all our endeavours, whether we are doctors, nurses, occupational therapists or belong to any other specialty, is our patient's well-being. And it is vital to remember that, however incapacitated, patients have rights.

The Right to Know (Thompson 1983b)

In some circumstances there may be an obvious conflict between the patient's right to know and the professional's duty to protect her from painful knowledge which she could not handle, e.g. where the patient is dying, has a mental illness or where accurate technical explanations may unnecessarily alarm the patient. Nevertheless, it is important to recognise that the patient has a fundamental moral (and sometimes legal) right to know. Knowledge is power, and the converse is also true, that to be systematically deprived of information is to be kept in a state of induced impotence and dependency. Recognition of the patient's right to know means the professional sharing his knowledge and expertise to facilitate the autonomy of the patient or client.

The Right to Privacy (Thompson 1983b)

Because patients are vulnerable and expose that vulnerability when they entrust themselves into the care of doctors and nurses, they have a right to expect that health professionals will protect their vulnerability. The right to privacy correlates with the duty of professionals to protect the personal dignity and confidences of those committed into their care. The right to protection of one's personal dignity may relate to the issue of physical privacy, protection of one's nakedness or protection from undue exposure to investigators or students; it also relates to respect for the particular cultural or religious practices or dietary requirements of patients.

The Right to Treatment (Thompson 1983b)

The right to treatment is normally interpreted as meaning that the patient has a right to be informed and consulted about the treatment options being offered, the right to set some limits to what is acceptable treatment, and the right to refuse treatment. The right to refuse treatment is an absolute right in law and if a patient is treated against her express wishes (unless she is mentally disordered or incompetent) the staff involved may theoretically be charged with assault. In practice, the courts tend to assume that staff are acting beneficently in the patient's best interests. However, this does not mean that the right to refuse treatment can be lightly disregarded. Further, professionals should consider whether the physical weakness of the patient or the position of being institutionalised does not prevent patients in some situations from exercising their right to refuse treatment when they are entitled to do so.

As occupational therapists, we are frequently aware of rights of the elderly: a patient's refusal to be hospitalised, her refusal to leave hospital, committal to hospital under the Mental Health Act, property rights, use of the Court of Protection for the confused, and so forth. It is inevitable in our day-to-day treatment of old people that we should have to consider all of these matters; (see Hospital patients and the law, below). What is crucial is the need to try and act in the patient's best interests at all times. We have to weigh up her wishes together with her physical capabilities and hope to find mutually acceptable solutions to her problems.

HOSPITAL PATIENTS AND THE LAW

B. Hunter and E. McPake

Hospital patients can be divided into innu-merable categories depending on the classifi-cation required. There are those who are bed-ridden and those who can get about, short-term and long-stay, in- and out-patients, surgical and medical cases, all of which can be seen at a glance or ascertained by simple questions. For present purposes the division is between those whose mental condition is relatively normal and who are capable of making decisions for themselves and those whose mental condition is in doubt or who have been diagnosed as suffering from mental disorder.

The former patients (those considered normal) are in the same position as anyone else in any field of activity. They may decide for themselves on any matter affecting their affairs; they may enter the hospital voluntarily and discharge themselves at will with or without the doctor's permission, and consent or not in their own discretion to the treatment offered. In this connection, it is the case these days that the question of whether or not consent has been truly given is coming before the Courts increasingly often both in this country and abroad, particularly in the U.S.A., and the medical profession is understandably concerned about this development. In general terms, consent must be free (i.e. obtained without coercion) and informed (i.e. the risks involved must be explained to the patient). Just what information should be offered to the patient has been differently judged in a variety of legal jurisdictions.

While in hospital the normal patient may, of course, continue to manage her business or financial affairs so long as she feels physically able to do so. If she feels that her illness may interfere with this management, she may appoint an attorney to act for her during her disability. The document dealing with this appointment is known as a Power of Attorney and is best drawn up by a solicitor, although, in England, a short statutory form of general power of attorney is available. The powers granted should be wide enough to encompass all possible contingencies and the attorney appointed should obviously be a person in whom the grantor has complete faith. The granting of the power does not prevent the grantor from acting simultaneously on her own account and the power may be withdrawn at any time solely at the discretion of the grantor, although notice of this action must be given to anyone to whom the power has been exhibited. Should the grantor at any time become mentally incapable of managing her affairs the power is automatically revoked, although in practice it will be found that its use is often continued as a matter of convenience. It is unusual, although not unknown, for the doctor in charge of a patient who has granted a power of attorney to initiate the recall, where he considers that the power is being abused. A recent development in this field has been the creation of a new (statutory) form of power of attorney which has come to be known as an enduring power of attorney. This will enable the person, who so wishes, to grant this power with a view to its indefinite continuation even should the grantor no longer be capable of acting inde-pendently. So far this is to be available only in England, but is being considered for Scotland.

Although in Scotland there may be a small number of technical cases in which married persons may be better off if their spouses do not make a will, in general, everyone having the necessary mental capacity should make a will. Obviously this advice has particular application for those contemplating serious surgery or suffering, from an incurable illness. Although in Scotland a will is valid if entirely written in the testator's own handwriting, dated and signed, it is preferable to have the will professionally drawn up and properly witnessed by two witnesses. The solicitor consulted then has the opportunity to offer advice on the consequences of the will from the point of view of the beneficiaries as well as of taxation, where appropriate. It should be noted that in Scotland spouses and children have a claim on the estate of their husband/wife/parent which cannot be defeated by testamentary provisions. In England, application to the Court can be made for an award (in the discretion of the Court for the benefit of dependants including divorced wives/husbands) where it is considered reasonable provision has not been made.

The second category of patients, where the mental capacity is in question, presents far greater difficulties. Here, further subdivision is required into those whose mental condition has led them to be detained in hospital under powers created by the Mental Health Acts or who have been sent there by Court order. These involuntary patients cannot leave the hospital of their own volition, whether or not they are considered able to make decisions for themselves, although many will eventually be discharged. The provisions of the Mental Health Acts govern their admission, detention, consent to treatment and release, along with allied matters, and should be consulted for their terms. Whether these patients are capable of managing their affairs outside the hospital will be a matter of fact and there may even be some who will be considered capable at some times and not at others. Delusions relating to a specific aspect of a person's life are not necessarily a bar to rational decisions in other fields.

It is with voluntary (so-called) mentally ill and confused elderly patients that the greatest difficulties are to be encountered. If such a development can be foreseen, there are steps which can be taken to mitigate the effects on financial and business arrangements. As previously mentioned, the power of attorney falls, where the person who granted it is no longer able to acknowledge its existence and or a mandate to the manager, allowing the relative to operate the patient's account, will remain valid. Where a bank manager knows the circumstances, he will usually co-operate in paying accounts which he knows to be genuine and which are instructed by a solicitor or close relative. If substantial investments are involved an arrangement to have the portfolio transferred into the nominee name of a bank or stockbroker can be made, which allows the management of the investments to continue without the intervention of the patient. In this way sales and reinvestments may proceed which would otherwise have to cease for want of consent.

The principal instrument whereby the management of the affairs of persons unable to deal with them on their own account is carried on, is, in Scotland, the appointment of a curator bonis. This is effected by application either to the Sheriff Court of the area in which the patient (known in this context as 'the incapax' or 'the ward') resides or to the Court of Session in Edinburgh. The person appointed is usually a professional, either an accountant or solicitor, but can be an appropriate member of the family.

Notice of the petition to appoint a curator has to be served on all near relatives who thus have an opportunity to oppose the appointment either in general or with regard to the proposed appointee. Where a sale of a house or land in the patient's name is intended, there is no way of dealing with the matter other than by such an appointment, but the procedure is an expensive one and not generally considered justified unless the estate to be administered exceeds £4000 or so in value. There is thus a very large number of small estates which are uneconomic to administer during the incapacity of their owner and it is for these that the proposed enduring power of attorney may have the greatest application. In England, a Receiver (usually the nearest relative) appointed by and acting under the supervision of the Court of Protection (a department of the High Court) performs a similar function to that of the curator in Scotland. Incidentally the court of

Protection has power to authorise the making of a will for the patient.

The curator is concerned only with the financial affairs of his ward and has no power over the person. As the person manipulating the purse-strings the curator is very often in a position to influence a decision as to where the patient shall reside, but has no legal right to make this decision. Since the patient, by definition, cannot make this decision for herself, there is an ill-defined area of difficulty here relating, for example, to the elderly patient confined to nursing home, hospital or old people's home, who tries to discharge herself. The Mental Health Acts again provide for a guardian to be appointed in suitable cases (which may well not include the confused elderly, since the criterion is 'mental disorder') and the guardian is then able to say where the patient is to reside and to compel the patient to attend for treatment or to see a medical practitioner.

It goes without saying that a curator cannot give consent for treatment to be given to his ward. Indeed, the power of the guardian in this field does not extend to this but only, as mentioned above, to requiring the patient to attend for treatment. The question of consent to treatment is, therefore, with patients in this category, one of the most difficult to resolve and one for which, with numbers of elderly confused and other so-called voluntary patients liable to increase greatly, further legislation appears necessary. Meantime, medical and legal practitioners are left to grapple with this problem on an individual basis wherever it arises. In short, the Mental Health Acts do not deal with the problems most frequently encountered, but these are, fortunately, now being looked at by a number of voluntary bodies.

In conclusion, it may be worth referring to the provisions of S.47 of the National Assistance Act 1948. This authorises, quite apart from the provisons of the Mental Health Acts, the compulsory and, if necessary, forcible removal from his home of a person who is not mentally disabled and who has committed no criminal offence. The section is rarely invoked but exists to secure care and attention for persons suffering from grave, chronic disease or being aged, infirm or physically incapacitated and living in insanitary conditions and who cannot devote to themselves or obtain the necessary care and attention. This is not to be regarded as a passport to the removal of a difficult neighbour and the section is very narrowly interpreted. It is mentioned here only that readers may be aware of its existence.

The above is intended as a general outline of some of the legal aspects relating to patients in hospital. The old saying that circumstances alter cases is nowhere more applicable than to this subject, and anyone with a specific problem should read this with this reservation in mind.

From what has been said so far, it may well be deduced that caring for the elderly is a complicated nuisance. Nothing could be further from the truth. The majority are very remarkable people, possessing tremendous fortitude and determination; and, contrary to the common view, they have strong recuperative powers which make it possible for a high proportion of them to lead independent lives, particularly if they are given the right stimulus and encouragement by their occupational therapist.

The occupational therapist who can take a genuine interest in her patient's life, not just in her clinical improvement, may well find herself doubly rewarded: firstly, by the patient recognising through the occupational therapist's interest that she is still a useful member of the community; and secondly, by what she, the occupational therapist, may learn about life from the patient. In this way occupational therapy is a most satisfying profession and, because of the multiplicity of problems involved in rehabilitating elderly patients, it is undoubtedly a most challenging one.

REFERENCES

Brocklehurst J 1978 Aging and health. In: Hobman D (ed) The social challenge of ageing. Croom Helm, London, pt 2, pp 149–172

Davis A J 1981 Ethical issues in gerontological nursing. In: Copp L A (ed) Care of the aging. Churchill Livingstone, Edinburgh, pp 38–46

Duncan A A, Dunstan G R, Welbourn R M 1977 Hippocratic oath. In: Dictionary of medical ethics. Darton Longman & Todd, London

Elderly population future dimension UK 1980 Office of Population Consensus and Surveys. Population trends 22 Winter. HMSO, London

Evers H K 1981 Tender loving care? Patients and nurses in geriatric wards. In: Copp L A (ed) Care of the aging. Churchill Livingstone, Edinburgh, pp 46–75

Harris A 1971 Handicapped and impaired in Great Britain. HMSO, London

Kayser-Jones J 1981 Old alone and neglected: care of the aged in Scotland and the United States. University of California Press, Berkeley.

MacIntyre S 1977 Old age as a social problem. In:

Dingwall R Health C, Reid M, Stacey M (eds) Health care and health knowledge. Croom Helm, London

Rossiter C, Wicks M 1982 Crisis or challenge? Study Commission on the family, London

Thompson I E 1983a Ethical issues in community based psychiatry. In: Reed J, Lomas G (eds) Psychiatric service in the community: developments and innovation. Croom Helm, London and Canberra, pp 45–46

Thompson I E 1983b Personal rights and public policy: dilemmas of health education and prevention. Paper given at the 12th World Conference on Health Education, Health Education Bureau, Dublin

Townsend P 1962 The last refuge — a survey of residential institutions and homes for the aged in England and Wales Routledge and Kegan Paul, London

US Dept of Health, Education and Welfare 1978 The Belmont Report: Ethical principles and Guidelines for the protection of human subjects of research. US DHEW Publication No (05) 78-0012

Williamson J et al 1964 Old people at home — their unpublished needs. The Lancet i: 1117–20

1

Theories of ageing and current attitudes to old age
M. Helm

THEORIES

Improved health care and living conditions in the developed world allow people the opportunity to complete their expected lifespan of more than seventy years. Women tend to live on average five years longer than men.

Gerontologists have produced several theories on what determines longevity. Leonard Hayflick (1980) of Stamford University, California has shown that certain human cells grown outside the body can only reproduce themselves accurately about 55 times. This sets a time limit on the length of human life.

The immune system of cells and antibodies protects us from disease, but this becomes less efficient as we age, and diseases such as influenza and pneumonia can kill old people.

As we get older our auto-immune system also becomes less efficient: that is to say, the body's ability to recognise its own cells can become impaired and, if it does, the body will destroy its own healthy tissue. Auto-immune disorders like carcinoma, degenerative joint disease and systemic lupus erythematosus are common in people over 65 years.

The clock theory of ageing suggests a programmer, possibly situated in the hypothalmus, which switches on and off various stages of our lives at the appropriate times. The cells of the body may have their own clocks — especially important cells being neurones which cannot reproduce and have to last a lifetime.

HABITS

Studies have been made of the habits of different races who live longer than average. Renee Taylor (1974) studied the Hunza people who live in an inaccessible valley in the Himalayas. She calls it the Valley of Eternal Youth. The Hunza people have evolved a way of living, eating and thinking which has lengthened lifespan and reduced susceptibility to most illnesses. David Davies, (1975) of the Gerontological Unit of University College, London spent two years studying the people of Vilcabamba, Ecuador, one of the longest living groups of people in the world. His book *Centenarians of the Andes* summarises his findings, and these are his tips for longevity:

1. Keep working steadily after retirement that is, if you have to retire.
2. Have absorbing hobbies to take over your mental activity after retirement.
3. Don't talk about growing old — try to avoid those who are depressed about the idea.
4. Drink and smoke in moderation — if at all.
5. Get plenty of natural sleep.
6. Avoid all forms of stress — at least learn to cope with stress if you cannot avoid it.
7. Don't worry about your children.
8. Walk at least one mile a day as this is the best form of exercise. Gardening is another good form of exercise.
9. Eat as little meat as possible.
10. Eat as much raw food and as little processed food as possible.

In our professional lives as occupational therapists we rarely meet someone who lives by these disciplines. We are more likely to be referred the type of person whom Benjamin Franklin described in 1749, when he estimated that nine out of ten people suffered from

Chronic Suicide, a label for long-term self-destruction. This condition is unrecognised officially but is being considered increasingly by psychologists and suicide researchers. It includes compulsive behaviour in the form of drug abuse, overeating, alcoholism and smoking. The degree of unconscious behaviour is hard to define but often people persist with their compulsive habits when they are aware that these are damaging their health — surely a form of suicide.

PERSONALITY

Havinghurst (1968) wrote in *The Gerontologist* that 'aging is better viewed from a social psychological perspective, not as process of engagement or disengagement but as a process of adaptation in which personality is the key element.' A study was carried out by Reichard et al (1962) in New York, to assess men's reactions to retirement. Those who adapted well were the mature, rocking-chair, armoured types: those who did badly were the angry and self-hating types. Neugarten (1968) in her study on *Patterns of Ageing* describes eight distinct personality types of elderly people. These are: the reorganiser, the focused, the disengaged, the holding-on, the constructed, the succorance seekers, the apathetic, and the disorganised.

Doubtless all therapists and health care workers will recognise which of these types will be a problem to rehabilitate, and equally which will co-operate and make every effort to regain their independence after illness or disability. Furthermore it is sobering to study that list and to consider which group we ourselves are destined for!

ATTITUDES

Dr Alex Comfort (1967) in his article 'On Gerontophobia' compares some doctors' attitudes towards ailing, crazy and dying old people to the anti-Semitic. They are either patronised or jollied along, but in both cases the falsity comes through. He warns of 'ageism' in his book *A Good Age* (1977) and encourages older people to stand up for themselves. Ageism, like racism, is based on ignorance and fear, and the weapons needed to defeat it are contradiction and accurate information to dispel hearsay and prejudice.

Unfortunately, health professionals' attitudes to the elderly are not always positive. We have all heard remarks from medical practitioners such as 'they're blocking my beds' or 'please see to her disposal — I need that bed' in the belief that their hospital beds are for those under the age of 65 and who have curable conditions. Dr Brooke studied psychiatrists in training (1973) and found that many indicated they would rather emigrate than practise in psychogeriatrics! Gale and Livesley (1974) conducted a survey at King's Hospital, London which compared the attitudes of clinical medical students with junior hospital medical staff on the subject of geriatrics. The students' attitudes were much more favourable than those of the hospital staff. The researchers believed this to be due to a deterioration of attitude after graduation, the students being 'patient/treatment orientated' whereas the junior hospital staff became 'education/career orientated'. Geriatrics was not viewed as an important speciality.

Baker (1978) looked at nurses' attitudes to care of the elderly in a Manchester hospital. She found that nurses practising routine geriatric nursing had a view of their patients as being less than fully responsible adults for whom the routinised provision of a minimal level of physical care was seen as appropriate, even inevitable, particularly in the light of the denial of status and deprivation of resources to which the wards where they worked were subjected. She noted that this style contrasted sharply with officially recommended policies but received the implicit and, in some cases, explicit approval of nursing management and medical staff. Gunter (1971) looked at student attitudes towards geriatric nursing and found that before they took a course in this subject 11% of the students stated that they had a strong interest, but by the end of the course only 4% said they had a major interest in this area. Futrell and Jones (1977) studied attitudes of physicians, nurses and social workers in Massachusetts. One of their findings showed that 'the relationship between attitudes toward the elderly and the length of time practising their profession appeared significantly negative for social workers and physicians, but positive for nurses.' They advise the social work and medical professions to find a way to keep the young inexperienced worker interested in solving the health problems of the elderly.

What about our own attitudes to treating elderly people? As therapists we should frequently examine our motives and make sure that we are seen to be positive and enthusiastic in our approach to the elderly, so that students working with us will also adopt such an attitude. Hedley Peach (1978) of Wales studied 'Career Plans of Rehabilitation Therapists regarding Geriatric medicine.' Out of 62 student physiotherapists, 35 estimated that they had been involved with elderly patients for more than half of their training; 52 thought physiotherapy was important in the care of the elderly but only 7 felt that it was very rewarding to give physiotherapy to elderly patients; only 10 gave a high or very high consideration to a career involving solely elderly people, and 7 would not consider it at all. Out of 100 occupational therapy students, only 7 estimated that they had been involved with elderly people for more than half their training; 95 thought that occupational therapy was important in the care of the elderly but only 9 thought it was very rewarding; only 16 gave a high or very high consideration to a career involving solely elderly people and 11 would not consider it at all. Professors of geriatric medicine are slowly convincing their local medical schools that specific training for medical students in the field of geriatrics is essential, and this specific training is now helping to modify previous 'dyed in the wool' attitudes. The same is happening with physiotherapists and occupational therapists who now undergo some of their training working with professionals in special geriatric units. A positive, knowledgeable approach to this challenging field is thus fostered.

General attitudes of the population towards ageing have been mentioned in the introduction. Novak (1979) described a widely held fear of ageing associated with a stereotyped image of 'sterility, loss of vital power and death.' Other fears he lists are those of being weak or sick, tired or ugly, stupid or mocked. The alternative to being old is to commit suicide. Butler (1977) reports that a quarter of all the suicides in the USA occur in people who are over 65 years. This is a horrific statistic which illustrates widespread inability to accept and adjust to growing old.

Attitudes to entering a geriatric medical assessment unit

In 1982, C. Joan McAlpine, Consultant Physician in Geriatric Medicine, and Zena J. Wright, Research Psychologist to the Department of Geriatric Medicine, Paisley, Scotland, conducted a special study into the attitudes of elderly patients on admission to a geriatric medical assessment unit. One hundred consecutively admitted patients were interviewed within two to eight days of coming to the unit: the grossly demented and those too physically ill were omitted from the study which amounted to approximately half of all admissions within the period of study. The questionnaire was concerned with the following areas
— The patient's self-reported reaction to the prospect of admission
— Her awareness of the nature of the unit
— Her reaction to being in a ward for the elderly
— Her expectation of the immediate future
— Her views on Local Authority Eventide Homes.
The results are based on what the patients were willing to admit at the time of interview. Additionally, a close relative or caring friend of each patient was given a brief 'multiple choice ' questionnaire to complete at the end

of the patient's visit to the unit, covering the following:
— The patient's willingness to be admitted
— The relative's willingness to have the patient in the unit
— The relative's view of the patient's anxieties associated with being in a geriatric ward, if any
— The relative's views on geriatric hospitals.
The researchers found that the anticipated reluctance to be admitted to a geriatric medical assessment unit was not present. Only two patients spontaneously mentioned their own ageing as a problem. To others, the matter seemed irrelevant or a fact long accepted. A high percentage in each group regarded their admission as being for purely medical reasons: they thought they were in the right place in a ward for the elderly. Interestingly, they were in general not pessimistic about the outcome of admission, and about half said they had no worries about hospitalisation. 53% expected to be in hospital for days or weeks, 43% had no idea how long they might be there, and 65% expected to go home on discharge.

About a quarter of patients in each case (a) compared the ward unfavourably with a previous hospital admission, (b) were distressed by the presence of confused patients, (c) were disappointed on entering the ward, (d) were uncommitted about the outcome of admission. 43% of patients were low in spirits at interview and only 23% reported having improved since admission. Younger patients (i.e. less than 79 years) more often reported improved mood shortly after admission (P = 0.03).

Patients in Social Classes I and II tended to react unfavourably in that they were more concerned at being in a geriatric ward and were disturbed by the presence of confused patients (P = 0.02). They were also less willing to be admitted in the first place (P = 0.04) and fewer were pleasantly surprised by the ward (P = 0.04). None compared the ward favourably with a previous hospital admission and they tended to be more pessimistic about the outcome.

Many patients became distressed when the

topic (mainly hypothetical) of Eventide Home admission was discussed. Only one third claimed they would have no anxieties about such admission and 39% could think of no advantages at all in entering a Home. The main problem was that of leaving their own homes and losing independence (24%), and the main gain was that of being looked after (20%).

Eighty-eight relatives returned the multiple choice questionnaire. Nearly all (96%) professed to be happy about the patient's admission and none reported changing their views for the worse. About one-fifth admitted they had regarded geriatric units as long-stay institutions for hopeless cases but later 52% thought they were geared to the special needs of the elderly and to getting them home. The relative's assessment of whether or not the patient had anxieties about being in a geriatric hospital was fairly accurate, but of the 18 patients who described themselves as unwilling to come into hospital, more than half of their relatives described them as willing. Depression is the most frequently found mood change in the elderly (Williamson 1978) and it is not surprising that almost half of those admitted confessed to being in low spirits on admission.

The strongest impression was that confused patients diminish the quality of social contact in the wards. This is particularly true of the lucid patient who is intelligent or who is socially isolated with no relatives or who is living alone. Confusion may be part of an acute process and may be reversible, or there may be an acute medical problem superimposed on a chronic dementing process. It is therefore inevitable that a certain proportion of patients with confusion will be admitted to a geriatric medical assessment unit.

Personal attitudes

As professionals we are trained to look at human problems with clinical detachment and objectivity which come from learning theories and facts. Ageing is subjective — it happens to us all. While training and working we should consider how well we are likely to adjust to being 'that age' and consequently endeavour to be more in tune with our patients' emotions and fears. We would also do well to consider how we ourselves might avoid some of the pitfalls of old age by adapting personal habits now and taking preventative measures to improve our prospects of a vigorous, rewarding and healthy old age. For example, by giving up smoking, eating sensibly and drinking alcohol in moderation we can avoid the double standard of advising one thing and doing the other.

Most of us lay down the problem (or solutions to) old age through habits acquired before we reach 40. We ought to be prepared to face up to our views of and attitudes to our own old age now: and in so doing we will be in a position to offer more constructive and useful advice to our patients on how to cope with theirs.

REFERENCES

Baker D E 1978 Attitudes of nurses to the care of the elderly, Manchester University thesis (PLD)
Brooke P 1973 Psychiatrists in training. British Journal of Psychiatry Special Publication (7) Headley Ashford
Butler R N 1977 Successful aging and the role of the life review. In: Zarit S H (ed) Reading in aging and death: contemporary perspectives. Harper and Row, New York, p 16
Comfort A 1967 On gerontophobia. Medical Opinion Review September: 31–37
Comfort A 1977 A good age. Mitchell Beazley, London
Davies D 1975 Centenarians of the Andes. Barrie & Jenkins, London
Futrell M, Jones W 1977 Attitudes of physicians, nurses and social workers toward the elderly and health maintenance service and for the aged: implications for healthy manpower. Journal of Gerontological Nursing 3(3): 42–46
Gale J, Livesley B 1974 Attitudes towards geriatrics: A report of the King's survey. Age and Ageing 3: 49–53
Gunter L M 1971 Students' attitude towards geriatric nursing. Nursing Outlook 19(7): 466–69
Havinghurst R J 1968 A social-psychological perspective on aging. Gerontologist 8: 67–71
Hayflick L 1980 The role of cell biology in aging research and education. Gerontological Geriatric Education (Winter) 1(2): 149–52
Lewis S C 1981 The mature years. Charles B Slack, New Jersey
Loebel J P, Eisdorfer C 1984 Psychological and psychiatric factors in the rehabilitation of the elderly. In: Williams Franklin T (ed) Rehabilitation in the aging. Raven Press, New York p 41–59
McAlpine C J, Wright Z J 1982 Attitudes and anxieties of

elderly patients on admission to a geriatric assessment unit. Age and Ageing 11: 35–41.

Neugarten B L, Havinghurst R J, Tobin S S 1968 Personality and patterns of aging. In: Neugarten B L (ed) Middle age and ageing. University of Chicago Press, Chicago, pp 173–177

Novak M 1979 Thinking about ageing: a critique of liberal social gerontology. Age and Ageing 8(4): 209–215

Peach H 1978 Career plans of student physical therapists regarding geriatric medicine. Age and ageing 7: 57–61

Pitt Brice 1982 Ageing and its problems. Professional attitudes. In: Psychogeriatrics: an introduction to the psychiatry of old age. Churchill Livingstone, Edinburgh, chs 2 and 3, p 6–37

Reichard S, Livson T, Petersen P G 1962 Aging and personality. Wiley, New York

Taylor R 1974 Hunza health secrets. Tandem, London

Wallechinsky D, Wallace I and A 1977 The book of lists. Cassell Corgi, London

Williamson J 1978 Depression in the elderly. Age and Ageing 7 Supplement: 35–40

2

Geriatric medical assessment units

M. Helm

These special units for elderly people have been opening for several decades in the United Kingdom on a large scale. During the last decade they have opened similar units in much smaller numbers in the United States, Canada, Australia and New Zealand.

Before they came into existence elderly patients were referred to general medical or surgical wards, where the primary reason for referral was treated but other existing problems were largely ignored. It was common in these general wards for over-worked nurses to undertake their elderly patients' basic functions, to avoid interfering with the set routine of the ward. In other words, they would get the patients up, wash them, dress them in night attire, occasionally even feed them (if they were slow eaters), put them on commodes, and sit them down next to their beds for the rest of the day. If the patient was apt to wander, a table would be fixed across her 'geriatric' chair, or she might be given a sedative or tranquiliser. Not surprisingly, many such patients soon became totally dependent and institutionalised, lacking will, motivation or any interest in their future.

In 1982 a study was carried out by Popplewell in Flinders Medical Centre, South Australia, to make a comparison of the treatment of 50 elderly people in geriatric medical assessment units with that of 50 elderly people in medical units, and to measure the difference in outcome of two groups of elderly patients. In the geriatric unit the mean age was 81.8 years (range 66–94): in the medical unit the mean age was 81.3 years (range 75–85).

The medical reason for admission and the profile of associated diseases were similar in both groups.

A comparison of drugs on admission and discharge was made: 54% of the patients admitted to the geriatric unit were on four drugs on admission compared to 52% on admission to the medical unit. In the geriatric unit 50% of drugs were withdrawn or other medication substituted, as opposed to 16% in the medical unit. On discharge the mean number of drugs prescribed was significantly less (P = 0.05 Mann Whitney).

The mean length of stay in the geriatric unit was 9.8 days, as compared to 10.9 days in the medical unit.

Fourteen patients from institutions (nursing homes or hostels) were admitted to the geriatric unit compared with ten to the medical unit. At discharge a further three went to institutional care from the geriatric unit, whereas an additional twelve patients went to institutional care from the medical unit.

This disparity in the rates of discharge to long-term care facilities supports the need for careful assessment of the health care needs of each patient. This is more successfully carried out by the multiprofessional team in the geriatric unit, and is reflected in Table 2.1.

Table 2.1 Utilisation of services at Flinders

Service	GMAU	OMU	P value (chi squared)
District nursing	12	3	0.02
Domiciliary care	20	6	0.01
Outpatient department follow-up	28	15	0.02
Medical consultations	15	5	0.03
Social worker	34	6	0.001
Remedial therapy (Physio, OT, etc.)	41	1	0.001

In British and US hospitals it has been shown that the attachment of a consultant in geriatric medicine to general medical wards meant:

1. shorter mean and median length of stay
2. more patients going directly home
3. reduction in the necessity for convalescent care.

(Burley et al 1979, Barker et al 1985)

A number of doctors have given many good reasons for the setting up of geriatric medical assessment units. Dr S. J. Brody (1976) of Philadelphia, states the following: 'A geriatric medical assessment unit is an interventive mechanism to avoid inappropriate placement of many elderly people both within and outside of the long-term care institutions . . . in order to contain costs, rationalise placement and ensure care for ageing, which enables them to achieve and maintain maximum independence and dignity.'

Dr Gabriel Pickar (Brody et al 1976) of New Brunswick, New Jersey, called his unit for the elderly 'SCAT' — Supplemental Care and Treatment Unit (based on concepts fostered by Cosin's Cowley Road Hospital, Oxford), and states these purposes:

1. Assess the individual's functional health status
2. Identify the service needs required to ameliorate her functional health problems
3. Determine appropriate referral to institutional or community-based resources for satisfaction of those needs, and
4. Provide short-term medical, health and social services, when necessary within the centre, prior to referral, with the objective of maintaining the aged in the communities served, at the highest level of independence appropriate to their individual abilities to function.

Dr Duncan Robertson (1982) who runs a geriatric medical assessment unit in Saskatoon, Canada, gives this explanation: 'For older persons who present with complex health problems, a geriatric medical assessment unit provides an environment for comprehensive assessment, treatment and rehabilitation. A thorough assessment at, or preferably before, the point at which their health breaks down, enables older people to return to and remain in the community and helps to prevent them from being admitted to an institution while they are still able to function with reasonable independence.'

Then there is the question of which patients are suitable for referral to geriatric medical assessment units. Professor Brocklehurst (1978) of Manchester applies the following judgements: 'Usually those with highly complex problems involving the effects of ageing, accumulated pathological changes, and a precipitating cause of breakdown which may constitute either an acute medical or an acute social problem.'

Brody (1976) states that: 'It is characteristic of this group that multiple disabilities are often clustered and interact to mask and exacerbate each other.'

Dr Popplewell (1982) describes his admission criteria in these terms: 'The unit is not linked to an admission roster but receives patients at any time from admitting areas, when the following criteria are fulfilled:

1. They are over 75 years of age (patients less than this are occasionally admitted when multiple medical problems producing continuing dependency indicate they would best be cared for in the multidisciplinary setting of the assessment unit)

2. They do not have a medical condition better handled by any other specialty clinic at the time: (such as surgical conditions, certain disturbances of cardiac rhythm etc.)'

The main function of a geriatric medical assessment unit can therefore be summed up in the following way: to afford a spell of in-patient care in order to identify all problems which can be resolved by short-term physical, mental and social treatment, and thus lead to the rehabilitation of the patient as early as is practicable. This message is continuously reinforced to patients and their families by all professional staff in the geriatric medical assessment unit who encourage patients to carry out all daily living functions on their own in order to make them increasingly self-reliant. It has been observed that patients who have received such treatment remain more active and better orientated, thus improving their chances of returning to their homes.

Geriatric medical assessment units offer support for carers and when necessary, respite admissions for their dependants. Table 2.2 gives examples of the diagnostic categories of patients referred to such a unit in Edinburgh, Scotland.

The staffing of a geriatric medical assessment unit will vary from unit to unit, the number of beds being one criterion. The population of over 65- or 75-year-olds served has to be ascertained. Number of admissions per month and year, average length of stay,

Table 2.2 All referrals to a geriatric medical assessment unit City Hospital, Edinburgh for 1983

System affected	Male	(%)	Female	(%)	Total	(%)
Musculoskeletal	112	(27.7)	451	(51.0)	563	(43.6)
Cardiovascular	115	(38.3)	335	(37.9)	490	(37.9)
Dementia	131	(32.3)	313	(35.4)	444	(34.4)
Gastrointestinal	103	(25.4)	221	(25.0)	324	(25.1)
Genitourinary	112	(27.7)	208	(23.5)	320	(24.8)
Respiratory	146	(36.0)	152	(17.2)	298	(23.1)
Vision	71	(17.5)	180	(20.3)	251	(19.4)
Hearing	76	(18.8)	175	(19.8)	251	(19.4)
Stroke	104	(25.7)	147	(16.6)	251	(19.4)
CNS	69	(17.0)	104	(11.8)	173	(13.4)
Depression	37	(9.1)	129	(14.6)	166	(12.9)
Endocrine	23	(5.7)	101	(11.4)	124	(9.6)
Other	33	(8.1)	90	(10.2)	123	(9.5)
Parkinsonism	43	(10.6)	66	(7.5)	109	(8.4)
Other psychiatric	26	(6.4)	63	(7.1)	89	(6.9)

discharge and death rate all have to be taken into consideration, as well as whether the unit has a fast, slow or moderate turnover.

For a high turnover, 40-bedded unit, staff might be as follows: Nine doctors (this may seem a high figure but often they have additional responsibilities, e.g. continuing care wards, consultative commitments to general medical or surgical wards and day hospitals); two occupational therapists plus two OT helpers; two physiotherapists (the two latter categories normally have additional responsibilities to continuing care wards); one social worker; one dietician; part-time speech therapist.

Nursing establishments vary but information from Pinel and Seriki (1976) indicates that number of beds/nurses in post = establishment. This works out at one nurse to every 1.4 beds and appears adequate until the figures are analysed in terms of shifts involved, bearing in mind a working week of 40 hours; the enhanced holidays provided by the Halsbury Report 1974, sickness, absence, management courses, seminars and study days for trainee nurses, have been calculated by Cormack and Fraser (1975) as representing 14% of the total training time.

The need for overlap between shifts for communicating information relating to patients' treatment must also be taken into account. Rogers (1981) quotes a total of 47 nurses for the Hammersmith Hospital Geriatric Medical Assessment Unit of 56 beds: a ratio of 1.2 patients per nurse. The nurses include differing numbers of the following groups: sister, charge-nurse, state registered nurse, state enrolled nurse, student, pupil, and nursing auxiliary.

The great value of geriatric medical assessment units is the multidisciplinary team of professionals which is brought together for the patients' benefit. This team, together with a link person from the community such as a health visitor or district nurse, hold weekly case conferences. Each member will contribute suggestions for resolving patients' difficulties and the team will arrive at jointly agreed plans for their future. This close liaison is essential to ensure that everyone involved, including most particularly patients and their families, knows exactly what strategy has been adopted for the patients' improvement. Where it is likely that patients will be sent home, it is imperative that the family is involved in whatever rehabilitation and management processes are required to bring this about.

The general practitioner also has a crucial role to play. It is he who makes the initial referral to the geriatrician, who knows the patient's medical and social background and so can advise what that individual's needs and difficulties are likely to be. Similarly, the GP will be kept fully informed of all that the geriatric medical assessment unit is arranging for the rehabilitation of his patient.

The role of the occupational therapist

Most elderly people referred to a geriatric medical assessment unit, as we have shown above, suffer from an amalgam of different complaints, so the team must adopt a 'holistic' approach when recommending plans for their treatment. All the varying factors in a person's life, and not just the clinical ones, must be taken into consideration when agreeing a strategy for her future, and this is where the occupational therapist has a special contribution to make. While in the hospital she provides a detailed assessment of all the daily-living activities, i.e., transferring from bed and chair, walking, washing, using the toilet, dressing, and eating. She may also have to assess the patient's ability to transfer from bath or shower, her safety in the OT kitchen, and, where applicable, her wheelchair independence.

There are several accepted assessments of daily living activity indices which are a matter of personal choice. Assessment reports should be retained in the patient's file after hospital discharge in order to compare present with previous functional ability, should the patient be readmitted.

In commenting upon the suitability of functional assessment instruments, the late Dr

Philip Nichols (1976) gave the following advice:

1. The ADL index needs to be comprehensive in its coverage of activities but as short and concise as possible
2. It should be simple enough to be carried out by any member of staff
3. It must be suitable for the assessment of all degrees of impairment
4. It must be constructed in such a way that it can be used for assessment of patients as individuals and must delineate their needs for care
5. It must be completely objective.

Long, complicated assessment procedures are inadvisable when working with old people: too many questions may make them suspicious, resulting in a loss of trust and co-operation, not to mention concentration. Items such as length of attention span, sequencing (ability to perform activities in logical order), concrete and abstract thought, can be noted while assessing and treating, but need not be tested routinely.

Together with activities of daily living and cognition, the occupational therapist must investigate the patient's domestic circumstances: the type, standard, condition and suitability of her accommodation; whether she lives alone or with relatives; if she receives support from local community services. Naturally, an elderly patient who lives in the context of a caring family will not have to achieve the same level of independence as one living totally on her own; nevertheless the family should not be seen as a substitute for professional care or as a prop for the patient to lean on. Relatives have their own lives to lead, so the occupational therapist must discover the attitude of the patient to her family and vice versa, as these can often differ markedly.

Once all of these factors have been assimilated and added to the clinical diagnoses together with reports from other professionals, the geriatric medical assessment unit team is ready to formulate a suitable plan for the patient's future, and a realistic treatment programme is immediately initiated.

Specific treatment for various conditions will be included in Chapters 3–10, but there are some general points which should be kept in mind when treating elderly people.

1. It is often not possible to improve function radically in elderly patients with chronic conditions. An optimum level can be achieved and maintained by allowing them to practise activities of daily living using suitable aids and home adaptations, whether they be new or well tried.

2. The patient's previous level of personal independence before illness should be regarded as a suitable treatment goal if total rehabilitation is not possible.

3. Initially, there may be set-backs not necessarily connected with the patient's medical status. For instance, admission to hospital can affect bodily functions such as sleeping, eating, bowel function and orientation.

4. Patients can suffer temporary acute confusion after being brought to hospital. This is particularly true when infection is present, or following anaesthesia.

5. Elderly patients must be allowed to take part in daily living activities at their own speed. It is a temptation for well-meaning helpers to step in to speed up the proceedings.

6. Old people should be encouraged to perform as many household duties as they did before coming to hospital. Fortunately there is home help support for those who might not otherwise be able to continue to live at home.

7. The majority of elderly people come to hospital with multiple problems, including gradual deterioration of mobility, memory, sight and hearing. Spectacles, hearing-aid, teeth and walking aid must always be used during treatment.

8. Hospital staff should try not to impose their standards on the way older people live.

9. Bathing is not an essential activity for the elderly. Often it is dangerous for unsteady disabled people, and severe loss of confidence is induced after a fall or 'being stuck in the bath.' A strip-wash seated at a basin or the

use of a shower fitted with a (non-spring-loaded) flip-down seat are adequate substitutes.

10. Frequent discussion with the patient's relatives is important to keep them informed of progress in daily living activities and other treatment.

THE ROLES OF OTHER HOSPITAL PERSONNEL WHO SEE AN ELDERLY PERSON IN A GERIATRIC MEDICAL ASSESSMENT UNIT

The following short descriptions illustrate the parts played by various personnel who work with elderly people. All are important and it should be borne in mind that the multidisciplinary team can only work effectively if there is mutual understanding and respect for each other's role.

The dietician

The dietician is responsible for customary or prescribed forms of feeding for the patient. She is concerned with what the patient eats in hospital and at home.

Often the elderly person, reluctant to spend much money on food, needs to be shown how to have a cheap, well-balanced diet. This may be implemented within the hospital where the dietician can assist a patient choose her menu. Before discharge she may plan menus for home, advise on the value of convenience foods and explain the necessity to have stocked cupboards for emergency supplies. She will discuss food prices with the patient, family or carers. She may be involved with the occupational therapist during kitchen practice for those patients disinterested in or unaccustomed to cooking.

The control of patients' feeding for therapeutic purposes is termed diet therapy. Therapeutic diets are planned and their provision is supervised by the hospital dietician, low-fat, soft, salt-free, high-protein, reducing or diabetic diets being the most common.

In these cases the dietician has to assess the diet by collating dietary history, obtaining a seven-day eating pattern and noting the amounts of specific nutrients. The dietician is responsible for explaining to the patient, carer, nursing and medical staff about foods allowed. This again must be continued after discharge. She may have to advise on nasogastric feeding and explain to nurses the types and amounts of food to be given.

Dieticians sometimes assume responsibility for general catering arrangements within the hospital and may work in the canteen advising on diet and instructing the cooks on the special diets listed above.

The doctor

Following an incident to an elderly person at home, the general practitioner is alerted and, if he feels the community services can no longer cope, he may refer to the geriatrician. The latter initially makes an assessment of the patient in her own environment and determines whether acute admission is necessary or not. He may be able to prevent admission by use of out-patient services. He is therefore involved in both the hospital and the community which it serves. Where he is involved in admitting a patient to hospital, the geriatrician will examine the patient physically and mentally and try to determine a diagnosis. He will catalogue her previous medical history, her social history and home situation, and prescribe medical management.

A multidisciplinary team is only effective if it has a co-ordinator, and the doctor usually performs this role. He is ultimately responsible for the patient's management in hospital and refers to other relevant disciplines shortly after admission.

The doctor ensures that adequate communication exists between these disciplines — he is responsible for holding regular meetings to enable all members of the team to contribute their assessments and observations of the patient and to encourage discussion amongst all responsible for her well-being. The aim of the meeting is to plan for the future care of the patient. Often other disciplines can offer advice on a patient's level of independence and the follow-up care necessary for successful discharge.

The doctor is responsible for all pharmacological care given to patients and discusses with the patient her symptoms, drug therapy and future plans. He monitors the patient's progress and explains her medical condition and likely prognosis. He may have to reassure the patient and her family about the future and try to instil in her realistic goals she may expect to achieve.

He may have to explain to the family how much the patient will be able to do when discharged, and he may be involved in arranging respites to share the care of dependent patients with their families.

He may be asked to assess an elderly person in a general medical ward to advise on management and on the involvement of other professions to allow for successful discharge. In continuing care, the doctor provides a supportive role and manages on-going or new problems, helping to minimise troublesome symptoms.

The electrocardiography technician

The role of the electrocardiography technician is to take electrocardiograms of most patients admitted to the geriatric wards or day hospital. By doing this, the technicians provide a recording of the heart rate and thus assist doctors to diagnose any abnormalities. Electrocardiography gives information on the general physical condition of the patient.

Special interest is taken when the patient complains of dizziness, drop attacks or falls. These symptoms may be vague and after an electrocardiogram the cause may be easily noted and suitably treated.

When a doctor wishes to record a reading for a longer period of time to note any fluctuation throughout a day, a 24-hour tape may be fitted. This permits a patient to participate in normal activities and and the heart function can be recorded during this time. These tests take a short time to carry out but reassurance is necessary. Patients often become quite anxious at this prospect and do not fully understand what is expected of them. The electrocardiography technician spends time explaining the procedure but does not give the result to the patient. The doctor looks at recordings and makes a diagnosis on the basis of those.

The nurse

The nurse's contribution and role remain constant, as each ward has nursing staff who are on duty 24 hours a day, seven days a week. The nurse, therefore has the most contact with patients and the greatest opportunity to observe and monitor progress, and is able to alert the doctor if the patient's condition alters. She is often in the best position to assess the patient's behaviour throughout the day and monitor performance. Without her, no other discipline could function. She is responsible for the patient's comfort, prevention of pressure damage, maintenance of nutrition and the issuing of drugs. She is also responsible for monitoring the patient's elimination processes and often for administering ways of trying to maintain continence. She may be the main person involved in the care of the terminally ill patient and tries to maintain the comfort and dignity of the dying person.

She constantly assesses the patient's need for care and often collaborates with doctors and all other health professionals. She is able to observe responses to therapy introduced by other team members and is often expected to carry on some of the responsibilities of other professionals when they are not there. The nurse is frequently the co-ordinator of care and is involved in planning the patient's care and daily routine through liaison with other professionals.

She is the person most likely to meet relatives and visitors on the ward and may have to discuss a patient's general condition and progress with them and to offer psychological support. She is able to observe the relatives' attitude to the patient during these visits.

She is involved in planning patient's

discharge and is frequently responsible for organising follow-up care.

The occupational therapy helper

The occupational therapy helper assists the qualified occupational therapist and is able to provide continuity in work with elderly patients. She works under supervision of and advice from the occupational therapist. She may assist in acute wards where full assessment has been carried out by the occupational therapist, but further practice in activities of daily living may benefit the patients and help maintain their level of independence. She will work closely with the occupational therapist and should be able to report all patients' progress to the therapist in charge. She is also responsible for mentally stimulating her patients by providing various activities on a daily basis. She may be involved in individual or group work to provide domestic, social, physical or intellectual activities. Not only does this work give the patients an interest and purpose to their day, but it may also enable them to participate in a programme which would otherwise be denied to them.

The occupational therapy helper may be able to introduce the patients to other elderly patients from other wards and frequently friendships may develop. The occupational therapy helper herself can establish relationships with patients as she develops their interests and skills. Often an outing or visit away from the ward organised by a helper may be enough to give patients an interest and topic of discussion when they return to the ward or when talking to relatives.

The physiotherapist

The physiotherapist's main concern with the elderly is the patient's mobility. She fully assesses the patient's condition and teaches her to become mobile again, providing a suitable aid as necessary. She encourages the patient to become independent and to increase her confidence and exercise tolerance in hospital and at home. She is respon-sible for the application and fitting of orthotics and prosthetics, and may issue surgical collars, corsets, splints or footwear. These will assist patients to attain maximum function and improved comfort, and their use must be carefully explained to relatives and other carers. She will make a clinical assessment of patients with new physical disorders and will note the nature of the disability, muscle power and joint mobility. Following a stroke she will aim to encourage postural control, return of muscle power, and controlled range of movement in bilateral use of limbs. During treatment she will try to improve balance and co-ordination, inhibit spasticity and prevent contractures. She will note sensory or perceptual loss and encourage body awareness.

She may give passive movements to paralysed or weak limbs following immobilisation through illness. She may also be asked to monitor the effect of drug therapy on patients' functional general mobility, e.g. Parkinson's disease. She may have to administer specialised treatments for isolated areas of discomfort using ice, heat or ultrasound, and she may have to provide chest physiotherapy for patients with chest infections.

Teaching correct positioning and lifting techniques to nurses/carers is often the responsibility of the physiotherapist. During any contact with patients, the physiotherapist will note the patient's personality, mood, morale and motivation, all of which can alter her rate of progress. To be effective, rehabilitation has to have the patient's co-operation and that of her family.

The physiotherapy helper

The physiotherapy helper is supervised by a qualified physiotherapist and is very useful for working with the elderly, but she is not always employed in geriatric units. She is not involved in assessing or treating patients but may help to maintain patients at the highest levels of independence possible. She may be involved with patients who have a long-standing illness and try to maintain their range of movement and tone in all muscles. She will encourage mobility and transfers, and report to the physiotherapist any deterioration in a patient's condition.

She may work on an individual basis with the patient to practise particular tasks given by a qualified therapist or in groups of patients with similar problems. She may take classes of music to movement or exercise patterns to promote participation and encourage general fitness. She may boost morale and be of great psychological support to those who no longer receive treatment by a qualified physiotherapist.

The porter

Porters provide the essential service of moving patients and equipment around the hospital. This varies from ward to ward but includes meal trolleys, mail within the hospital, laundry, mortuary boxes etc.

Porters are frequently required to take frail elderly patients for appointments at various departments. Often X-ray, physiotherapy, speech therapy and occupational therapy departments are dependent upon porters to bring patients and take them back to their wards throughout the day. The porters are expected to assist with transferring patients from wheelchairs.

The radiographer

The job of the radiographer is to X-ray the patient following referral from the doctor. The doctor will specify the part of the body to be examined.

Frequently, the radiographer explains the X-ray procedure and assists with transferring the patient onto the necessary apparatus, then takes and develops the required X-rays. A hydraulic table which can be switched to various heights is often used to ease transfers for the elderly patient who should never be left unattended.

A radiologist will report a diagnosis and the X-rays will then be available for the ward doctors.

The social worker

The social worker is involved in assessing the patient's needs and in providing her colleagues with information about the patient's home circumstances. She may be asked to deal with social problems that are worrying the patient. Her work may include tasks such as making arrangments for pets to be looked after, and attending to bills, rent or other domestic matters if there are no relatives to do this. She will also advise on matters such as re-housing and Social Security benefits, and co-ordinate Social Services on the patient's discharge. These are most likely to be a home help and meals-on-wheels but may include attendance at a day centre or organising an emergency alarm service.

Most elderly people live in the community but many depend on family, friends or neighbours for daily help so that they can remain at home. It is important that these carers (who may be elderly themselves) receive as much help as possible. The social worker may be involved in monitoring the home situation and arranging respite admissions to hospital, a residential home or, if available, a foster family in the community. Some carers need help to let the patient remain in care when they can no longer be supported in the community without unacceptable physical or emotional cost to the carer. They may experience a grief-like reaction and need appropriate support at this time.

For the patient who is unable to return home, the social worker will be responsible for arranging residential care or, where this is not appropriate, helping her adjust to the prospect of continuing hospital care. Similarly, the patient's relatives may need sensitive support and practical advice as they adjust to this major change in their lives.

The social worker will advise the patient about giving up her house and disposing of her belongings where there are no relatives, and may be actively involved in doing this for the patient. Helping patients and their carers cope with loss is a major theme in hospital social work, when couples become separated by illness or death or their relationship changes through disability, or when patients face loss of privacy, independence, their sense of identity and perhaps their home. Social workers are often called on to give emotional support to patients and their carers at such times.

The speech therapist

The speech therapist treats patients who have language disorders or swallowing difficulties. She may offer assistance with diagnosis and differentiate between dementia and dysphasia. The main problems with the elderly occur following a stroke, or in Parkinson's disease, or bulbar palsy.

She is able to assess fully patients' speech abilities, their ability to comprehend and their ability to read and write. She has to decide on the best means of functional communication. She is able to explain to the patient and other staff about the disability and how best to manage this to reinforce her treatment programme.

She will explain what she is doing to encourage communication and how others can best assist the patient. She is usually involved with relatives or those who know the patient well and who can tell of interests and level of function prior to the illness. She may have to counsel patients and help them come to terms with the loss of speech. She may have to encourage them to be realistic and to find alternative means of communication by use of gestures. She will try to reduce anxiety, fear and frustration. The speech therapist may well be involved in treatment after the patient is discharged from hospital, as speech problems seldom detain a patient.

She may involve her in stroke or social clubs which are sometimes run by volunteers or self-help groups, in which case all necessary information can be transferred from the speech therapist to volunteers. She aims to sustain motivation in individuals or groups and tries overall to prevent their social isolation.

The untrained nurse

The role of the untrained or auxiliary nurse is to assist trained staff in patient care on the ward. Auxiliary nurses, always supervised by qualified staff, are accountable to the nurse in charge.

The untrained nurse is much involved in patient care in elderly care units where she may supervise bathing and help wash and dress patients in the mornings. She may also help transfer and mobilise patients. The auxiliary nurse is often responsible for administering patients' tea, giving out meals and helping patients to eat. She may also have duties around the ward of tidying ward areas, i.e. lockers, linen room and sluice. She may be responsible for putting away clean linen and stores. She is expected to be adaptable, to fit into ward routine and be observant, so that she can report on patients' progress.

The ward domestic

The domestic is responsible for the general cleanliness and hygiene of the ward. She follows a daily plan of cleaning for each area in the ward and its surrounding offices. She is responsible for cleaning toilet areas and ensuring that all accessories are available. She makes tea for the patients and prepares the trolley with cups and saucers. She sets the tables for lunch and collects patients' lunch trays afterwards. She ensures that patients have clean water jugs and tumblers on their lockers daily.

The ward domestic is in regular contact with patients as she works around them; she may often befriend patients who may well confide, to this non-professional, things they would be reluctant to impart to a professional.

SUMMARY

As geriatric medicine becomes more widely recognised, a multidisciplinary team approach has been adopted by doctors to deal with the complex problems of the elderly. However, this is only possible if there are common goals, co-operative relationships and co-ordinated activities and efforts. In a geriatric medical assessment unit, there will inevitably be much overlapping of roles. Effective communication within the team and also with patients and their families is therefore imperative: competition between different elements of the team is totally counter-productive.

APPENDIX I

VARIOUS THEORETICAL APPROACHES TO
OCCUPATIONAL THERAPY TREATMENT
(abridged from Trombly & Scott, 1977)

1. The rehabilitative approach considers the
   capacities of each individual, ie, physical,
   emotional, cognitive, social, cultural, vo-
   cational and environmental factors. The goal
   to be achieved is the patient's recognition
   of strengths and limitations, and her adjustment to these.
2. The behavioural approach seeks to eliminate maladaptive responses, and improved
   desired behaviour is rewarded and
   reinforced.
3. The humanistic approach examines how
   the individual experiences her environment
   and if she is in control of it. It gauges the
   patient's self-awareness, attitude and mood.
4. The biomechanical approach is for patients
   suffering from musculoskeletal problems.
   It seeks to improve range of movement,
   strength, endurance and stamina.
5. The neurodevelopmental approach concerns
   brain damage resulting from stroke or head
   injury where patients lack voluntary control
   over muscle groups. The treatment attempts
   to modify abnormal patterns of movement
   by placing patients in anti-spastic positions.

APPENDIX II

VARIOUS ADL INDICES WHICH MIGHT BE
USED WHEN ASSESSING ELDERLY PATIENTS

The simplest and most comprehensive test
amongst the plethora of ADL indices is from
the Department of Neurology, Winnipeg,
Canada (Newman 1972) — a fifteen point functional 'score' as follows — one point awarded
for each function achieved.

Transfers: (3 pts)	Bed to chair with assistance Bed to chair without assistance All transfers safe, unassisted
Wheelchair: (1 pt)	Wheelchair management
Walking: (4 pts)	In parallel bars With walking aid and assistance With walking aid and no assistance Safe gait with even stride
Stairs: (2 pts)	With one person's assistance With aid of rail only
Dressing: (3 pts)	Upper garments Upper and lower garments Unaided, including fastenings
Toilet: (2 pts)	Urinary continence Independent use of WC and ability to wash

An even more concise version of this functional evaluation might be used in the ward to
chart a patient's progress.

Amongst the longer ADL indices, the most
useful ones would seem to be:

1. The Northwick Park ADL index (Benjamin
1976) which uses a three point score:

    a. Total
       independence   — performing an
                     activity without
                     supervision, with
                     or without an aid

    b. Partial
       dependence   — patient can
                     perform the
                     activity but
                     requires physical

	verbal assistance or supervision to complete the activity
c. Total dependence	— (if a patient refuses to co-operate, even though she is deemed able, she is given a (c) score).

(The timed tests they suggest are inappropriate when assessing elderly people.)

2. The Edinburgh Stroke Rehabilitation Assessment is a useful form used by Margaret Smith (1977), Research OT. She has recently amended it to a five point scale. This is a valuable way of pinpointing how much physical help a patient will require and how safe she will be at home: but nuances of change are not shown up on this scale.

3. The Barthel Index of Independence (Mahoney & Barthel 1965) was developed in a hospital for the chronically ill. The aim was to assess the ability of patients with neuromuscular and musculoskeletal problems to be self-sufficient. Emphasis is on continence and mobility, as this test is designed to gauge nursing levels required for the care of the chronically disabled. One of the advantages of this test is that it measures patients' independence before, during and after treatment. Its scoring system is worked out in fives: a score of one hundred means total independence. This test does not measure a patient's ability to cope at home.

4. The Katz Index of Independence (Katz et al 1970) was designed for stroke patients. Through observation, the following activities are assessed: bathing; dressing; toileting: transferring: continence: feeding.

There are seven stages to choose from between 'A' = Independent and 'G' = Dependent.

5. Kenny Self Care Evaluation Index (Shoening et al 1965) looks at six items: bed transfers; locomotion; dressing; personal hygiene; feeding. The scale is 0 to 24 — the latter being top score for independence.

6. A useful and well-constructed index is to be found in Ann Turner's *The Practice of Occupational Therapy* (1981). This is more appropriate for community OTs, as it includes home pursuits such as gardening and caring for pets and/or grandchildren.

It must be remembered that, however good the indices are, each patient is an individual, and the ability to list the exact problems together with the means of overcoming them is an essential part of the skill of the therapist. The index should be accompanied by a short report which lists precise difficulties present at the test time, and gives an indication of how the patient and her family feel about her condition.

As well as ADL, it is important to assess an elderly patient's cognitive function, including memory, orientation and ability to solve problems. Attributes like mood and personality will be observed during treatment; these intangibles are often useful predictors of recovery and outcome. Several cognitive tests have been standardised for the normal elderly population. Three notable ones are:

1. Clifton Assessment Procedures For The Elderly (CAPE), devised by A. H. Pattie and C. J. Gilleard (1979). This battery of tests can be split up so that individual components can be used in isolation.

2. The Mini-Mental State (Folstein et al) which includes eleven questions requires only five to ten minutes to administer, and 'is reliable on 24 hour or 28 day retest by single or multiple examiners.

3. The Short Portable Mental Status Questionnaire (SPMSQ) was published by E. Pfeiffer (1975), having been given to a sample of one thousand elderly people. He arrived at four score categories: 0–2 errors means intact mental functioning; more than 7 errors represents severe organic impairment: this test constitutes ten questions.

Other well-known and well-used cognitive tests are the Isaacs-Walkey Mental Impairment Measurement (Isaacs & Walkey 1963) and the Crichton Intellectual Rating Scale (Robinson 1977). There are numerous other tests which evaluate ability to communicate, mental state, mood and behaviour, as well as cognition. These are designed more for psychogeriatric patients, and some of them are described more fully in Paul Brewer's (1984) useful article.

REFERENCES

Barker et al 1985 Geriatric consultation teams in acute hospitals: impact on back up of elderly patients. Journal of the American Geriatric Society 33(6)

Benjamin J 1976 The Northwick Park ADL Index. British Journal of Occupational Therapy 39: 301–8

Brewer P 1984 Brief assessments for the elderly mentally infirm. British Journal of Occupational Therapy 47(6): 168–72

Brocklehurst J C 1978 The evolution of geriatric medicine. Journal of American Geriatric Society 26: 433–439

Brody S J, Balatan D J, Pickar G, Vermeiren J C 1976 Diagnostic and treatment centre for the aging: a program of pre-placement intervention. Gerontologist 16 Feb. 47–51 (Pt 1)

Burley L E, Currie C T, Smith R G, Williamson J 1979 Contribution from geriatric medicine within acute medical wards. British Medical Journal 2:90

Folstein M F, Folstein S E, McHugh P R 1975 'Mini Mental State.' Journal of Psychiatric Research 12: 189–199

Katz S, Thomas D, Downs T D, Cash H R, Grotz R C 1970 Progress in development of the index ADL. Gerontologist 10: 20–30

Cormack D, Fraser D 1975 The nurse's role in psychiatric institutions (part II). Nursing Times (occasional papers), p 29

Isaacs B, Walkey F A 1963 Assessments of the mental state of elderly hospital patients using a sample questionnaire. Americal Journal of Psychiatry 120:173

Mahoney F I, Barthel D W 1965 Functional evaluation: The Barthel Index. Maryland State Medical Journal 14: 61–5

Newman M 1972 The process of recovery after hemiplegia Stroke 3: 701–10

Nichols P J R 1976 Are ADL indices of any value? British Journal of Occupational Therapy 39: 160–3

Pattie A H, Gilleard G J 1979 Manual of the Clifton Assessment procedures for the elderly. Hodder and Stoughton, Sevenoaks

Pfeiffer E 1975, A short portable mental status questionnaire for the assessment of brain deficit in the elderly. Journal of the American Geriatric Society 23: 433–41

Pinel C, and Seriki C 1976 Nursing establishments in geriatric hospitals, Nursing times 72: 850–3

Popplewell 1982 Acute admissions to a geriatric assessment unit. Medical Journal of Australia. 17th April: 343–4

Popplewell P Y, Henschke P J 1983 What is the value of a geriatric assessment unit in a teaching hospital? Australian Health Review 6 (2) May

Riley C G 1974 A geriatric assessment unit: The first 12 months. The New Zealand Medical Journal 80 Nov 27: 435–442

Robertson D, Christ L W A C, Stalder L J 1982 Geriatric assessment unit in a teaching hospital. Canadian Medical Association Journal 126 1st May: 1060–4

Robinson R A 1977 Differential diagnosis and assessment in brain failure. Age and Ageing 6 (suppl):42–9

Rogers P J 1981 A new concept — The new geriatric acute assessment unit at Hammersmith Hospital. Nursing Focus 2 10 June: 356–7

Shoening H A, Aderegg L, Berstrom D, Fonda M, Steike N, Ulrich P 1965 Numerical scoring of self-care status patients (Kenny). Archives Physical Medicine Rehabilitation 46: 689–97

Smith M et al 1977 Measuring the outcome of stroke rehabilitation. British Journal of Occupational Therapy 40: 51–3

Turner A ADL 1981 In: The practice of occupational therapy. Churchill Livingstone, Edinburgh, p 34–35

Trombly C A, Scott A D 1977 Occupational therapy for physical dysfunction. Williams and Wilkins, Baltimore

3

Osteoarthritis and rheumatoid arthritis

J. Caspers
E. Ostle

According to the British League against Rheumatism (Wood 1977), estimated statistical figures of sufferers of rheumatic disorders in the UK published in 1977 were as follows:

osteoarthritis	— 5 000 000
rheumatoid arthritis	— 500 000

Estimated disabilities from rheumatic disorders, especially the severe arthritides, were as follows:

significant impairment of function	— 1 000 000
severe disability	— 200 000
housebound	— 143 000
confined to bed, chair or wheelchair	— 51 000

By retirement age it is estimated that 80% of the population has some rheumatic complaint (Kolodny & Klipper 1976) and one third of geriatric patients attending day hospitals have arthritis (Brocklehurst 1978). Similarly, Acheson (1982) showed that osteoarthritis is one of the commonest of all chronic diseases in North America.

OSTEOARTHRITIS

Osteoarthritis, also known as osteoarthrosis, is a degenerative joint disease in which there is a progressive loss of articular cartilage accompanied by new bone formation and capsular fibrosis. It is usually classified as either (a) primary — having no definite aetiology and either localised or generalised; or (b) secondary — having a known cause which is local or systemic (those latter causes being most commonly, traumatic, infectious, congenital, inflammatory, metabolic or vascular in nature). The disease is often polyarticular and symmetrical, with the hand being the most commonly affected site. Besides the distal interphalangeal joint and first metacarpal joint of the hand, the next most frequently affected joints are the hip, knee, first metatarsal, lumbrosacral spine and cervical spine (Kale & Jones 1981).

In the elderly patient without secondary complications, osteoarthritis of the large weight-bearing joints, the hip and the knee, are often the most disabling conditions. Usually the hand, when affected by osteoarthritis, becomes painless in the latter stages, leaving the affected joints deformed and stiff. There is little loss of functional ability because there is not much loss of muscle strength. This is in marked contrast to the patient with rheumatoid arthritis where the disease is systemic, often producing unstable joints as well as severe muscular weakness which greatly reduces the functional ability of the hand. Therefore the remainder of this section on osteoarthritis will deal specifically with the treatment of the elderly patient with hip and/or knee joint problems.

Signs and symptoms

The most commonly reported clinical features, both at the hip and the knee, are pain, general stiffness, deformity and diminished range of movement. In addition, there may also be symptoms of swelling, 'locking', or giving way at the knee. X-rays will usually show loss of joint space, subarticular sclerosis, bone cysts, and osteophytes. What is important to know is that the clinical symptoms and the patient's ability to perform activities of daily living are not always related to the severity of the radio-logical changes. Therefore, these patients should ideally be managed by a team of professionals including the physician, orthopaedic surgeon, occupational therapist, physiotherapist, social worker and nurse in order to get an accurate picture of how the patient is affected by the disease. The patient should be seen at regular intervals to enable the team to monitor her progress. This way, appropriate help can be provided at the most opportune time in order to maintain the patient at home for as long as possible with maximum independence.

Conservative management

Pain relief

Unfortunately there is no pharmaceutical cure for osteoarthritis and therefore the drugs used are primarily symptom suppressant. They are aimed mainly at pain relief and relief of swelling.

Rest for short periods of time can also be an important way to reduce pain. But unfortunately, rest in bed for the customary eight hours can exacerbate pain. As a result the patient can have difficulty sleeping and may also be prescribed night sedation. In the elderly this can have a disastrous effect, especially if the patient needs to use the toilet during the night (see Ch. 4, e.g. reasons for falling). Another problem facing the patient with osteoarthritis is that prolonged periods of rest in a position of least pain can lead to stiffness and eventually loss of joint range of movement and deformity. However it is often the case that once the joint has become completely stiff or arthrodesed, it is no longer painful as discussed earlier about the hand. But when the weight-bearing joints become fused or unstable in an 'unfavourable position' they cause undue stress to be placed upon compensatory joints, and wear and tear damage to these joints can further complicate the overall disease picture. For example, a hip that becomes fused in greater than 70 degrees of flexion will put a great deal of stress on the knee of the same leg, the opposite hip and the lumbar spine, probably causing backache.

It is therefore important for the patient with joints that are prone to be stiff to understand the above information so that she can be persuaded to spend some time each day lying in a prone position when resting with her feet hanging over the end of the bed so that her knees and hips can be stretched out straight in extension to help prevent the formation of disabling contractures at those joints.

Mobilisation

The patient should be instructed in a programme of passive, nonstressful range of movement exercise by the physiotherapist which can be continued at home. These exercises are aimed at strengthening the muscles that surround the joint and maintaining or increasing the joint range of movement. This will help to stabilise the joint.

Joint stiffness and protective muscle spasm can be relieved by warmth which is applied locally. Adequate heating in the patient's home is therefore also important to help keep her as mobile and as independent as possible.

Load reduction

Although the evidence is not clear, many physicians and surgeons feel that excessive weight will aggravate the symptoms of a degenerative weight-bearing joint and recommend a reduction to normal body weight for the obese patient. Other means of load reduction at the hip and knee are by joint protection with the use of assistive devices (i.e. sticks, splints, braces, and shock-absorbing heel pads) and by teaching the patient to use good body mechanics while performing activities of daily living.

Factors that aggravate symptoms and stress the joints unnecessarily can often be revealed by finding out about the patient's manner of doing housework, the type of furniture used in the house and how a patient uses her leisure time. For example, a person with osteoarthritis of the knees may find it very difficult to get up from a low armchair. The provision of a high chair will put her in a position of mechanical advantage.

Restoration/maintenance of independence in activities of daily living

As the patient becomes more disabled through pain, loss of joint range of movement and deformity, the occupational therapist's role in the management of the osteoarthritic patient becomes increasingly important to help maintain the patient in the community and keep her from becoming totally dependent. The patient should be assessed in her home to find out about specific difficulties with activities of daily living so that domestic furniture and household activities can be rearranged, as stated previously, and essential

Table 3.1 Problem-solving list for degenerative weight-bearing joints

Problems	Solutions
On/off bed	raise bed height, use firmer mattress
On/off chair	raise chair height, firmer cushion, use ejector seat
On/off toilet	raise toilet height (*Fig. 3.1*) provide grab rail
Getting to the toilet at night after bedtime	provide commode next to bed
In/out bath	provide bath aids, change to shower, provide shower chair
Dressing lower half of body	provide long shoe-horn, elastic shoe laces, sock/stocking aid (*Fig. 3.2*) tights aid, helping hand, suggest wearing slip-on shoes
Picking up items off floor	provide reacher or helping hand (*Fig. 3.3*)
Up/down stairs	provide extra bannister, grab rails, stair-lift, half-step
Walking indoors	provide walking frame or stick/s
Walking outdoors	provide wheelchair for relatives and friends to take patient on outings
Carrying items from one room to another when using walking frame or 2 sticks	provide walking frame bag for carrying objects, trolley
Standing for any length of time	provide suitable seating where necessary (i.e. kitchen, telephone, wash hand basin, etc)

adaptive equipment supplied. Please see Table 3.1 for a list of common problems and suggested solutions.

It may also be part of the occupational therapist's role to involve the services of home care agencies and other community services to help with shopping, cleaning and cooking, depending on the needs of the patient and the amount of family support.

It can be seen from Table 3.1 that it is of great importance that the elderly, in order to remain independent, should be living in suit-able and sensible housing (i.e. ground floor, near friends and relatives, easy access to shops, etc.). If possible, the elderly person should be made to consider this before it becomes a necessity and while she is still fit enough to cope with a move.

Surgical management

When the patient's pain can no longer be managed satisfactorily using the conservative methods outlined above and her quality of life is greatly reduced, surgery is usually indi-

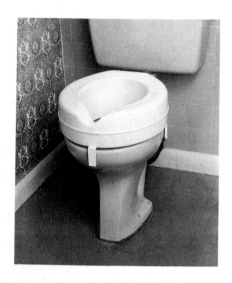

Fig. 3.1 Raised toilet seat

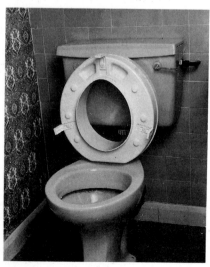

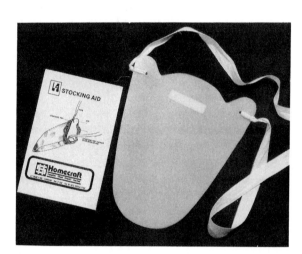

Fig. 3.2 Stocking aid

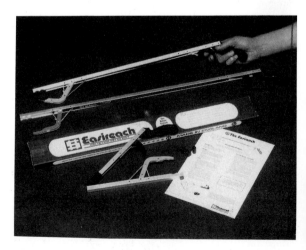

Fig. 3.3 Easireach

cated. Age is no barrier to surgery, but the patient's medical condition must be good enough to withstand the effects of an anaesthetic.

Most sources agree that the type of surgical management for the patient over the age of 55 with osteoarthritis of the hip is the total joint replacement or arthroplasty. The choice of surgery at the knee joint is less clear since the long-term results of the knee replacement have not yet been fully evaluated. However, many sources agree that the patient should have a knee arthroplasty if there is advanced degeneration, if osteotomy has failed and if the patient's activities will not be very excessive post-operatively. Knee arthrodesis is seldom used in the elderly except as a last resort. Both the hip replacement and the knee replacement allow the patient to be mobilised quickly post-operatively which is ideal for the elderly.

As the different types of artificial hip and knee joints and the surgical techniques are described in detail in other sources as well as being constantly redesigned and revised, it will be superfluous to describe them all here. (See the recommended reading list at the end of this chapter.)

Post-operative management of the knee replacement

Management for the knee replacement mainly involves physiotherapy. The aim is to get a minimum of 90 degrees of flexion and maximum strength when fully extending the knee in order to achieve stable weight-bearing. There is normally very little occupational therapy involvement in the form of giving advice on the use of adaptive equipment as the patient is usually very much better post-operatively by the time she is discharged and well able to transfer from beds and chairs. There may be some problems if the patient's disease is polyarticular or the knee replacement has failed and a knee fusion is being attempted. Should one be faced with a person in these circumstances, see Table 3.1 for help in solving specific problems.

Post-operative management of the hip replacement

Many surgeons recommend that patients limit the movements at their hips post-operatively for 6–12 weeks to reduce the risk of dislocation. This is usually associated with reduced stability at the joint in the first few weeks following surgery until soft tissue healing can take place and full muscle control at the hip is restored. Much depends upon the surgeon's approach, technique and type of joint used. It is therefore essential to find out from the surgeon what his post-operative regime consists of and exactly which movements will need to be restricted. Most commonly, hip flexion of more than 90 degrees, hip rotation, hip adduction and, in particular, any combination of these movements will need to be restricted for a period post-operatively. It can be helpful to patients with memory problems and their relatives for written guidelines to be supplied to back up instructions given in the hospital on how to perform activities of daily living while avoiding restricted movements. Since the patient's hospital stay is normally 10 days to 3 weeks, the occupational therapist should try to see the patient pre-operatively to find out about the patient's home situation (e.g. type of housing, barriers to access, height of furniture, availability of family and friends, household responsibilities and pre-operative level of independence) and other medical and orthopaedic problems. This will help the therapist to plan the patient's post-operative rehabilitation. Before being discharged, the occupational therapist should demonstrate to the patients and supervise them in the use of any assistive equipment to make sure that the patients know how to use the equipment safely.

Excision arthroplasty or pseudoarthodesis of the hip

When dealing with the elderly, it may be necessary to treat a patient post-operatively for an excision arthroplasty of the femoral head and neck, first introduced by Girdlestone in 1943 for the management of sepsis in the hip joint. In recent years this procedure has been used as a last resort where other surgical attempts (i.e. hip replacement) have failed due to implant loosening and deep sepsis, which normally occurs months or years post-operatively.

The limb is normally managed in traction for a period of 2–6 weeks post-operatively, followed by mobilisation using a walking frame and a shoe raise as the leg is often shorter. Sometimes a weight-bearing caliper will be necessary where there is excessive movement between the femur and the pelvis.

The aim of this surgery is mainly to relieve pain at the hip and to allow the patient to walk for some distance. Many patients will require a walking frame or two sticks permanently and will need the help of assistive devices and adaptations made to the home in order to be independent in activities of daily living. A home visit is usually recommended. See Table 3.1 for help with solving specific problems.

RHEUMATOID ARTHRITIS

As can be seen by the statistics given, osteoarthritis is much more prevalent than rheumatoid arthritis but, from the point of view of the occupational therapist, the sufferers from rheumatoid arthritis require more time, energy and mechanical aids per person and must be considered accordingly. Rheumatoid arthritis is the most common and serious type of inflammatory polyarthritis. The inflammation affects primarily synovium and may lead to severe joint destruction. Although the brunt of the disease falls on the joints, it is a systemic condition and, together with disorders such as systemic lupus erythematosous, ranks as a systemic connective tissue disease (Currey 1983).

Various studies have been made about the sexual bias of incidence of rheumatoid arthritis; one by Ehrlich et al (1970) reports patients who contact the disease before the age of 60 years with the ratio of male:female as 5:1 which changes to 2.5:1 in those whose onset is after 60 years; while the Empire Rheumatism Council in 1950 and Short et al in 1957 report that 1% of the male population and 3% of the female population in the UK suffer from rheumatoid disease in one form or another.

The disease is progressive and widely varying in its severity. In the most common forms it runs a course of exacerbation and remissions, eventually leading to some degree of deformity. The initial symptoms are the same in the young and the elderly. The onset can be acute and rapidly progressive; occasionally the disease may be monarticular or affect a few joints, but more commonly there is polyarthritis. The main symptoms are morning stiffness, joint pain and tenderness, fatigue and general malaise along with the signs of hot swollen joints, muscle and tendon weakness. There may also be restricted joint movement, contractures, impaired mobility and function with possible nodule formation. Sometimes there are arteritic and neuritic changes indicating systemic involvement. A fairly common additional symptom which the therapist should be aware of is Sjogren's syndrome which is a disease of the lacrimal and parotid glands, resulting in dry eyes and mouth. Many patients with this problem have difficulty in administering the necessary artificial tears because of limited functional ability in the upper extremities.

Rheumatoid arthritis may start at any age and because of the chronicity of the disease many patients who develop the disease in earlier life carry it with them into old age when they may already be suffering from degenerative changes and other illnesses; whilst others may manifest the disease for the first time in old age. Once the initial signs and symptoms are exhibited and an accurate diagnosis has been made, the medical treatment plan should begin embracing all the available resources, i.e. the 'team approach'.

The general aims of treatment are:

1. relief of pain
2. maintenance of function
3. prevention and correction of deformities
4. control of the disease process.

The requirement is one of continuous re-appraisal and assessment, since changes in the patient's state of health necessitate different members of the team bringing their expertise to bear upon the problems as they arise.

The occupational therapist should be involved not just within the hospital or in the community after a hospital admission, but also after initial diagnosis and when surgery may be indicated but not yet possible due to long waiting lists or for any other reason. This will be referred to later on in the chapter.

The treatment of patients suffering from rheumatoid arthritis ranges from mild chemo-therapy to the most advanced forms of replacement surgery, but the majority of patients fall within these two extremes. At the time of the initial diagnosis the patient is usually prescribed medication: this is possibly the beginning of a lengthy association with drug therapy. In the main, these drugs will come from one of the following groups:

— non-steroid anti-inflammatory drugs (NSAID). These include the salycilates, e.g. asprin, which if taken in the prescribed dosage may control the inflammation
— intrasynovial steroid injections which may provide localised suppression of inflam-mation in one joint
— remission-inducing drugs which include gold, penicillamine and antimalarial drugs
— steroids: these can prove most efficacious but may have many serious side-effects
— analgesics which are purely for the relief of pain and may have no effect upon the progress or state of the disease.

At the time the patient starts to require medication it is of value as a 'back-up' service for her to receive advice concerning joint protection techniques and correct resting positions; and a line of communication should be set up so that the patient can approach the pertinent therapist if and when further problems arise. Initially the help may be as minor as demonstrating the ease of turning a tap with a tap-turner, but care should be taken by the therapist not to fore-cast too gloomy a future (which, indeed, is impossible with any degree of accuracy) whilst at the same time delivering the message that steps taken to prevent deformity are easier than those required later when deformities have already formed.

Joint protection techniques

Although joint protection techniques are not accepted 100% by all rheumatologists, enough has been written to warrant a mention in this chapter since they cost nothing and almost certainly are efficacious in the overall manage-ment of a rheumatoid arthritis patient of any age. The principles are as follows:

1. to have respect for pain
2. to balance activity and rest
3. to maintain muscle strength in joint range of movement
4. to reduce effort which includes work simplification
5. to avoid positions of deformity
6. to use stronger/larger joints where possible
7. to use each joint in its most stable, anatomical and functional plane
8. to avoid staying too long in one position
9. to avoid activities that cannot be stopped or interrupted
10. to use assistive equipment and splints when such are indicated.

In order to be effective it must be stressed that these principles should be discussed individually with each patient so that the patient clearly understands the point of the regime and so that it can be tailored to the individual's own requirements. The rheuma-toid arthritis patients have limited energy at their disposal, and whilst it is psychologically good to be as independent as possible, there may come a time when it is wise to get prior-ities right — to use that limited energy for the better things in life and accept help from others to do the more mundane tasks.

Positions of rest

When the body aches, it is the most natural thing to curl up in the most comfortable position, but, as stated earlier in this chapter, it is important that the patient is educated to rest with the joints in proper alignment, otherwise contracture deformities arise which not only mean loss of range of movement, but consequent loss of function and, particularly in weight-bearing joints, the formation of deformities in other joints as a compensatory mechanism. The knees should be straight — never have a pillow underneath — the feet supported at right angles to the tibia and protected from the weight of the bed clothes. If the knee joint is affected it can be in a resting splint which affords the patient some relief from the pain, particularly during sleep. Attention should be paid to the wrist; if the disease is currently causing pain there, splinting can ease the pain and support tendons under stress. Splinting is performed by many members of staff, depending on the facilities available. Obviously a trained orthotist with experience is the ideal person for this job, but in less than ideal situations many others may have to acquire the specific skill, including the occupational therapist. Whatever the working environment, it behoves the occupational therapist to know of the potential problems, warning signs and to whom to relay this relevant information so that suitable action can be taken.

Functional classification

Assessment of the patient both before and after medical and surgical treatment should form a major part of the occupational therapist's role, and in order to make these findings meaningful the following classifications can be useful, American in origin, they have come to be almost universally understood and accepted:

Class I = patient able to perform all activities without handicap

Class II = patient able to perform adequately for all normal activities despite discomfort

Class III = not able to do very much, can live on her own but needs help from others and assistive equipment

Class IV = completely incapacitated, bedridden or confined to wheelchair.

Having classified the patient after assessment, many problems will emerge to be solved. Table 3.2 gives some of these and their solutions. It will be noted that many of those problems are common to both the osteoarthritic and the rheumatoid arthritic, but for the purposes of expediency, please refer to Table 3.1 for difficulties involving the weight-bearing joints of hips and knees.

Table 3.2 Problem-solving list for rheumatoid patients

Problems	Solutions
Feeding	
Unable to use ordinary utensils	use built-up handles — possibly with angled shafts
Unable to use ordinary cup	use lightweight mug with handle deep enough to enclose 4 digits — possibly thermal so that two hands can be used without fear of burns on supportive hand
Dressing	
Refer to chapter on clothing	
Toileting	
Unable to use toilet paper	use special appliance for holding paper or make a 'wipe' from sponge on coat hanger
Unable to flush toilet	extend handle of toilet lever
Unable to cope with garments	see Chapter 19
Washing	
Unable to clean face	use 'spontex' sponge or flannel on wooden spoon
Unable to clean neck	use manufactured strip of towelling with plastic bangles at either end
Unable to clean underarms	use spontex sponge
Unable to clean feet	use long-handled sponge
Unable to clean teeth	extend and/or change toothbrush handle or use batteried brush
Unable to shave	extend razor handle; if electric a special casing can be contrived either with extended handle or loops for both hands
Unable to apply make-up	make extended holders for lipsticks, cotton buds, etc from dowelling
Unable to comb hair	use extended comb

Bathing

Unable to get in/out of bath	depending on severity of problems, use bath board, bath seat or mechanical device such as 'Mangar' or Ambilift. Alternatively use a shower.

Household activities

Unable to operate cooker	enlarge knobs or use contour grip turner
Unable to hold saucepan	use 2-handled lightweight pans, slide them, not lift, and use basket in pan to remove load from liquid in which it is cooked
Unable to hold teapot/kettle	use teapot tilt/one cup multi-boiler/'Air-pot' thermos flask
Unable to prepare vegetables	use food processor or cook first and slice later when soft or use 'Chop-a-lot'
Unable to slice bread/meat	purchase already sliced/use Styrex knife/electric knife
Unable to open tins	use electric can opener with lever action
Unable to open jars/bottles	use 'Beli-clamp' to immobilise jar/bottle and strongboy/Tigercrown opener to turn lid (*Fig. 3.4*)
Unable to extract electric plugs	use plugs with loops
Unable to use aerosol containers	rig up lever action depressor with 2 ice lolly sticks, one taped to container and other hinged with tape at right angles
Unable to turn taps	use lever taps/tap turners (*Fig. 3.5*)

Mobility

Difficulty getting in/out of car	put plastic on seat cover to reduce friction
Difficulty turning ignition key	extend key to include lever

Communications

Difficulty in holding pen/pencil	widen grip with foam or use propriety pen holder, N.B. felt tip pens are easier to use than ball points
Difficulty using regular telephone	check with telephone company re availability of suitable instrument. Alternatively, use telephone holder which has receiver on extended flexible arm.

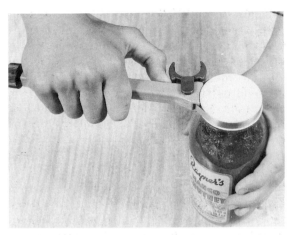

Fig. 3.4 Strongboy opener

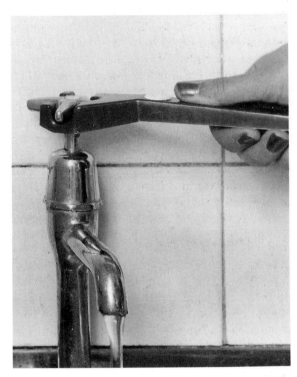

Fig. 3.5 Lever tap turner (photographs of aids to daily living supplied by Homecraft of London)

Preface to joint surgery in the elderly. When considering surgical treatment of the elderly patient, it is the overall health of the body rather than the longevity of the patient which is of importance. However, in the UK, the current length of waiting lists must obviously have some bearing on the choice of patient; if her life expectancy is going to be less than the length of the waiting list, then this may prove to be the deciding factor against surgery. With many elderly patients who are otherwise fit, surgery may prolong their independence at home and prevent them being demoted to the final functional classification which is total dependency.

In this chapter it is inappropriate to detail every available procedure for the various joints involved and the occupational therapist's role therewith. A brief resume will be given, mentioning the most common procedures. For more detailed information a suggested reading list is provided at the end of the chapter.

Cervical vertebrae

Affection of the cervical vertebrae is common and the aim of treatment is to prevent pressure on the spinal cord with its subsequent sensory and motor neurological involvement and possible subluxation. The conservative treatment consists of the use of cervical collars, the practice of joint protection techniques and traction. The last resort is surgical fusion of the spine, but this is approached with great caution and after much deliberation. No matter how severe or otherwise the cervical damage, all patients will require assistive devices to help with activities of daily living and other activities due to restricted neck movement and subsequent limited field of vision. The shoulder, elbow and wrist joints cannot be viewed in isolation since they are all vital links in the chain between the trunk and the hand. A functional hand is of little use to the patient who cannot place it where it is required.

Shoulder joint

This is one of the more difficult joints in which to achieve success in surgical intervention, due to the basic mechanics and shape of the articular surfaces involved. Good musculature around the joint is particularly necessary for success post-operatively since there is little else to provide stability. Conservative treatment of local injections into the joint are effective in relieving pain during the early stages. Later on in the state of degeneration, surgical measures may be necessary; these include synovectomy, bursectomy, interpositional arthroplasty, hemi-arthroplasty, total arthroplasty and osteotomy, the latter being

effective depending upon the site of the problem. The prime object of relief from pain is usually obtained but full range of motion will probably be limited. Translated into terms of occupational therapy this means a re-assessment of the need for assistive devices and advice to be given on safe use of the joint within its limitations. This is always a matter to be agreed upon with the surgeon and physiotherapist since individual cases vary.

Elbow joint

The conservative treatment is local injection to alleviate pain. Surgical measures are (1) synovectomy and (2) joint replacement. Synovectomy is a good procedure for relieving pain should it be performed at the right time — too late is ineffective — but it is a short-term measure. Total elbow arthroplasty is probably more applicable in the elderly patient. This is a joint which should be assessed as part of the total body, particularly since the rheumatoid arthritis patient may be currently undergoing lower limb surgery and need the upper limbs to lean on crutches, sticks or zimmer aids. The occupational therapist should be aware of the limits to activities imposed by these procedures, i.e. she should check with the surgeon as to his views on maximum weight loads and rotational stresses since the prostheses vary in their post-operative management and ultimate maximum abilities. There are usually constraints to activities following elbow arthroplasties such as vigorous hoeing in the garden when the jarring movement might loosen the prosthesis.

Wrist joint

The problems arising from wrist involvement can be caused by synovitis alone or synovitis leading to laxity of ligament with subsequent subluxation. Then the ultimate bony erosions and tendon ruptures may finally destroy the joint and render the hand useless unless there is surgical intervention. The following procedures are commonly used:

(i) wrist arthroplasty
(ii) wrist stabilisation
(iii) wrist arthrodesis
(iv) excision head of ulna
(v) decompression of carpal tunnel.

Following most wrist surgery there follows a period when the joint may be splinted, then comes the task of functional retraining which should be shared by both physio and occupational therapists.

Hand

The main deformities are ulnar drift and metacarpophalangeal subluxation; bout-toniére's and Swan-neck deformities of the fingers; 'Z' deformity of the thumb and ruptured tendons — most commonly the extensors to the ring and little fingers. The management of these problems requires a special skill since often these deformities may look appalling but the hand is still quite functional, and drastic alteration may improve appearance but cost the patient dearly in function. Pre-operatively it is important for the occupational therapist to give the surgeon a thorough assessment of the upper limbs' function as opposed to a series of measurements which, although accurate, may prove meaningless.

The most common surgical procedures include joint replacement, joint fusion in positions of optimal function, repair of tendons, tendon transfers. Post-operatively the occupational therapist's role usually includes re-education of the hand, splinting, teaching of joint protection techniques in addition to assessment for post-operative comparisons, to be followed by the usual activities of daily living training.

Hip and knee

These joints have been discussed earlier in the chapter under Osteoarthritis: management is similar in terms of the surgery involved, but the rehabilitation of rheumatoid patients is more difficult since they usually have involve-ment of the upper limbs which makes the use of walking aids more problematical. Usually the patient also has problems transferring and the period of caution after surgery tends to be longer since the rheumatoid patient's joints can be less stable due to muscle weakness.

Ankle joint

Rheumatoid arthritis involvement of the ankle can be treated conservatively by injections into the joint for pain relief, and sometimes a German leather anklet is enough to support the joint. The surgical measures which may be necessary are joint replacement and joint fusion.

Feet

Rheumatoid arthritis involvement of the foot is very common indeed, but only a small proportion of the patients require surgery. Conservative management includes much help from the chiropodist, the use of pertinent supportive in-soles and correct footwear. Surgically, the most common procedures are:

1. metatarsal head resection, which brings the toes down into alignment with the rest of the foot
2. ablation of toes. This is a most effective measure but many patients are understand-ably apprehensive about such an irreversible operation. However, to overcome this fear, it can help to have a former patient demonstrate the success of pain-free mobility using footwear with blocked toes.

Footwear. It may fall to the lot of the occupational therapist to help the patient find correct footwear. There are two main areas of difficulty: (1) finding shoes wide and deep enough to encompass the toes without pressure; (2) finding supportive shoes which the patient with deformed hands can fasten independently. Initially the choice may be made from wide fitting shoes 'off the shelf'; then the next stage, as the condition causes more deformity, is to try special orthopaedic shoes 'off the shelf'; and lastly, to have footwear made to measure. The last recourse is easily the most effective one, but two things must be borne in mind; firstly, the high cost and secondly, the appearance tends to be less than glamorous, even for the more elderly ladies.

In conclusion, it can be seen that one of the major roles of the occupational therapist is to bridge the gap between hospital and home. She is the team member who is in the unique position of being able to assess the patient in her own home prior to finalisation of plans for hospital discharge. But one must not forget the most central member of the team, the patient, without whose co-operation and understanding no plans can be successful for her adjustment to living with arthritis.

REFERENCES

Acheson R M 1982 Heberden Oration 1981 Aspects of the epidemiology of osteoarthrosis. Annals of Rheumatic Diseases 41: 325–334
Adler E 1966 Rheumatoid arthritis in old age. Israel Journal of Medical Science 2: 607–613
Brocklehurst J C 1978 Geriatric services and the day hospital. In: Brocklehurst J C (ed) Geriatric medicine and gerentology. Churchill Livingstone, London, p 747
Currey H L 1983 Essentials of rheumatology. Pitman Press, Bath
Ditunmo J, Ehrlich G E 1970 Care and training of elderly patients with rheumatoid arthritis. Geriatrics 25: 164–172
Ehrlich G E, Katz W A, Cohen S H 1970 Rheumatoid arthritis in the aged. Geriatrics 25: 103–113
Kale S A, Jones J V 1981 Rehabilitating the elderly arthritic. Geriatric Rehabilitation 36: 6: 101–106
Kolodny A L, Klipper A R 1976 Bone and joint diseases in the elderly. Hospital Practice 11: 91–101
Slaninka S C 1980 Difficult disease, difficult patient. Journal of Gerentological Nursing 6: 94–95
Wood P H (ed) 1977 The challenge of arthritis and rheumatism. The British League Against Rheumatism, London

RECOMMENDED READING

Apley A G, Solomon L 1982 Apley's system of orthopaedics and fractures, 6th edn. Butterworth, London
Brattstrom M 1975 Principles of joint protection in chronic rheumatic disease. Yearbook Medical Publishers, Chicago
Devas M (ed) 1977 Geriatric Orthopaedics. Academic Press, London
Fairburn S M 1985 Daily activities following hip replacement: A handout. British Journal of Occupational Therapy 48:6: 167–168
Goldstein L A (ed), Dickenson R C (ed) 1981 Atlas of orthopaedic surgery, 2nd edn. Mosby, St Louis
Harris N H (ed) 1983 Postgraduate Textbook of Clinical Orthopaedics. Wright, London
Haworth R J 1982 Use of aids during the first three months after total hip replacement. British Journal of Rheumatology 22:1: 29–35
Insall J N (ed) 1984 Surgery of the knee. Churchill Livingstone, New York
Melvin J L 1982 Rheumatic disease: occupational therapy and rehabilitation, 2nd edn. Davis, Philadelphia
Seegar M S, Fisher L A 1982 Adaptive equipment used in the rehabilitation of hip arthroplasty patients. The American Journal of Occupational Therapy 36:8: 503–508
Wigley F M 1984 Osteoarthritis: practical management in older patients. Geriatrics 39:3: 101–120

4

Falls, fractures and fixtures in geriatric orthopaedic rehabilitation units

C. Peterson

The geriatric orthopaedic rehabilitation unit, as its name suggests, is run on a combined care basis. The patients are looked after initially by both a consultant geriatrician and a consultant orthopaedic surgeon. However, as the patients' acute orthopaedic problems cease to require attention from the surgeons, their care is taken over solely by the geriatrician and his team.

Falls and subsequent fractures are one of the most common causes of admission to hospital in the elderly population and orthopaedic surgeons have found this type of unit an invaluable method of dealing with the problem of blocked beds. In one study, 13% (43) of 325 acute surgical and orthopaedic beds were found to be blocked by elderly patients, mostly women with fractured femurs who had previously been living alone (Murphy 1980).

The reasons for these blocked beds were many, but the main problem appeared to be that there had been no contact with the geriatrician, who is aware of the importance of the early establishment of aims of treatment and plans for resettlement in collaboration with other members of the multidisciplinary team, i.e. the occupational therapist, physiotherapist, medical social worker and nursing staff. In the above study, no long-term plans whatsoever had been made for 12 of the 43 patients.

Collaboration and teamwork are essential factors in successful rehabilitation of the elderly patient admitted with a fracture.

FALLS

As mentioned previously, falls are one of the main causes of admission to any geriatric medical assessment unit.

Many falls do not result in a fracture, but after examination and investigation an undetected underlying medical condition may be found and treated during a short period of assessment and rehabilitation in a geriatric medical assessment unit.

There are several ways of classifying the causes of falls. Poor lighting may be an environmental cause of a fall. Many old peoples' houses are badly lit for various reasons, e.g. use of low wattage light bulbs to save electricity, curtains kept closed because of fear of burglars or nosey neighbours. Another related cause is lack of bedside lighting, i.e. an old person may fall while walking across the bedroom in the dark to reach the light switch. A high proportion of falls occur when old ladies, with a history of osteoarthrosis, fall while getting out of bed to go to the toilet during the night.

Trips and slips can happen both indoors and outside. Rugs scattered throughout the house, a candlewick bedspread trailing on the floor, loose wires and toilet mats strategically placed on highly polished linoleum in the bathroom are a few of the many extrinsic hazards to be found in most homes belonging to the elderly. In cases where a fall has occurred indoors with no apparent trip or slip, the patient is investigated fully for any underlying condition, e.g. hypotension, osteoporosis.

Outdoors there are many dangers facing the elderly: traffic, impatient bus drivers, uneven kerbs, and of course the weather. There is often a marked increase in admissions to an accident and emergency unit following a high wind, and a steadier increase during snow and icy weather.

Defective vision can also be a cause of falls. Following a cerebral vascular accident a hemianopia, which is a defect in vision in half of the visual field, can develop. This, coupled with the more common visual problems found in the elderly, e.g. cataracts, glaucoma, macular degeneration, can transform a familiar living room into a hazardous obstacle course. Incorrect lenses in glasses can be equally dangerous. Some elderly people may not have visited an optician for several years because of poor mobility or fear that it may cost too much to have a new pair of glasses. Another reason often found is elderly people who wear glasses belonging to late spouses or well-meaning friends.

Drop attacks are commonly seen in the elderly. The cause of these attacks, where the elderly person suddenly falls to the ground with no warning and no signs of neurological deficit, is difficult to identify and therefore hard to treat. There are several theories suggesting that the attacks are caused by vertebral ischaemia with loss of postural reflexes. These attacks can occur at any time and are obviously extremely incapacitating and dangerous for the sufferer. Fractures are not always a result of one of these attacks, but sooner or later, as the sufferer becomes older and more frail, the likelihood of serious injury increases.

People suffering from Parkinson's disease are prone to falls which are mainly a result of the typical shuffling gait associated with the condition, but can also be caused by postural hypotension, another common feature of the disease.

Falls are also associated with transient ischaemic attacks. These episodic periods of cerebral ischaemia can lead to diplopia and vertigo which can lead to falls. Decreased blood flow to the brain can also be a feature of cervical spondylosis which is a degeneration of the cervical vertebrae, usually osteoarthritic in nature. The vertebral arteries become compressed as the neck's position is changed. This usually happens when the patient looks upwards, a common cause being looking up when drawing curtains. The compression and resulting decreased blood flow then leads to a fall.

Confusion and dementia are probably amongst the most common underlying causes of falls. Disorientation, clouding of consciousness, disturbances of thought processes all predispose to a general lack of awareness of hazards and particularly dangerous situations.

Hypotension in the elderly can predispose them to falls. The drop in blood pressure leads to a decrease in cerebral blood flow causing syncope. This drop in blood pressure can present as a feature of myocardial infarction or as a feature of haemorrhage from the gastrointestinal tract or of pulmonary emboli. These emboli are common in the elderly because an overall lack of mobility leads to venous thrombosis which, when repeated, can lead to frequent falls. Postural hypotension is often caused by drugs (see Ch. 15), mainly those used to treat hypertension, the major tranquillisers — phenothiazines or diuretics.

Certain gastrointestinal problems such as diarrhoea and constipation have been known to lead to falls. Severe episodes of diarrhoea can cause brief periods of loss of consciousness, and chronic diarrhoea can result in a deficiency of potassium and lead to muscle weakness and increased instability. Some patients with constipation have strained so hard on the toilet that they have lost consciousness.

Osteoarthrosis and rheumatoid arthritis (see Ch. 3), because of their debilitating nature, lead to generalised weakness and instability rendering the sufferers of these diseases prone to falls and fractures. Other musculo-skeletal conditions can lead to falls. Osteomalacia results in muscle weakness and chronic aching pain, causing general instability in an elderly person. Osteoporosis causes a reduction in the density of bone, allowing fractures to occur with little force. Often a sharp twisting of the body, usually seen when turning to answer the telephone for example, can cause a fracture which results in a fall

rather than the fall causing the fracture.

There are also metabolic causes of falls seen mainly in thyroid disease. Thyrotoxicosis may cause muscle weakness leading to instability, and myxoedema may cause ataxia, clumsiness and an overall lack of mobility.

As mentioned previously in the case of hypotension, drugs can be the cause of falls. Over-sedation and anticonvulsants, hypoglycaemia caused by drugs used in treating diabetes mellitus, and vertigo caused by use of certain types of antibiotics have all been noted as factors leading to certain falls.

An accurate clinical history is vital if underlying conditions are to be found and treated in order to prevent further falls.

Whatever the cause, falls can be very traumatic experiences for elderly people, leaving mental as well as physical scars. One of the most common complications seen is that of loss of confidence and fear of further falls. Other complications of falls are: loss of mobility, bruising, subdural haematoma (see Ch. 8) burns, hypothermia, dehydration, bronchopneumonia, pressure sores and fractures (Coni et al 1980).

FRACTURES

The most traumatic outcome of a fall for any elderly person is a fracture.

For most people this results in several weeks or months in hospital — a first time for many. Some are deeply shocked by this experience and never really regain their confidence. Another common reaction to the injury and subsequent hospitalisation is that of anger and bitterness that 'this should happen to me at this stage of my life'. Surgical intervention and internal fixation are considered the most appropriate forms of treatment for the elderly. This limits the length of time the elderly patient spends in bed, and thus prevents complications arising such as pressure sores and bronchopneumonia. The most commonly seen fractures in the elderly in acute orthopaedic wards and geriatric orthopaedic rehabilitation units are: fractures of the femur, pelvic fractures, fractures of the patella, tibial fractures, fractures of the humerus, Colles' fracture.

1. Fractures of the femur

(i) Subcapital fractures

These are normally caused by a fall in which the foot or leg becomes twisted and the femoral neck is broken by rotational force. There can be a considerable amount of displacement which is measured using Garden's classification (Apley 1977):

> Grade 1 — incomplete
> Grade 2 — complete without displacement
> Grade 3 — complete with partial displacement
> Grade 4 — complete with full displacement.

The preferred method of treatment of these fractures varies from unit to unit. Some may still use internal fixation, such as a nail, threaded pin or lag screw, which fails in about 30% of patients (Devas et al 1977). Other surgeons' first choice is one of replacement arthroplasty, such as the Thompson prothesis or Hastings prosthesis (see Fig. 4.1).

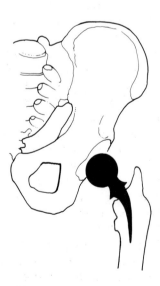

Fig. 4.1 Hemiarthroplasty

(ii) Trochanteric fractures

Early internal fixation is again vital with these fractures. The method in these cases is to insert pin and plate or screw and plate devices, e.g. McLaughlin pin and plate, Richards screw and plate (see Fig. 4.2).

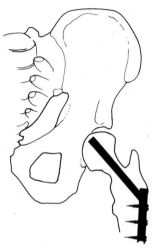

Fig. 4.2 Screw and plate fixation

(iii) Fractures of the shaft of femur

These are often caused by a violent force, e.g. falling down stairs. If the fracture occurs in the upper part of the femur then the same procedure is used as with trochanteric fractures, that of pin and plate. However, if the fracture is in the lower part of the femur an intramedullary nail or pin is used. Again, the operation should be carried out within 24 hours of the trauma.

(iv) Supracondylar fractures

These are usually found in the very frail, osteoporotic elderly patient who has probably suffered one or more previous fractures. Therefore, internal fixation and early mobilisation are vital. The fractures can be fixed using either intramedullary nails (Rush) or a specially designed nail plate.

Falls, fractures and fixtures / 47

2. Fractures of the pelvis

These painful and quite disabling fractures, when isolated and not involving any pelvic ring disruptions, can be seen in three sections of the pelvis: fractures of the (a) ilium (b) floor of the acetabulum and (c) pubic rami. Isolated fractures are normally treated by bed-rest followed by gentle mobilisation. Unstable fractures, rare in the elderly, can be treated by external fixation using screws fixed into the ilium and a turnbuckle crossbar which allows the patient to get up and walk short distances. The fixation is normally removed three weeks later.

3. Patellar fractures

These are usually caused by a direct blow to the patella, but can occur in the elderly with little force. If the patella is cracked but not fragmented then a crêpe bandage or light-weight plastercast is applied to allow immediate mobilisation. Often, if movement is painful, a lightweight full length plaster cylinder or backslab can be used — light enough to allow mobilisation and gentle quadriceps exercises. A stellate fracture can be treated by wiring the fragments, or if there is displacement, a patellectomy may be necessary.

4. Fractures of the tibia and fibula

(i) Tibial plateau — internal fixation using bolts and washers, or conservatively a plaster cylinder may be used.

(ii) Upper tibia — reduction and plaster cylinder are usually used; often the patient may be partial or touch weightbearing initially.

(iii) Shaft of tibia — intramedullary nails may be used to walk. If the fracture is found in the lower part of the tibia then the treatment is more conservative — generally a plaster from below knee to toes.

5. Fractures of the humerus

A fracture of the neck of the humerus is common in the elderly population. The patient usually falls on her outstretched hand and the upward thrust breaks the surgical neck of the humerus.

Treatment can be conservative, wearing a collar and cuff sling, or operative — insertion of an intramedullary Rush pin. The latter often means that the patient has a more pain-free range of movement, allowing her to reach maximum independence more quickly. This fracture can be quite disabling for an elderly person who would find most activities of daily living painful and awkward. Such patients can be admitted to a geriatric orthopaedic rehabilitation unit purely as a 'social admission' if they have no support at home, either from family, friends or social services.

6. Colles' fracture

This is one of the most common fractures seen in the elderly. It is usually caused by a fall on the outstretched hand or, if bilateral, hands. The fracture is generally reduced under a general anaesthetic and a plaster cast applied. Normal movement of fingers, elbow and shoulder is encouraged. Union usually occurs at six weeks when the plaster is removed or bivalved and active movement of the wrist commences. Many people are left with a slight deformity at the wrist but early return of function is more important than cosmetic appearance.

There are obviously many other fractures seen in geriatric orthopaedic rehabilitation units — too many to mention here, but which are described fully in most books on orthopaedic surgery (see p. 49).

The day after these operations the patient is expected to be able to be out of bed for a couple of hours, sitting in a chair, standing and doing a little walking with the supervision of a physiotherapist. The length of time out of bed is gradually increased as is the distance to be walked each day.

Depending on the progress made in the first few days, decisions are made as to the patient's future. Some patients may be discharged directly home if they have become independent in the ward and they have adequate support from family and friends. Others may be considered by the geriatrician attached to the orthopaedic wards to be suitable candidates for rehabilitation and transferred a few days post-operatively to the geriatric orthopaedic rehabilitation unit.

Complications of fractures

There are many complications presenting in the unit following fractures: some are directly related to the fracture, e.g. avascular necrosis, non-union which, if it occurs in the head of femur after a subcapital fracture, can result in the removal of the head and replacement arthroplasty or excision arthroplasty (Girdlestone pseudoarthrosis, see Fig. 4.3) being carried out, leaving the patient more disabled and very frightened. Other more general complications are incontinence, pressure sores, confusion, wound infection etc. It is here that the geriatrician and his team with their varied skills and expertise can take over from the orthopaedic surgeons and begin the rehabilitation process. Geriatric orthopaedic rehabilitation units are a relatively recent innovation; many of them are based on the Hastings model (Devas et al 1977).

One example of this type of unit is found in the Astley Ainslie Hospital, Edinburgh, Scotland. It is a twenty-bedded ward in which all patients are female, over sixty years old and have suffered one fracture or more. The ward is run on the previously described continuous care basis, involving orthopaedic care, geriatric assessment and rehabilitation. The team consists of: consultant geriatrician, consultant orthopaedic surgeon, general practitioner, senior house officer, nursing staff, occupational therapist, physiotherapist, and medical social worker. A health visitor attends the weekly ward round for information on discharged patients for follow-up visits; a chiropodist treats patients once weekly; and a hairdresser is available two mornings each week.

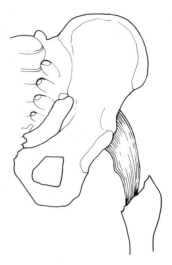

Fig. 4.3 Girdlestone pseudoarthrosis

All the beds in the ward are, in theory, allocated for short-term assessment and rehabilitation. However, there is a problem of 'blocked beds' as in other geriatric units. Usually about a quarter of the beds are blocked at any given time, with most patients waiting up to nine months or a year for long-term care, psychogeriatric care, part IV (III) accommodation, or a shorter period if they are being discharged to a nursing home. A side ward has been converted into a predischarge unit (see Ch. 12). The ward has a catchment area of half of south Edinburgh and Midlothian.

All patients who come to the ward are first admitted to the Royal Infirmary of Edinburgh at the time of their injury. A few days after their treatment, usually an internal fixation, a geriatrician visits the orthopaedic wards to assess the patients and decide which ones are to be transferred to the rehabilitation ward. The emphasis is then on independence in all areas of self-care and mobilisation. Patients' progress is discussed at the weekly case conference and ward round, and decisions reached regarding their discharge and resettlement.

APPENDIX
Outline of occupational therapy programme

Introduction	— explain role and place in the team to the patient and tell her what will be expected of her in the ward programme.
Initial assessment	— usually takes the form of an informal chat, mainly to find out how the patient was coping prior to the fall, e.g. family support, stairs in the house, whether she was housebound.
ADL Assessment	— dressing assessment and practice, toilet and self-care assessments, mobility and transfers — in conjunction with physiotherapist. Kitchen assessment and practice.
Home visits	— approximately 75% of patients have home visits — liaise with community occupational therapist, family, home care organiser, district nurses etc.
Social activities	— organised with help from nursing staff — baking, bingo, outings etc.
Resettlement	— including home visits, Part IV (III) accommodation, nursing homes, long-stay units — assess both patient and placement suitability.

REFERENCES

Adams J Crawford 1981 Outline of orthopaedics, 9th edn. Churchill Livingstone, Edinburgh

Apley A 1977 System of orthopaedics and fractures, 5th edn. Butterworths, London

Coatley Davis 1982 Establishing a geriatric service. Croom Helm, London.

Coni N, Davison W, Webster S 1980 Lecture notes on geriatrics, 2nd edn. Blackwell Scientific Publications, Oxford.

Devas et al 1977 Geriatric orthopaedics. Academic Press, London.

Murphy F W 1980 Organising orthopaedic services. DHSS, London

Webb J T 1985 Notes on orthopaedic nursing, 2nd edn. Churchill Livingstone, Edinburgh

5

Smoking-related diseases

M. Helm
R. Trevan

CHRONIC OBSTRUCTIVE AIRWAYS DISEASE

M. Helm

Very little has been written for occupational therapists on this subject. This is surprising as acute chest infection in elderly people suffering from chronic obstructive airways disease (COAD) frequently precipitates hospital admission. Confusion resulting from acute infection, in the absence of domestic support, is the principal reason for admission.

Chronic bronchitis and emphysema

These are frequently found together in the same patient, although their aetiology and pathology are different. These chronic conditions are found in males more frequently than females. Sufferers rarely survive beyond 75 and many die well before.

Chronic bronchitis is characterised by excessive production of mucus in the tracheo-bronchial tree, that is to say more than 100 ml per day during a minimum of three months of the year and for at least two consecutive years. The bronchi are narrowed by long-standing irritation, usually from cigarette smoking. As a result of narrowing and increased secretion of mucus, airflow and gas exchange is hindered. This makes the patient prone to mucus plugging and secondary infection. Air has difficulty in passing freely in and out of the lungs during respiration; some of the air is trapped and the lungs become distended.

Emphysema is another disease usually associated with cigarette smoking. It damages the lung tissue itself but not the air passages. The alveolar walls are destroyed, thus reducing the number of alveoli and the area of the pulmonary membrane, and dilatation of lung tissue distal to the terminal bronchioles. Destruction of the alveolar walls produces distended air sacs separated by fibrous septa which gradually replace normal lung tissue. When lung tissue is damaged in this way ability to exchange oxygen and carbon dioxide is impeded; therefore it is more difficult for oxygen to pass into the bloodstream. Consequently people with emphysema become breathless.

Five levels of functioning in COAD patients are described in Chest 77 3rd March 1980 in a special report by Dudley, Glaser, Jorgenson and Logan of the USA

1. Patient with recognised disease, with no restriction, is able to do what peers can do, continues usual life pattern.
2. Patient with minimal or moderately restricted activity, is able to do productive work, has some difficulty keeping up with peers, has begun to modify life pattern.
3. Patient with markedly restricted activity, is not homebound, may not be able to do productive work, but is able to care for himself.
4. Patient with severely restricted activity, is not able to do productive work, is essentially homebound but is able to care for himself.
5. Patient with very severely restricted activity is homebound or in an institution, is not able to care for himself.

Medical treatment

Antibiotics are prescribed during an exacerbation of bronchitis. At this stage physiothera-

pists are very helpful as, using techiques of clapping, rib-springing and shaking, they clear the bronchi of thick purulent sputum. Bronchodilators are routinely prescribed for COAD patients in Groups 3, 4 and 5.

People with COAD present with the following physical symptoms:

— Breathless on slight exertion
— Susceptibility to respiratory infection
— Tire easily
— Inability to walk for any distance
— Cough and sputum
— Difficulty in climbing the smallest hill.

People with COAD present with the following psychological symptoms brought on by their physical state

— Loss of confidence and self-esteem
— Inability to relax
— Limited concentration
— Disturbed sleep pattern
— Tendency to be anxious and irritable
— Low spirits leading to feeling of hopelessness and finally depression.

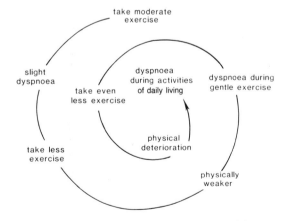

Fig. 5.1 Respiratory impairment cycle (adapted from Haas et al 1979)

People with COAD tend to react in this way, becoming less and less active and more and more incapacitated. The occupational therapist's role, along with the rest of the multidisciplinary team, is to try to reverse the spiral illustrated above. Agle et al (1973) found at least seven factors which produced improved psychological state and performance.

1. Progressive exercise leading to a decrease in unrealistic fear of activity and dyspnoea
2. Education in self-care leading to increased autonomy in the control of symptoms
3. Staff attitudes stressing that the patient is worth the effort
4. The setting of realistic goals leading to improved self-esteem
5. Monthly follow-up to consolidate gains
6. Mutual support from group interaction
7. The psychosocial factors within the patient that lead to strong motivation.

Occupational therapy treatment

This can be divided into health education, improvement of dyspnoea, improvement of mobility and general muscle power, reduction of anxiety including phobic reaction to dyspnoea.

Health education

Health education on the subject of how the lungs work and what happens to them when infection is present is useful and gives the patient a greater understanding of his condition. A description of how we breathe enables the patient to appreciate why he becomes breathless on exertion. Advice on the damage smoking causes is not given in a nagging way but objectively and factually, for example:

1. In the UK in 1983, 100 000 people died from smoking-related diseases
2. 95% of people with chronic chest disease are or have been smokers
3. The average smoker doubles the risk of coronary heart disease
4. Carbon monoxide is absorbed by haemoglobin more easily than oxygen and is not released, therefore efficient use of red blood cells is reduced. Carbon monoxide is present in cigarette smoke.

5. Non-smokers' health may suffer if they breathe in other peoples' smoke
6. If you smoke 20 cigarettes a day your chances of dying from a smoking-related disease are 1:25.

Simple hand-outs with diagrams should be given so that patients can read and assimilate the information at their leisure. Publications on chronic bronchitis are available from the Chest, Heart and Stroke Association. These can be used as the basis for a discussion group. Diet and nutrition can also be covered in this way, with the therapist advising on vitamin content in different foods and which vitamins help protect against infection (vitamins A, C and D) and which can reduce anxiety (vitamin B).

Improvement of dyspnoea

1. Positions to adopt either sitting or standing when dyspnoeic should be taught to bronchitics. The emphasis being to encourage the patient to lean forward and breathe deeply through the nose to cure the panic reaction of taking shallow gasps of air through an open mouth with the neck extended.

2. Teach breathing exercises to improve lung function (see Figs. 5.2 and 5.3). People in Groups 3 and 4 may have difficulty in carrying out the supine exercises and those in Group 5 should not attempt them. If patients find certain exercises distressing leave them out.

3. *Diaphragmatic breathing* should be taught to the patient or to a group for economy and mutual encouragement. Give a simple handout to remind the patient how to do it when she wants to practise at home so that she learns the correct method. This type of breathing is used in co-ordination with relaxation exercises but is best learnt first as deep breathing puts you into a relaxed state of mind.

Improvement of mobility and general muscle power

Any simple exercise plan can be adopted. I have used the most basic of the Canadian Air

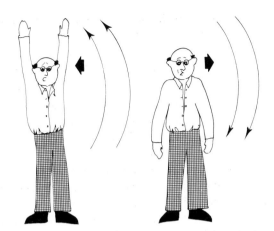

Fig. 5.2 *Arm raising*. Lift your arms as you breathe in. Lower them slowly as you breathe out

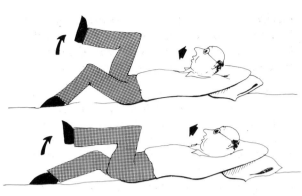

Fig. 5.5 *Knee raising*. Lying down, lift your right knee toward your chest as you breathe out. Breathe in as you lower your leg. Note: If it's easier for you, you may breathe in while raising your leg and breathe out while lowering it

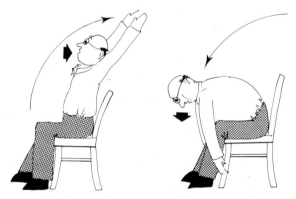

Fig. 5.3 *Forward bending*. Sit in a chair, lean back, and lift your arms as you breathe in. Lean forward slowly, tuck your chin into your chest, and let your head fall forward as you breathe out

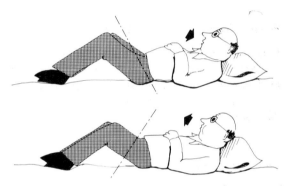

Fig. 5.6 *Pelvic Tilt*. Lying down. Tighten the muscles of your stomach and buttocks as you breathe in relax as you breathe out

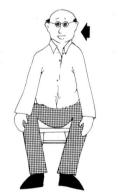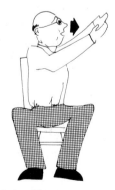

Fig. 5.4 *Trunk turning*. Sit in a chair with your shoulders relaxed and breathe in. As you breathe out slowly, turn your trunk to the left, raise your arms over your left shoulder, as if you were reaching behind you. Bring your arms up and down a few times. Rest, and repeat on the other side

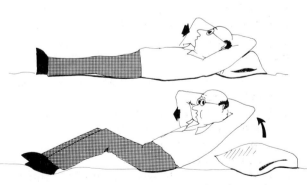

Fig. 5.7 *Head and shoulder raising*. Lying down, place your hands behind your head and breathe in. Breathe out while you lift your head and shoulders as far as you can. Feel your stomach muscles tighten. (You don't have to raise yourself to a sitting position.)

Force Plans for breathless pensioners. Indirect exercise is often more popular. Activity in the OT department can be graded and chosen to suit individual abilities and preferences. Projects might include macrame (using cotton twine not jute), typing, printing, woodwork, stoolseating, stained glasswork. Group efforts can achieve bookshelves, coffee tables, dolls' houses and furniture, model railways etc. Achievements gained in the OT department improve self-esteem and concentration as well as stamina and muscle power.

Reduction of anxiety and phobic reaction

1. *Hand and shoulder massage.* Tension is a very obvious presenting symptom in a patient with chronic chest disease. Patients often complain of cramp in the hands and stiff shoulders and neck. I have found that gentle neck and shoulder massage prepares the patient for relaxation, and along with neck exercises and shoulder shrugs loosens up this part of the body most prone to stress. Relatives can be shown how to massage the neck and shoulders safely. The patient is taught how to massage his hands — this is a modified form of reflexology which I have not felt appropriate for elderly dyspnoeic people for whom lying prone is virtually impossible.

2. *Relaxation.* Dr Edmond Jacobsen in his 1938 book *Progressive Relaxation* said 'Rest does not correspond to relaxation — usually people have to be taught to relax'. When teaching relaxation to people with chronic chest conditions it is better to teach them seated, as they find lying uncomfortable unless propped up with pillows: and since one is teaching a method which should be for use under any circumstances, sitting or standing are most appropriate.

There are many different methods of teaching relaxation. I have found the more structured method developed by Jacobsen suitable for use with elderly people. In his method the individual is taught to recognise the presence of muscle contraction and then to let go and feel the tension disappear. The therapist practises with the patients tightening

and releasing large groups of muscles, starting with the face or the feet, depending on which she finds more satisfactory. Patients' limbs are tested by the therapist, and if this is performed in a group one half of the group will test the other half, and also test the therapist's limbs, to learn what relaxation feels like in another person. It is important that the therapist joins in the relaxation to demonstrate the methods being taught.

Diaphragmatic breathing is co-ordinated with the tensing and releasing of muscle groups. After people learn how to relax they need no longer do the muscle tightening exercises but simply think themselves relaxed and so become relaxed. Imagery and visualisation techniques can also be used to teach relaxation, for example:

1. Think of the time when you had no breathing problems, you are warm and comfortable without a care, perhaps you are at home in a comfortable chair or on holiday in the sun.

2. Sit for a while with your eyes closed and your head falling forward slightly, concentrate on your breathing. Imagine the breath coming in through your nose, filling up parts of your lungs that haven't been used efficiently for some time, then let the breath out again to make room for more clean air.

General advice — compiled by a group of patients with COAD Research by Helm and Prince (1984)

1. Do not smoke. Avoid smoky atmospheres.
2. Breathing and relaxation exercises should be done two or three times daily. Start a routine.
3. Don't do them immediately after a meal.
4. Loosen any tight clothing which might restrict the movement round your waist, lower chest and neck.
5. While doing the exercises, keep warm. So do not do them in a cold, draughty place,
6. The first exercises in the morning are best practised sometime after you have had breakfast.
7. Eat sensibly.
8. Try to arrange your daily activities to avoid needless hurry.
9. Be as active as possible but be aware of your limitations, e.g. do not run for a bus.
10. Turn on a low wattage heater to warm the bedroom before going to bed.
11. An electric blanket is essential for bronchitics. An over-blanket is the safer type.

12. Have a heater in the bathroom (heated towel rail or wired-in wall type.)
13. If you heat your house by electricity keep flat bowls of water in front of the heaters to humidify the air.
14. Do not open the windows unless the weather is warm.
15. Try not to go out on wet and windy days, keep warm.
16. If you have to go out on wet and windy days and you don't have a car, use a taxi. There may be cheaper taxis for disabled people in your area. Ask your doctor or therapist.
17. Wear a hat in cold weather and keep your feet warm.
18. Breathlessness is not a killer. You can learn to accept and control it. You don't have to let bronchitis rule your life.

PERIPHERAL VASCULAR DISEASE

M. Helm

Peripheral vascular disease is caused by atherosclerosis, arteriosclerosis embolism or venous thrombosis. Symptoms of ischaemia are produced by localised thrombosis and occasionally by stenosis: walking becomes painful because of intermittent claudication (muscular pain) which may be relieved by rest but will be reproduced with further exercise. Pain experienced at rest is more serious as it warns of the onset of gangrene (tissue necrosis). Another cause of lower limb ischaemia is diabetes; therefore before treatment begins, urine must be checked for sugar and blood for anaemia. Arteriography is carried out for patients requiring surgery.

Medical treatment

If diabetes or anaemia are diagnosed, they are treated immediately. Alcohol which is a vaso-dilator may be prescribed, but patients who smoke should be asked to stop as nicotine is a vasoconstrictor. Bed-rest, ensuring that the legs are kept horizontal, brings pain relief.

Operative treatment

This includes arterial grafting; lumbar sympath-ectomy for ischaemia, rest pain and Raynaud's changes; amputation for chronic pain, thrombosis and gangrene. The latter two procedures are most frequently carried out on elderly people. Lumbar sympathectomy is not considered whenever a limb is swollen and gangrene is present. Gangrene in diabetics is caused by the following factors:

Ischaemia. Atherosclerosis is likely to develop two years earlier in diabetics than in non-diabetics suffering from peripheral vascular disease.

Neuropathy. Diabetics may develop periph-eral neuritis making their extremities insensi-tive to touch. Consequently they are in danger of injury and abrasion leading to infection; untreated infection may result in gangrene. In such cases amputation of the toes and infected metatarsals may be adequate to reduce the risk of further trauma.

Levels of amputation are described as follows:

Transverse metatarsal	— through the foot
Syme's	— through the ankle
Below-knee	— through the calf
Gritti-Stokes	— through the knee
Above-knee	— through the thigh
Hip disarticulation	— through the hip

Occupational therapy treatment

One would think that the effects of lower limb amputation would be extremely difficult for elderly people to adjust to; however, due to the severity of the pre-operative pain, the majority adjust well as the worst symptom has been eradicated. Nevertheless, coming to terms with the loss of one or both lower limbs demands great courage and psychological strength.

Pre-operative. The therapist must counsel the patient about the operation and its conse-quences, explaining the level of personal independence she may be expected to achieve. The therapist must allow the patient to talk about the sense of loss that will inevi-tably follow the removal of a limb, and must reassure her and her family about the outcome of the operation. She must also keep the patient as active as her present mobility will allow and keep her upper limbs well exercised.

Post-operative. As soon as practicable, the therapist will adopt 'the rehabilitative approach' and teach the patients to be as independent as possible in the following ways: transferring from bed to wheelchair, on and off the WC, washing and dressing, sitting balance, standing tolerance, maintaining upper limb strength. Four or five days after the operation, once the patient is fitted with a Pneumatic Post Amputation Mobility aid (a PPAM aid), the therapist will incorporate into her programme activities designed to improve standing balance and posture, as well as to strengthen stump muscles.

Post-operative problems. The patient may have to contend with a number of post-operative complications, as follows:

1. Contractures of the hip or knee of the amputated limb — the physiotherapist will give preventative exercises and lying prone will minimise these problems.
2. Phantom pains which may range from tingling or numbness to severe pain. Tense patients who experience pain more acutely sometimes gain relief from prescribed tranquilisers.
3. Phantom limb. The memory of the lost limb may be so vivid that the patient may hallucinate and even try to walk on the absent limb. Firm bandaging will help to lessen this sensation.
4. Care of the sound limb. Sometimes so much attention is given to the stump that care of the remaining limb is neglected. It is essential that this limb is kept healthy and well exercised.
5. Relating disorders and other ailments. It is important that patients with conditions such as anaemia, rheumatoid arthritis and diabetes should continue to be treated for these conditions.

Specific occupational therapy for below-knee amputees

This can be divided into the following categories:

1. The promotion of independence in all transfers and daily living activities.

2. The improvement of sitting balance: by sitting in a wheelchair with the sides removed, patients can play games like skittles and bowls.
3. The improvement of standing balance and tolerance. This can be achieved through the use of activities such as printing gardening, stool seating, woodwork bench work and floor games.
4. The strengthening of the amputated limb. It is most important that the quadriceps group of muscles be exercised actively to prevent contractures and be made strong enough for walking with an artificial limb.

The following are examples of:

Static quadriceps exercise. The patient sits on a Camden stool with the amputated limb in a sling and her hip at 90°, and operates a treadle sewing-machine or foot-loom using the remaining lower limb.

Active quadriceps exercise

a. A temporary pylon is fitted to the stump, allowing the patient to use a rug loom or treadle sewing machine.
b. The patient sits on a Camden stool or bicycle seat with her hip at 90°, and operates a 'quadriceps switch.' (see figure in Ann Turner's *The Practice of Occupational Therapy*, p. 157). The stump is supported in a metal cup and a pressure-pad filled with air is placed under the thigh. The switch is then attached to an electrical appliance (which can operate in short bursts), such as a sewing machine, typewriter, soldering-iron or even a train set. When the patient contracts the quadriceps isometrically, the action of the thigh being pushed down on to the pressure-pad completes an electrical circuit: when the quadriceps is relaxed and the pressure released, the circuit is broken again.

The above exercises are also appropriate for above-knee amputees to increase the strength of hip extensors in order to prevent contractures.

Specific occupational therapy for bilateral amputees

All the foregoing activities are also applicable for these patients, with the addition of activities for upper limb strengthening and exercising of remaining lower limb joints, using both static and active activities. Elderly patients who have the misfortune to loose both limbs will have to spend most or all of their days in a wheelchair; therefore great emphasis will be put on wheelchair training. Transfers using a short board, and front transfers on and off the WC, will be particularly important to practise.

Specific occupational therapy activities for the prosthetic stage

It is extremely unusual for an elderly person to be fitted with bilateral artificial limbs; therefore this section applies to unilateral above and below-knee amputees. The principal OT functions are: to improve posture with limb fitted; tolerance to wearing the limb; standing tolerance; to maintain upper limb strengthening; to improve strength and co-ordination of lower prosthetic limb, using electric bicycle, treadle sewing machine and wobble-board once the patient has sufficient confidence; to practise daily living activities including kitchen work, housework, laundry, shopping and most particularly dressing — the patient is taught at which stage in the order of dressing to put on her artificial limb (see Ann Turner's *The Practice of Occupational Therapy*, p. 247).

Functional outcome to be expected from elderly amputees

Below-knee amputation — Good, with the patient walking using the artificial limb plus a stick or zimmer walking frame. She should become independent in all aspects of daily living, learning to use aids for WC, bath and kitchen.

Above-knee amputation — Good, as for below-knee amputees, with these minor differences. Firstly, elderly amputees are given 'locking' knee joints, not pneumatic swinging joints, so 'vaulting' is evident when rising from the sitting position or when swinging the artificial limb forward in walking. Secondly, when walking, steps are shorter as the remaining leg is brought through more quickly than in normal gait.

Bilateral below-knee amputation — These patients will probably spend part of the day in a wheelchair but can become independent in daily living activities using aids. Most will lose one leg for a while before they lose the other, and can adjust to coping with one artificial limb before having to manage with two. With successful rehabilitation the patient will learn to use a zimmer frame for walking.

Bilateral above-knee amputation — These patients are likely to rely totally on a wheelchair unless very fit and highly motivated. Some may manage to walk with a zimmer or with crutches for short distances as this is exhausting; for the very few, artificial limbs will be prescribed — these will be two or three inches shorter than the patient's own legs. Elderly patients who are frail, obese or with other disabilities will be unlikely to achieve independence and will probably be referred to continuing care wards because of their inability to transfer without help.

Home visits

Once the patient is rehabilitated and independent, either with or without a wheelchair, a home visit will be made to assess for aids and adaptations which will be required in the patient's home. Usually these constitute bath aids, toilet rails, ramps or rails at the front and back door, and an armchair of the same height as the wheelchair. A home care supervisor should be present during the home visit to assess the patient's need for home help and meals-on-wheels. Day centre attendance will be of great help to amputees, and the OT should ensure that relatives are aware of how they can be of most help and support to the patient.

Prognosis

Where the reason for amputation was ischaemia or diabetic gangrene, an elderly patient has a one-in-ten chance of losing the other leg during the following year. The lifespan for an elderly amputee suffering from peripheral vascular disease is five years.

CORONARY ARTERY DISEASE AND THE ELDERLY PATIENT

R. Trevan

The coronary arteries are the arteries of supply to the heart which arise from the aorta, just beyond the aortic valve, and through which the blood is delivered to the muscle of the heart (Black's Medical Dictionary Thomson 1983). With advancing years the coronary arteries, as with other arteries in the body, may be affected by arteriosclerosis and atheroma. The narrowed lumen results in a diminished blood supply and subsequent shortage of oxygen to the heart muscle. This often presents as angina pectoris but may lead to myocardial infarction.

These conditions are rarely seen in isolation they are part of the ageing process. Coronary artery disease (CAD) may be one of the multiple conditions with which the elderly may present. Although the incidents of CAD is greater in men than women below the age of 60, the incidence evens out with the increase of age.

ANGINA PECTORIS

Angina pectoris is characterised by pain, often severe and sudden. It usually presents post-sternally, and may radiate into the left arm, side of the neck and/or chin. Often the patient complains of 'tightness in the chest' and a feeling of suffocation. The pain varies in intensity and location from individual to individual.

The pain is caused by an inability of the coronary arteries to supply the heart muscle with the blood supply it demands, especially when the demand is altered with a change in muscular activity or a change in external temperature (whilst maintaining body temperature), hence the term angina of effort.

MYOCARDIAL INFARCTION

Patients who suffer a myocardial infarction from an occlusion of a large artery may die suddenly. More commonly the patient will survive, and the area of heart muscle that has been deprived of oxygen will form a fibrous scar area. Usually this is firm and strong and the functional ability of the heart is near normal. A large area of scar tissue may become stretched and an aneurysm in the heart wall may form. A small aneursym could lead to only minimal impairment of cardiac output. If the area is large or if the surrounding heart muscle is not sufficiently strong the cardiac output may be grossly impaired, and congestive cardiac failure may occur.

CONGESTIVE CARDIAC FAILURE

Where there is extensive damage to the left ventricle and a reduced ability of the pumping mechanism, strain will ultimately be felt by the right side of the heart. The rest of the heart will, to some extent, become damaged. For the left ventricle to provide extra force and adequate output the muscle of the left atrium hypertrophies. This may provide sufficient power for adequate circulation to be maintained; when it does not a 'back-log' of blood occurs through the heart and to the lungs, causing the lungs to be 'flooded'.

The patient presents with shortness of breath (dyspnoea on exertion), complains of sudden breathless attacks at night (paroxysmal nocturnal dyspnoea) and cyanosis.

REHABILITATION

Most of the existing rehabilitation programmes for patients suffering coronary artery disease cater for the younger patient with the emphasis placed on return to work.

The needs of the elderly patient with similar medical problems must not be forgotten. An occupational therapist should be concerned with the three main areas of activity — self-maintenance, useful activity and leisure. Shortness of breath, pain and discomfort and fear of death can have an effect in all these areas. The principles of enabling the patient to maximise her potential are common throughout. Not only will the occupational therapist help the patient learn to recognise the physical limitations and advise on how to work within or to them, but of equal importance is the patient's psychological adjustment and acceptance of those limitations.

PSYCHOLOGICAL FACTORS

At Northwick Park Hospital we have observed that patients with chronic heart disease demonstrate bereavement. In her book Elizabeth Kubler-Ross (1970) describes this process of grieving. This process of coming to terms with a loss may be observed in patients who have recently begun to experience angina pain, who have had a myocardial infarction or a coronary artery by-pass graft. The psychological acceptance is equally as important as learning to cope with the physical symptoms associated with this disease.

It is important that the family or carers are involved at an early stage and throughout the rehabilitation process. Education — the provision of information both verbally and written — and advice comprise the two elements of their involvement.

Information should be given about the aetiology of the disease, its effect on the physical and psychological functioning of the patient and risk factors. The carers and family should be advised and encouraged to prevent the production of a 'cardiac invalid', by the patient's response or an over-protective attitude of the carers. A healthy balance is essential.

The grieving process

Patients need to be helped through the stages of grieving. They may respond in one of three ways:
a. reject the limitations — 'I'm not going to be beaten'
b. enjoy the attention — 'I've worked all my life and now someone can look after me'
c. have a healthy and sensible approach — 'In what ways do I need to change?'

Many people find it difficult to change methods of performing tasks. This difficulty is often greater when attempting to change the habits of a lifetime. It is quite natural for a patient to deny the need for change or express anger or resentment at the need. The patient may become depressed and withdraw from family, friends or therapists, and need explanations, re-assurance and encouragement to persevere. As she begins to accept her physical problems she may begin to bargain. Subjects for bargaining may be activities, diet, smoking, or alcohol intake. It is essential to give a constant response at this stage. It is not enough for the patient to accept her 'lot'. She will, with time, have hope for a meaningful life, which may be demonstrated through a graded programme of activities relating to her self care and leisure interests.

ACTIVITY PROGRAMME

Self-maintenance or activities of daily living must be the first area of intervention. This will involve ergonomic advice rather than the provision of a large number of aids. Sequencing of activities, elimination of excessive use of stairs and carrying of heavy objects without major disruption of the normal routine are required.

In some instances it may be necessary to provide aids or adaptations or services when these reduce the effort required to perform the task. The ability of the carer (spouse, sibling, other relatives, friend or neighbour) to contribute should be taken into account during the assessment for the provision of services which should be aimed at maintaining the individual's independence. Taking a shower requires less effort than bathing. Similarly, using a trolley around the house for carrying items from room to room or indeed within a room reduces effort. Where function is greatly reduced the provision of home care workers to undertake some tasks such as shopping and cleaning may allow the elderly person to continue independent living.

For most elderly patients this may be all they require. The more active person will require this advice and treatment programme to extend to their leisure activities. A programme of graded activities within the department will help to demonstrate the extent of the patient's physical function. The therapist also uses these sessions to teach sequencing and pacing of activities and recognition of warning symptoms and self-monitoring. These activities should be related to the individual's leisure pursuits, and advice on alternatives should be provided where required.

Coronary artery disease in the elderly usually results in a degree of lost functional activity. It is the role of the occupational therapist to enable the patient and her carers to adjust to the altered life-style, maintaining as great a level of independence as possible, social activity and self respect.

REFERENCES

Agle D F, Pattison G M 1973 Group psychotherapy in patients with severe diffuse obstructive pulmonary syndrome. Psychosomatic Medicine 35: 41–49

Bronchitis and emphysema 20 Qs and As. Breathing exercises for chronic bronchitis and emphysema. Chest, Heart and Stroke Association

College committee on Thoracic Medicine 1981 Royal College of Physicians: Disabling chest disease — prevention and care. Journal of the Royal College of Physicians 15(2)

Crofton E 1972 Questions people ask about smoking. The Health Education Dept, Greater Glasgow Health Board.

Dudley D L, Glaser E M, Jorgenson Betty, Logan D L 1980 Psychosocial concomitants to rehabilitation in chronic obstructive pulmonary disease. Chest 77: 413–420; 544–551; 677–684

Haas A, Pineda H, Haas F, Axen K 1979 Pulmonary therapy and rehabilitation. Williams and Wilkins, Baltimore

Helm M, Prince K 1984 Unpublished

Houston J C, Joiner C L, Trounce J R 1982 A short textbook of medicine, 7th ed. Hodder and Stoughton, London

Hrehorow Z 1984 Better breathing for health fitness. Winslow Press, Buckinghamshire

Jacobsen E 1938 Progressive relaxation. University of Chicago Press

Kubler-Ross E 1970 On death and dying. Macmillan, New York

Macleod J (ed) 1984 Davidson's principles and practice of medicine 14th ed. Churchill Livingstone, Edinburgh

Rosser R, Gus A 1981 Psychological approaches to breathlessness and its treatment. Journal of psychosomatic research 25: 439–447

Sears W G Winarood R S 1975 Medicine for nurses. Arnold, London

Taylor S, Cotton L 1968 Diseases of the arteries, A short textbook of surgery, 2nd ed. Unibooks, London, ch 8, p 73–84

Thomson W A R 1983 Black's Medical Dictionary. Black, Adam and Charles, London

Troup I M, Wood M A 1982 Total care of the lower limb Pitman, London

Turner A 1981 Amputation. In: The practice of occupational therapy. Churchill Livingstone, Edinburgh, ch 14, p 237–260

Yarrow A 1975 So now you know about smoking, A family doctor booklet published by B M A, London

6

Strokes

S. Grindlay

INTRODUCTION

Occupational therapists spend a great deal of their time in trying to rehabilitate elderly stroke patients. It is very difficult to predict accurately how many weeks' treatment will be required, before a stroke patient is able to move home. Twelve weeks is a good average recovery time for an elderly patient; however total recovery is unusual; for example only 10% regain full use of the affected hand although 90% of patients walk again (Garraway et al 1982). Of those who survive a major stroke, Andrews (1982) predicts that one third will live at home alone, one third with a carer, and one third will require institutional care.

Epidemiology

Mortality rates for stroke in the United Kingdom and the United States of America have fallen over the last 30 years. Results fron Minnesota suggest that this is mainly due to a decline in the incidence (Whisnant 1984). Annual statistics for a population of 760 000 illustrate this trend (see Table 6.1).

Aetiology

Minor strokes or transient ischaemic attacks (TIA) are indicators of cerebrovascular disease. They are episodes of temporary and focal cerebral dysfunction of vascular origin, leaving no persistent neurological deficit and lasting

Table 6.1 Lothian Health Board Annual Stastistical Report — Mortality for Cerebrovascular Disease 1979 and 1983

Year	1979		1983	
Age	65–74	75+	65–74	75+
Male	167	225	113	231
Female	186	584	114	571

Table 6.2 Results of arterial occlusion

Artery	Signs and symptoms following occlusion
Internal carotid	Contralateral motor and sensory deficits Contralateral homonymous hemianopia Aphasia (dominant lobe) Disorders of body image and neglect (non-dominant lobe) Apraxia Ipsilateral blindness (transitory) = Amaurosis fugax Altered conscious level if damage is diffuse
Middle cerebral	Contralateral motor and sensory deficits Contralateral homonymous hemianopia Aphasia (dominant lobe) Disorders of body image and neglect (non-dominant lobe)
Anterior cerebral	Contralateral motor and sensory deficits affecting lower limb more than upper Dyspraxia Dysphasia Flat affect Urinary incontinence
Posterior cerebral	Contralateral homonymous hemianopia
Posterior inferior cerebellar	Vertigo Ipsilateral ataxia Contralateral sensory loss in the limbs and ipsilateral loss on the face Nystagmus Ipsilateral Horner's syndrome
Vertebrobasilar	Bilateral motor and sensory deficits Vertigo Nystagmus Diplopia or blindness Ataxia Dysphagia Coma

less than 24 hours. They are often caused by temporary blockage of the cerebral circulation by microemboli. Results from TIAs are short lived but resemble those following a major stroke (to be described later).

Symptoms resulting from cerebrovascular disease are caused by cerebral ischaemia. The brain requires a constant supply of oxygen and nutrients and if these supplies are cut off for more than 3 minutes, neurones are permanently destroyed.

In the majority of strokes affecting elderly people cerebral ischaemia is caused by atherosclerosis. Atherosclerosis is an accumulation of fatty deposits upon which a thrombus forms, blocking an artery and causing an infarct. An embolus is a clot, often formed in the valves of a damaged heart, which travels to a cerebral vessel and through blocking it causes an infarct in the same way as a thrombus.

The third cause of stroke is cerebral haemorrhage which is strongly associated with hypertension and a weakness in an artery wall or both. When an artery ruptures, blood escapes into the brain tissue and destroys it. Prognosis for patients who have had a cerebral haemorrhage is worse than for those who have sustained a thrombosis or embolism. Many die rapidly; others remain unconscious for a while: if they survive they often have serious permanent disabilities.

Occlusion of an artery causes ischaemia followed by infarction. Dependent upon which artery is affected signs and symptoms are as indicated in Table 6.2.

The signs and symptoms listed refer to damage on either side of the brain. As a general rule damage to the left side of the brain is more likely to result in:

— Right hemiplegia/hemiparesis
— Right hemianaesthesia
— Right homonymous hemianopia
— Dysphasia/aphasia (expressive, receptive or global)
— Apraxia

— Loss of balance reflexes
(with parietal lobe damage Gerstmann's syndrome and language perseveration).

Damage to the right side of the brain is more likely to result in:

— Left hemiplegia/hemiparesis
— Left hemianaesthesia
— Left homonymous hemianopia
— Disturbances of body image and the ability to judge and discriminate
— Reject/neglect syndrome
— Anosognosia
— Visual agnosia
— Impairment of postural reflexes
— Astereognosis.

Stroke patients' memory and concentration span may also be affected which prevents them from learning how to cope with and accommodate for their many disabilities.

Factors affecting outcome

With advancing age there is progressive loss of cerebral neurones, and by the age of 65 years 20% of the brain cells present at birth will have died. The speed at which this happens varies. Cognitive changes in the elderly may manifest themselves as disorientation in time, place or person, short-term memory impairment, or difficulties with judgement and reasoning.

Treatment of elderly stroke patients may be complicated by the presence of another disability, for example a chest or heart condition, osteoarthritis, Parkinsonism. Helm (1981) found that psychological and mood disorders were barriers but that most were amenable to therapy.

Stroke units or general medical wards

Not all stroke patients are admitted to hospital for treatment, many are treated at home. They may receive domiciliary physiotherapy and advice on aids to daily living and home adaptations from a community occupational therapist.

Of those admitted to hospital, most are referred to general medical wards but some are treated in units especially designed for stroke patients. It might be expected that the latter group would improve more quickly with more intensive therapy.

In the report of the Geriatrics Committee Working Group on Strokes (1974) to the Royal College of Physicians, London, it was proposed 'that it was not enough to show that patients do well in a stroke unit, they must be shown to have done better than they would have if treated elsewhere'.

The Edinburgh Study (Garraway et al 1980) provided evidence that despite patients' early improvement in a stroke unit, there was a 'levelling out' effect following discharge home. This was perhaps due to the withdrawal of the stroke unit's intensive rehabilitation programme. After a year patients from a stroke unit and those from medical wards produced identical results when assessed for activities of daily living.

Approaches to the treatment of strokes

Not so many years ago a patient would have been immediately encouraged to compensate for unilateral loss of movement by using her unaffected limbs. We now know that this limits the patient's potential for recovery and increases spasm in the muscles paralysed by the stroke.

To date there is no scientific evidence to back a particular treatment method. Neuro-developmental theories have been adopted as a basis for treatment. The work of practitioners such as Ayres, Brunnstrom, Bobath, Johnstone, Knott and Voss is well recognised and references for their books are listed at the end of the chapter. Most are described in *Occupational Therapy for Physical Dysfunction* by Trombly and Scott (1977).

TREATMENT

The rehabilitation team

Before going on to discuss treatment, it is important to state that the occupational therapist is only one member of a team. As Mrs

Bobath was once reported to have said: 'Rehabilitation should take place twenty-four hours a day'. The co-ordinated team approach to rehabilitation was identified as an important factor in the achievement of independence in self-care by Smith et al (1982). The various members of the team are identified and their roles elaborated upon in Chapter 2.

In the early stages of recovery a little treatment often is usually the maxim. This provides stimulation for the patient and affords the therapeutic team the opportunity to establish a basis of good treatment (Figs. 6.1 & 6.2).

Close involvement with the patient's relatives or carers is also vital. If this is initiated early it gives carers greater understanding and confidence to cope when they are with the patient at home.

The occupational therapist

Her role is to enable the patient to function as fully as possible in a given environment. She must encourage purposeful movement. Where movement and power are lacking the therapist has to assist the patient (Fig. 6.3).

Treatment by occupational therapy

When planning a treatment programme for an elderly stroke patient one should bear in mind the suitability of activities which are to be presented. The stroke patient may find it difficult to adjust to hospital life and so to confront her with unfamiliar tasks will not be productive. Therefore a case should be made for using activities of daily living both in assesment and treatment. They are necessary and familiar and involve all the components for everyday living. Successful rehabilitation

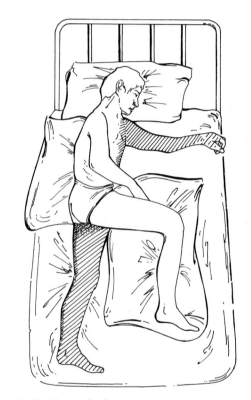

Fig. 6.2 Position in bed

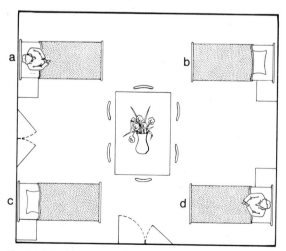

Fig. 6.1 Position in ward of patient with right hemiplegia (a and d)

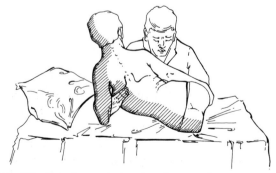

Fig. 6.3 Transfer: note hand under scapula

depends upon the patient's independence in ADL. An example of a daily living activity analysis is as follows:

Dressing evaluates:

— Comprehension
— Concentration
— Memory
— Equilibrium reactions
— Righting mechanisms
— Head alignment
— Trunk rotation
— Ability to weightbear on the affected side
— Proprioception
— Sensation (superficial)
— Spatial relationships
— Body scheme
— Vision, if present pre-morbidly.

Those of us in good health dress ourselves automatically, but for the stroke patient with sensory difficulties and/or loss of function in her preferred hand, dressing presents as a complex activity. Repeated practice with special attention to proprioception is probably the most helpful approach to those with sensory loss.

Principles of treatment — suggestions

Having provided a quiet and comfortable environment for the patient, one should begin treatment with the following points in mind:

— Make sure you are within the patient's visual field
— Talk simply and slowly to the patient
— Explain one step at a time
— Allow time for absorption and interpretation of instructions
— Allow sufficient time for each movement
— Reinforce by demonstration but keep it simple.

One of the complications of treating stroke patients may be that of poor communication. The speech therapist will advise as to the best approach. Aphasia is a complex problem and very distressing for the patient. In addition, the therapist should make sure that the elderly patient is hearing her properly. If she has been provided with a hearing aid, it should be worn; this also applies to spectacles.

Suggested guidelines for treatment (positioning)

When the central nervous system is damaged, loss of motor control may result: muscle tone may be flaccid initially but spasticity usually develops. This abnormal condition is treated by the physiotherapist.

Table 6.3 Abnormal posture following a stroke

Lateral flexion of the trunk to the affected side
Retraction of the affected shoulder with depression and internal rotation
Flexion of the forearm
Pronation of the forearm
Flexion of the fingers
Adduction of the fingers
Retraction of the pelvis
External rotation of the affected leg
Extension of the hip, knee and ankle.

The abnormal position should be inhibited by facillitating normal movement (Table 6.4).

Orientate the patient towards her affected side by placing objects and by approaching her from that side, but always within her visual field. Use of a long mirror may help the patient to maintain a good sitting position.

All activities should start and finish from a symmetrical position. The patient should try to weightbear on the affected side. The head should be slightly rotated towards the affected side of the body.

Table 6.4 How to position a patient to overcome abnormal posture

Elongation of the trunk on the affected side
Protraction of the scapula
External rotation of the arm
Extension of the forearm
Supination of the forearm
Extension of the fingers
Abduction of the fingers
Protraction of the pelvis
Internal rotation of the leg
Flexion of the hip, knee and ankle

Balance and symmetry are basic principles for rehabilitation and encouragement of these is the first priority of treatment. If unable to weightbear on the affected side a patient will not have a true perception of herself. This position sense is known as proprioception and is fundamental to the way one moves. A change in position is a proprioceptive change.

The therapist should work with open hands when touching the patient, making sure that her skin temperature is as close to the patient's as possible, because some stroke patients have increased sensitivity to touch. Pain or discomfort may result in increased muscle tone.

Patients whose sitting balance is impaired have to be washed and dressed by the therapist/nurse who will encourage the patient in the ways indicated in Table 6.5.

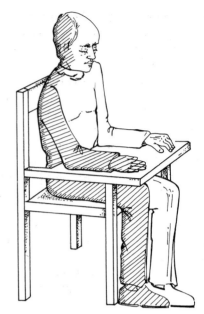

Fig. 6.4 Patient sits right back in the chair with ankle, knee and hip at 90°. Patient is symmetrical. Affected arm is protracted at the shoulder and supported

Table 6.5 Position to improve sitting balance

Sit well into the chair flexed 90° at the hips

Place both feet firmly on the floor

Work towards an upright position remembering the head

Rotate trunk towards the affected side

Weightbear on the affected lower limb to prevent spasticity

Stretch the affected arm

Position the affected arm, protracted at the shoulder, with elbow extended, forearm supinated, wrist extended, thumb abducted and fingers extended

The patient should sit positioned (Fig. 6.4) between treatment sessions and for activities such as feeding and writing. If a wheelchair is being used it should have a table fixed across the front where the arm can be placed within the visual field.

Progression 1

During dressing practice the therapist sits on the affected side and dresses the patient. At this stage in treatment the patient is encouraged to shift her centre of gravity as she flexes forward or leans sideways, always returning to the symmetrical upright position. The thera-pist must observe, noting normal movement and identifying and inhibiting abnormal movement.

Progression 2

The second aim of treatment is to encourage the patient to participate actively in dressing. Clothes are fed onto the extended affected upper limb at first by the therapist and then by the patient who completes the dressing of a particular garment. Top garments should be put on one after the other to provide repetition of the patterns of movement. Once the upper half is dressed and the patient can maintain good sitting balance, the lower half may be dressed. She dresses the affected leg first, crossing it over the supporting leg.

If dressing appears to be a great effort and produces increased tone in the upper limb, there should be a pause in the activity while the therapist facilitates extension in the patient's hand and upper limb providing maximum stretch, encouraging her to weight-bear on that arm into the therapist's hand.

The present generation of elderly patients

are, in the main, extremely modest. Washing and dressing are intensely personal activities and the therapist should be appropriately sensitive in her approach.

Suitable clothing is dealt with in Chapter 19. People often do not possess 'easy-to-manage' clothing, but it is theirs and familiar to them. Early clothing adaptations may remove some of that feeling of familiarity. The provision of aids such as a long-handled shoehorn should be made after careful assessment, especially for those patients suffering from perceptual disabilities.

The patient should be given an indication of the possibility of independence. The therapist should encourage the patient by pointing out improvements, however small. The patient must feel that she has progressed a little every day.

In an assessment of independence in activities of daily living, Smith et al (1982) found that 53% of patients in a stroke unit, and 38% of those in medical units, achieved independence in spite of impaired arm function. Only 30% and 23%, respectively, of those with proprioceptive loss, attained the same level of independence.

Progression 3

Standing will be introduced naturally as part of dressing, along with transfers from bed to chair, chair to chair and on and off the WC. Great care must be taken when the patient stands to prevent her thrusting back in extension.

Sitting to standing method

— The patient should rock forward from the back of the chair until both feet are placed firmly on the ground.
— She should then lean forward until the head is vertically above the feet.
— She should not use her 'good' arm to push up on, as this upsets symmetry.
— The affected arm is held in extension by the therapist who supports the patient by placing her arm against the patient's ribs

(*not under the axilla*). Some therapists encourage the patient to clasp her hands, pushing her arms out in front.
— Place the affected leg a little behind the other as this encourages early weightbearing. Weightbearing must be through the hip, knee and heel.
— Before standing, practise lifting the buttocks just off the chair.

Progression 4

Patients who have suffered a stroke are best treated individually at first, as this allows for greater concentration. They must also function socially — eating, communicating and sharing the environment with others. This is the time to involve the patient in remedial games or group treatments.

Remedial games

The choice of games should, if possible, relate to the patient's former interests. The ability to play games requiring numerical skill is usually unimpaired. These activities may be graded in the following ways:

a. A position may be changed to encourage increased range of movement and improved position sense. One should remember that if the same stimulus is applied over a degree of time a process of adaptation or habituation occurs and synaptic activity diminishes.
b. The equipment may be adapted for size of grip or for bimanual activity.
c. Games may be played on a one-to-one basis or in a group. Check the patient's position in the group.

Games are useful for augmenting the activities of daily living and provide stimulation and variety for the patient. Return of function should be utilised in the correct order. For example, the ability to place and hold the shoulder, then the elbow, with pronation and supination of the forearm, should be established before wrist flexion and individual finger movements. Mass movement should be discouraged because it consists of complex movements which change the position of a limb from flexion to extension.

Feeding

The patient should be seated as shown in Figure 6.4 with the affected arm supported on a table of the correct height. A non-slip mat and a plate with raised sides are helpful at this stage.

As recovery takes place and grasp is achieved, cutlery with enlarged handles provide tactile stimulation and give the patient more independence. Yoghurt is an excellent food for early practice as it is not mucous forming. Chewing and swallowing difficulties are treated by the speech therapist (Ch. 7).

Mobility:

Once stability in standing is achieved, the physiotherapist will work to improve mobility, walking the patient, first with the support of two people and then with one person and a stick. It is not desirable to use a tripod, as this encourages the patient to weightbear on the sound side, thus contravening the rules of symmetry. It is possible for a stroke patient to walk with a rollator. The affected hand may be fixed by a removable strap but the patient must have good shoulder control.

Writing

The occupational therapist is responsible for retraining the patient in the mechanics of writing, the other components being dealt with by the speech therapist. The written word is not a substitute for the spoken word in those patients suffering from aphasia, and unless the elderly person has a clear wish to write, it need not be regarded as a priority.

The substitution of speech by the use of picture or symbol boards is not necessarily the answer for the aphasic patient. There may be difficulties with interpretation and with understanding visual as well as auditory clues.

If writing requires to be practised the patient should be seated, properly positioned and given graded writing exercises using the non-preferred hand, and suitable or built-up pencils for the recovering stroke hand.

Perceptual testing

Problems of sensation further complicate recovery from stroke. These may be identified as neglect, sensory inattention, defects of visual spatial perception, apraxia, asterognosis and right/left orientation.

Andrews et al (1980) discuss the value of simple picture drawing as an early prognostic tool. The elderly appear to be more likely to draw abnormal pictures and demonstrate inattention and perplexity.

On the other hand, Rasmussen et al (1983) concluded that the Barthel Index (see Ch. 2) was the most reliable prediction as to whether the patient should be able to return home. Cognitive testing was more effective in determining that continuing care would be necessary.

If a therapist feels that formal perceptual testing is appropriate, she should remember that the rules of positioning are still fundamental and that testing does not constitute treatment. The therapist must also make allowances for the tests being strange and therefore perplexing to the elderly patient (Whiting et al 1984).

Apraxic patients will often improve if allowed to perform tasks of daily living automatically (subcortically). Such patients will respond well if engaged in conversation while carrying out familiar activities such as washing or dressing.

Orientation

Orientation for time and place should be an integral part of the treatment programme. Stimulation should occur naturally in conversation, as should questions about home and family background. Information is often gathered more fruitfully in an informal way but is no less valuable when an assessment of cognition is being made. Close liaison with the rest of the team should provide a general picture of the patient. This is important before resolution can take place.

RESOLUTION

There is an equation of resolution: the degree of functional independence balanced against the amount of support in the environment. For those patients who do not make a full recovery, a supportive spouse or family, and aids to daily living (Table 6.6), make life possible in the community.

Table 6.6 Aids and adaptations which promote independence for stroke patients

Problem	Solution
Mobility	
Getting about outside	Rails at front or back door, adapted car, buggy, scooter, electric wheelchair
in the house	wheelchair — narrower the better walking stick, occasionally zimmer or tripod
stairs	extra bannister rail, stair lift
carrying items about	trolley, zimmer with bag
Living room	Height of armchair, raise level of sockets, electric plugs with loops top controls for gas/electric fires push button telephone, Holdaphone
Writing	Built up pen (fibre) electric typewriter clipboard and non-slip mat
Dressing	Velcro fastenings elastic bra Boxer shorts stockings with elastic tops wool socks longhandled shoehorn elastic laces slip-on shoes sports shirts front fastening roomy dresses washable trousers helping hand aid
Bedroom	bed height same as armchair height commode for night use bedside light duvet
Feeding	non-slip mat plate guard Dynafork built up utensil handles/cutlery
Kitchen	Undoit (for jars) one handed tin opener Belliclamp, front knobs on cooker aid to hold pot handle firm one handled grill pan cook veg in wire basket grill pan with one handle cooker with front controls teapot tipper plastic kettle (safe & lightweight) kitchen stool
Bathroom	grab rail at side of WC Mowbray raise & rails bath seat & board board & tap spray Mangar bath hoist Autolift shower with flip down seat (if helper available) sponge for washing suction nail brush electric shaver (battery powered)

The hospital occupational therapist is responsible for assessing levels of function. Prior to discharge, close liaison with the community occupational therapist is essential for the smooth transition from hospital to home. A joint home visit is recommended. Home adaptations and the provision of aids are discussed in the Chapter 23.

Part IV Homes may pose problems for stroke patients with communication difficulties as they may feel rejected by their peers. Also there may be longish distances to walk. Sheltered housing may be a more suitable alternative. The advantages and limitations of special housing are examined in depth in Chapter 22. For the third of stroke patients who require continuing care in a hospital or nursing home (Andrews 1982), occupational therapy treatment should not stop; a programme to stimulate and maintain these patients at their maximum is described in Chapter 13.

REFERENCES

Andrews K, Brocklehurst L, Richards B, Haycock P J 1980 The prognostic value of picture drawings by stroke patients. Rheumatology and Rehabilitation 19: 180–185

Andrews K 1982 The recovery of the severely disabled

stroke patient. Rheumatology and rehabilitation.
Nov: 225–230

Garraway W M, Akhtar A J, Prescott R J et al 1980
Management of acute stroke in the elderly; results of
a controlled trial. British Medical Journal 280: 1040–3;
281: 827–9

Helm M 1981 A personal approach to rehabilitation
following brain damage in adults — treatment of
stroke patients in medical wards. British Journal of
Occupational Therapy 44(1): 19–20

Rasmussen G, Parsman V A, Gyling M D 1983 Own
home or nursing home? (a stroke assessment) First
European Conference, Research and Rehabilitation,
Edinburgh

Smith M E, Garraway W M, Smith D L, Akhtar A J 1982
The impact of therapy on functional outcome in a
controlled trial ol stroke rehabilitation. Archives of
Physical Medicine and Rehabilitation 63: 21–24

Whisnant J P 1984 The decline of stroke. Stroke
15: 160–8

Whiting S et al 1984 Rivermead Perceptual Assessment
battery. NFER-Nelson, Windsor

FURTHER READING

Ayres A J 1974 Integration of information. In: Henderson
et al (eds) The development of sensory integrative
therapy and practice. Kendall Hunt, Dubuque, Iowa

Bobath B 1978 Adult hemiplegia; evaluation and
treatment, 2nd edn. Heinemann, London

Brunnstrom S 1970 Movement therapy in hemiplegia.
Harper and Row, New York

Eggers O 1983 Occupational therapy in the treatment of
adult hemiplegia. Diebal C (trans). Heinemann,
London

Johnstone M 1987 Restoration of motor function in the
stroke patient, 3rd edn. Churchill Livingstone,
Edinburgh

Knott M, Voss D E 1956 Proprioceptive neuromuscular
facilitation; patterns all techniques. Harper add Row,
New York

Trombly C A, Scott A D 1977 Occupational therapy for
physical dysfunction. Williams and Wilkins, Baltimore,
ch 6, p 70

7

Communication
E. M. R. Ewing

NORMAL AGEING

Language

Change in language use appears to take place with increasing age. Maxim (1982) comments that 'more dysfluencies begin to appear, as do the use of 'indefinite' words. There is a divergence in the use of written and spoken language with a less frequent use of embedded sentences in spoken language, while written language becomes more formal in grammatical structure'.

Memory

In considering healthy elderly people, Smith and Fullerton (1981) suggest that while there is no difference between age groups in short-term memory capacity, the time required to respond does vary. Recall using episodic long-term memory may be affected by increasing age. The speed of retrieval of names from semantic memory also may be affected by age.

Hearing

Hearing loss, which has physical, psychological and social consequences, affects about one third of those over 65 years. It is a handicap which leads to loneliness and isolation.

There are many causes of conductive deafness and sensorineural deafness, but the most common amongst the elderly is presbycusis. In the older population this is considered as part of the ageing process and typically involves loss of sensitivity in the higher frequencies. The causes are varied, such as genetic defects, noise exposure, disorders of circulation, injury to the ear and cell death. Presbycusis tends to affect both ears equally and is more frequent in males than in females.

The difficulty for elderly people suffering from presbycusis may not be that of hearing people's voices — because their hearing of low frequencies is adequate — but will be understanding what is said. This is because they will be unable to hear many consonants in the high frequency range, e.g. s, sh, th, f, k. These consonants and others may be difficult to distinguish and produce confusion. A. Newby (1958) comments, the words 'fake', 'cake' and 'sake' may all be confused on the basis of hearing alone because the initial or final consonant may not be heard in any of the words. All the person may hear is the 'a' sound.

A conductive hearing loss is due to dysfunction of the outer or middle ear, the difficulty being that of conducting sound to the analysing system rather than the perception of sound. Sometimes the elderly person may speak very quietly due to the bone conduction mechanism being affected in the feedback of the speaker's voice.

People with conductive impairment do not hear well in noisy surroundings. This is an important factor when considering noise levels in a geriatric ward. Speech discrimination is relatively unimpaired for the person with a conductive deafness and she will understand what she hears. Recruitment and tinnitus are common, although tinnitus can occur without hearing loss.

If a hearing aid is to be provided to overcome the effects of presbycusis, it should be considered as a communication improver because of the condition's multiple problems. Hearing aids are least effective in noisy situations or in listening to groups of people; they are most useful in improving hearing in quiet, face-to-face conversations. Bamford (1981) comments that adequate counselling should be given over a period of time to both the wearer and her family, to help both parties adjust to living with a hearing aid as well as to the problem of hearing loss.

Many elderly people find the mechanics of a post-aural aid difficult to cope with and the device not easy to insert, especially if they have arthritic hands or hand tremor.

Hospital audiology departments and the Social Services are able to supply advice, information and a variety of devices, and manufacturers are always introducing new devices to help with amplification of telephones, television and radio.

In order to minimise the problems experienced by the elderly deaf person, others need to be much more aware of her needs. It is helpful to speak slowly, clearly but not too loudly, with pauses between sentences. It is important to face the the deaf person so that she can lip read while listening. Above all, she must continue to be included in family and social conversation, and be encouraged to take an active part in all such conversation.

Vision

Elderly people tend not to report their visual problems because they accept a lower standard of performance as an inevitable part of old age.

A variety of visual changes takes place in the ageing process which affect the amount of information an old person takes in. These include:

> astigmatic changes in the lens or cornea
> cataracts
> glaucoma
> muscular degeneration
> retinal changes.

A common feature of visual changes may be observed when an elderly person is seen holding a book at arm's length while reading. This can be due to the lens losing elasticity and so stiffening: discrimination of shape and colour may also be affected.

Poor vision can directly affect communication if a person is unable to lip read or see the speaker's facial expression. Inability to judge the distance between the speaker and herself may cause the deaf person to misjudge the voice volume needed for normal conversation.

Poor vision can be extremely frustrating to people who rely on reading and television for their main source of entertainment, or who correspond frequently with friends and relatives. Good, well-positioned lighting is essential and large print books are helpful.

Voice

Specific physiological changes in muscles and joints adversely affect agility and range of movements. Hence it is to be expected that respiration, vocal pitch, volume and resonance of voice will deteriorate with advancing years (Greene 1982).

Greene (1972) states that research shows that men's voices age more than women's voices, but do not change until the age of approximately 80 years.

The human ear is often an extremely good judge of the age, physical and emotional condition of a speaker. Elderly people who keep themselves fit, alert and mentally active reflect this in their voices.

Vocal strain may be experienced by elderly people who have to speak to deaf relatives or companions, or who have to compete against a background of noise. Care and attention should be paid to preserving vocal efficiency since this enables the elderly to continue playing an active role in the community. A hoarse, deteriorated voice makes an individual sound old and ineffective, possibly to herself as much as to a listener (Greene 1972).

COMMUNICATION AFFECTED BY STROKE

The most common cause of communication problems in the neurologically impaired elderly person is 'stroke' (see Ch. 6). A variety of problems may arise involving language, speech, voice articulation and swallowing.

Dysphasia

Dysphasia is an acquired impairment of language due to a focal lesion or cerebral vascular disease in the left hemisphere of the brain. In the early stages following 'stroke', the patient may be aphasic, that is, she may have no functional language either in understanding or expression. Usually her condition stabilises and she develops an incomplete language function, dysphasia.

The important feature of language recovery is to work on what the patient can achieve rather than on what has been lost.

Comprehension

There may be a loss of language comprehension. The dysphasic patient replies inappropriately or uses unintelligible jargon. She confuses 'yes' and 'no' in gesture as well as in speech. Difficulties with comprehension tend to confuse patients, and complications with reading and writing are also experienced.

Expression

Internal thought processes may be very confused, especially early on. Hopefully this stage settles to a point where the patient knows what she wants to say but may be unable to 'bring the word out'.

A variety of problems may be experienced:

(i) naming difficulties
(ii) word finding difficulties. The patient may be left with a language impairment involving grammatical structure, and the idea of structure — noun, verb, object — may be extremely difficult to produce
(iii) perseveration occurs when the patient keeps repeating the same word: this can be very frustrating to both speaker and listener
(iv) paraphasia can occur in speech, reading or writing and consists of omission or substitution of part or whole of a word
(v) circumlocution is talking round the subject matter and can help overcome the inability to name objects.

Reading

A patient's recovery of this ability depends on her pre-morbid use of reading. One of the principal difficulties is poor memory. Even if comprehension of the material is good, she may be unable to remember the start of a page or paragraph. In dysphasia, sentences, words and even letters may not be recognised, but often words are more easily recognised than letters because of their shape or the context in which they occur.

Writing

If recall and recognition of letters is difficult, immense frustration and anxiety arise when the elderly patient realises she cannot write fluently. Spelling and grammatical construction are often affected. In order to write at all, she may have to use her non-preferred hand, but, provided she has manual control and vision, this does not usually present many problems. Mood is a predictor of success or failure in recovering this skill.

Calculation

This involves mental arithmetic, time and money. If the patient is to return home to live on her own, it is essential that she is able to cope with rent, rates, pension book, housekeeping money etc. Time and recognition of a clockface are also important. It should be remembered that calculation is an abstract concept and, as such, is not easy for a dysphasic patient to cope with. Practice with money in everyday situations is vital if the patient is to return home without support.

Visual problems

In addition to those already mentioned, there are a number of commonly experienced visual difficulties:

(i) perceptual problems: due mainly to parietal lobe damage. This causes patients to see the world tilted through several degrees, or mirrorwise; and may make it impossible for them to interpret what they see. This is undoubtedly very alarming and bewildering for the elderly, and this writer believes that perceptual problems are much more disabling than language deficits

(ii) visual field defect (hemianopia) may be present, often showing up in reading when the patient consistently ignores the left or right side of the page, often reading without pause and failing to comprehend the subject

(iii) diplopia makes reading and writing difficult. Double vision can occur horizontally, vertically and diagonally and is very distressing to the patient. If there is sufficient vision in one eye, it may be alleviated by use of an eye patch on the other

(iv) nystagmus, or flitting vision, which occurs in cerebellar involvement, makes reading and writing almost impossible, drastically reducing a patient's ability to communicate

(v) following 'stroke', the prescription of previously worn spectacles may no longer be appropriate. It is usual to delay retesting vision until the patient is neurologically stable.

Memory, concentration and new learning ability

Both memory and concentration problems are often apparent following stroke and impede the recovery of communication skills. As attention span and concentration improves, so it becomes easier to assist the return of memory. This work may have to be done slowly, gradually and repetitively, with care and sensitivity to the individual's needs.

There are elderly patients who can learn despite neurological impairment and, if well motivated, they are often successful in coping with their communication problems. Much depends on their pre-morbid personality and state of health. Those who have no new learning ability, as well as having problems with 'old learning', are unlikely to succeed in adapting to alternative means of communication, so may have to be excluded from speech therapy.

The speech therapist's involvement

The speech therapist, working either in a hospital or in the community, will require to assess the patient's language skills and use of functional language in order to prescribe appropriate treatment. Short courses of intensive therapy appear to be more effective for the dysphasic elderly than infrequent longer sessions, particularly in the early stages.

The emphasis should be to encourage functional communication, and the speech therapist should work in conjunction with the occupational therapist, particularly in the area of daily living activities and social contacts. For those patients returning home, special activities should be organised in a true setting to assist with the problems of coping with time and money.

The speech therapist must explain to other staff how to encourage the patient to make efforts to communicate using speech, gesture, mime, eye pointing, writing and drawing.

A vital part of the speech therapist's role is to keep the patient's relatives fully informed about her condition, and to help them come to terms with and adapt to the difficulties confronting her.

Dysarthria

This is a neuromuscular disorder, including slurred, weak, laboured and other forms of distorted articulation; it also involves inco-ordination of phonation, respiration and articulation. Reflex behaviour, such as for swallowing and chewing, may also be affected. The type, level and severity of lesion determines the prognosis and treatment.

Brain (1956) described the main types of dysarthria:

1. Upper motor neurone or spastic dysarthria results from bilateral lesions in the pyramidal tracts. This type of lesion causes a paralysis of movement, and patients show difficulty in chewing, swallowing and coughing, as well as in speech which is slow, slurred and hypernasal with pitch alterations.

2. Cerebellar dysarthria results from lesions of the cerebellar vermis or its connection with the brain stem. This type of lesion causes speech to be slow and unco-ordinated with unnatural separation of syllables (scanning speech), and the voice is explosive with alteration in pitch.

3. Lower motor neurone dysarthria results from lesions of the cranial nerves supplying the cuticulatory muscles. The affected muscles show wasting and weakness, and quality of speech depends on which muscles are paralysed.

4. Extrapyramidal dysarthria results from lesions within the extrapyramidal system. This system influences muscle tone, co-ordination and speed of movement, and has an important role to play in the ability to initiate speech.

Swallowing

One area of particular concern in the elderly is difficulty with chewing and swallowing. Attention must be paid to dentition. If the patient has ill-fitting dentures, then these should be checked by a dentist. As it is the tongue muscle which 'holds' the lower denture in place, it is not surprising that a partly paralysed tongue will interfere with the 'bedding' of the denture.

A speech therapist cannot alter the swallow reflex, but to help the patient cope with this problem the following details must be checked:

a. oral hygiene before meals
b. posture — preferably sitting up, well supported, leaning slightly forward towards the table
c. diet (see Ch. 16) needs to be nutritious, have appropriate texture and temperature (heated plate), and be colourful and well presented. Taste is important: spices, herbs, lemon and/or orange flavour should be used to stimulate the taste buds
d. utensils and how to use them, where to

place food in the mouth and the appropriate quantity per mouthful

e. swallow technique (icing the tongue before meals may be helpful), talking the patient through the swallow process is known as the 'cognitive technique'

f. oral hygiene after meals

g. sitting upright for 15 minutes after meals.

Drooling

Drooling is another problem which can be helped by the patient having well-fitted dentures, a good posture and being constantly reminded to swallow. There are mechanical devices to remind patients to swallow, such as palatal lifts, and in the last resort certain operations can be carried out to overcome excessive drooling.

Voice volume

It is a feature of 'stroke' that the patient may be unable to control her voice volume. A loud booming staccato voice is common in cerebellar dysarthria and is socially unacceptable.

By working on breathing, face, lips, tongue and soft palate, the speech therapist may help the patient to cope with a permanent reduction in voice volume. There are also a number of voice amplifiers available on the market.

Aids to communication

There is a growing number of 'aid' to communication now available. These are almost all for patients with an articulation problem (i.e. dysarthria), but there are a few which are language-based, e.g. 'Vocaid' and 'Convaid'. Reasonable vision is required to operate these, as well as the ability to select one picture/diagram/word from several others. Severely dysphasic patients may not be able to do this reliably. The speech therapist should assess the patient's ability and requirement before an aid is bought.

Dyspraxia

This condition is the inability to perform purposeful movements in the absence of paralysis.

Although it can be regarded as an entity on its own, a verbal or articulatory dyspraxia is usually seen in conjunction with dysphasia: thus the elderly patient is doubly handicapped. When she does know what she wants to say, she may not know how to say it.

Orofacial dyspraxia is present when the normal movements of the face cannot be carried out to command, e.g. blowing (necessary as an egressive airstream for speech), sucking, licking the lips, whistling, winking, protruding the tongue etc.

Verbal dyspraxia is when the patient struggles to produce correct articulatory positions in sequence. There is usually difficulty in initiating speech, particularly the first sound or syllable. The inability to start off sequential movements is perhaps the most disabling factor in attempting speech. Some patients respond to words written down as a kind of 'prompt'. Often, dyspraxic patients can sing, even when they cannot speak. If successful, singing and chanting should be encouraged.

Problems involving calculation are common: the patient may be unable to sequence numbers, and this has adverse implications for those living independently and having to cope with money. The abstract concept of numbers is often difficult for dysphasic–dyspraxic patients to grasp.

If a writing dyspraxia is shown, alternative means of communication should be substituted, e.g. speech, mime or gesture.

Ideational dyspraxia involves putting ideas into logical sequences of actions, and may require repetition, the use of clues and gesture by the therapist.

Emotional problems associated with communication

Grieving for the loss of social and physical independence or of the use of a limb can directly affect the desire and motivation to work on communication problems. Depression is common following a 'stroke', when the patient recovers enough to appreciate what problems she is faced with. It is understandable that some feel unequal to the struggle and withdraw.

Excessive verbal and auditory stimulation is not the method to use for encouraging communication. Peace and quiet is needed, interspersed with appropriate activities designed to encourage speech. The elderly need time to recoup their physical and emotional resources.

Support groups

Both dysphasic and dysarthric patients can benefit from group activities. Penwill (1958), in describing group activities, found that they resulted in a reduction of anxiety and related tension, and thus helped to create optimum conditions for learning.

Small groups for supporting relatives of new strokes are suggested, to provide information and to discuss individual speech problems. These should be run by a speech therapist and a clinical psychologist (Fraser 1980).

'Speech after Stroke' Clubs and the Chest, Heart and Stroke Association also provide valuable groups for patients and support for relatives.

SENILE DEMENTIA AND COMMUNICATION

Lishman (1978) defines dementia as 'an acquired global impairment of consciousness'. Dementia can be regarded as a problem of cognitive function rather than a language problem, although at times it may resemble one.

The speech therapist Stevens (1985), in her 1981–83 pilot study of the language of dementia in the elderly, says that language structure, verbal fluency (except in very advanced cases), and the ability to cope with concrete familiar material and automatic tasks all appear to be broadly intact. All types of stimuli used with dementing patients need to be explicit, reducing the need for interpretation and inference. Working on improving language skills seems inappropriate if it is the ability to organise and use that language which is limited.

CONCLUSION

So far, there seems to be a scarcity of research into how normal ageing elderly people communicate. We know their use and style of language changes with age: the prosodic features of voice and speech are affected as may be vision and hearing. Life-style, social interaction and relationships are all affected by the standard of daily communication.

For the neurologically impaired, there is the added despair of language difficulty, of not understanding and not being understood, of increased loss of independence and dignity. There will be strong feelings which they cannot express.

It is of great benefit to the elderly to know that people care about and understand their problems and feelings.

'The need to communicate does not lessen in importance with age nor with an increase in physical disability. On the contrary, dependence upon the ability to communicate effectively becomes progressively more important to an elderly person if a level of social involvement is to be maintained.' (Le Ferre 1979)

ACKNOWLEDGEMENTS

My thanks to Patricia Bennett, Speech Therapist, Liberton Hospital, Edinburgh, and Audrey Jamieson, Speech Therapist, Balfour Pavilion, Astley Ainslie Hospital, Edinburgh.

REFERENCES

Bamford J M, Wilson I M, Alkinson D, Bench J 1981 Predicting speech — hearing from the audiogram. British Journal of Audiology 15:3. ex Mitchell J, 1982 Normal age — an overview. In: Edwards (ed) Communication changes in elderly people. The College of Speech Therapists, London

Brain R 1956 Diseases of the nervous system. Oxford University Press, Oxford

Fraser C (1980) Personal communication

Greene M 1972 The voice and its disorders, 3rd edn. Pitman Medical, London

Greene M 1982 Ageing of the voice: A review. In: Edwards M (ed) Communication changes in elderly people. The College of Speech Therapists, London

Le Ferre M 1959 Speech therapy for the geriatric patient In Geriatrics, Vol 12, no. 12. *ex* Mitchell J 1982 Normal age change — An overview. In: Edwards (ed) Communication changes in elderly people. The College of Speech Therapists, London

Lishman L A 1978 In: Organic psychiatry. Blackwell Scientific, Oxford. *ex* Mitchell J Normal age change — an overview. In: Edwards (ed) Communication changes in elderly people. The College of Speech Therapists, London

Maxim J 1982 Language change with increasing age. In: Edwards (ed) Communication changes in elderly people. The College of Speech Therapists, London

Newby H A 1958 Audiology. Vision Press, London

Penwill M 1958 An experiment with a heterogeneous group in a geriatric unit. Speech Pathology and Therapy, Feb

Smith D A, Fullerton A M 1981 Age differences. In: Beasley D S, Davis C A (ed) (ed Edwards) Episodic and semantic memory in ageing: Communication processes and disorders pub. Greene and Stratton *ex*

Mitchell J. Normal Age Change — An overview In: Edwards (ed) Communication changes in elderly people. The College of Speech Therapists, London

Stevens S 1985 The language of dementia in the elderly: A pilot study British Journal of Disorders of Communication 20(2)

SUGGESTED READING

Edwards M 1982 (ed) Communication changes in elderly people. The College of Speech Therapists, London

Lubinski R 1981 Language and ageing: An environmental approach to intervention in topics in language disorders.

Obler L K and A, Martin L 1980 Language and communication in the elderly. Heath and Co, Lexington, Mass.

Skinner C, Thomson I 1983 The assessment of clinical and functional language in the aged. Bulletin Audiophonology 16(8): 263–272

Walker S A 1984 The communication status of older people. International Rehabilitation Medicine 139–142

8

Neurological conditions

M. Helm

The most common neurological conditions to affect people over 70 years are strokes and brain failure leading to dementia. Occupational therapy treatment for these conditions is described in Chapters 6 and 9 respectively. Many people in the United Kingdom suffer from multiple sclerosis (one in 2000) but they rarely survive to the age of seventy. Support and management of people with this condition along with that for people with motor neurone disease belong in a book about the young disabled.

This chapter will concentrate on three common conditions affecting many elderly people: parkinsonism, head injury and herpes zoster (shingles).

PARKINSONISM

Parkinsonism comprises a collection of symptoms caused by impairment of voluntary movement. It is found in 1% of the over-60 population and is a progressive degenerative disorder affecting the basal ganglia. There is no known cause for parkinsonism in three-quarters of the people who suffer from it. Others may develop parkinsonism after using major tranquillizers (e.g. phenothiazines), following head injury, during or following a boxing career (punch drunk syndrome) or in association with mid-brain tumour. Extrapyramidal features may be found in patients with widespread cerebrovascular disease. The disease progresses more quickly if the cause for the condition is drug induced (by major tranquillizers, antiemetics or antivertigo agents (stemetil)).

Tremor

Tremor is often the first symptom in idiopathic parkinsonism. At first, one hand and forearm are affected, and then the condition eventually spreads to the leg and during the next year or two to the other limbs. Tremor is more exaggerated if the person is anxious or tired. It can be subdued by making purposeful movements and disappears when the person is asleep. Precise movements such as writing or picking up a cup or cutting up food may be hampered by tremor.

Rigidity

Rigidity is a common presenting symptom in elderly people and precedes tremor in postencephalitic parkinsonism (now a very uncommon condition). Muscle tone is increased, greater effort is required for any voluntary movement and all activities are slowed down. Resistance to passive movement may be smooth (plastic rigidity) or intermittent (cogwheel rigidity). Rigidity is often accompanied by muscular pain in the trunk, shoulder and pelvic girdles.

Hypo- or bradykinesia

Hypo- or bradykinesia, as well as rigidity, hamper free movement. These patients experience difficulty in initiating movements like rolling over in bed, rising from a chair, starting to walk, talk or write. All movements are smaller and slower than the person intends them to be. Muscle power and sensation are normal.

Speech is very quiet and often slurred but the content is usually lucid and patience is required to wait for answers. Writing is very small and often illegible. Involuntary movement is also affected, for example lack of facial animation, and associated movements, like swinging the arms when walking, are lost.

Lack of expression often makes the person look depressed or simple-minded — often she is neither but just has great difficulty in altering facial expression.

Mental changes

Depression is a common feature of parkinsonism and some say occurs in one in three elderly patients. Dementia is always a feature of postencephalitic parkinsonism but not necessarily an accompaniment of idiopathic parkinsonism.

Role of occupational therapy in treating parkinsonism

— To assess patients' independence in activities of daily living and provide aids to ensure its improvement.
— To encourage patients to be more mobile and increase the size of voluntary movement.
— To help patients' written communication and encourage clarity of speech.
— To perform hand function tests pre- and post drug therapy (for example Sinemet or Madopar).

Activities of daily living

People suffering from rigidity move very slowly and find each movement a great effort. It is therefore essential for the OT to simplify daily living activities, especially those requiring fine finger dexterity. This helps to prevent frustration and despair. The following lists illustrate ways in which this can be done.

Dressing

— Loose, light, warm clothing (for example track suits for the trendy of average build) can be worn
— Elastic waistbands or velcro fastenings instead of small buttons, hooks and eyes or trouser clips should be used
— Tabs on zippers are useful

— Elastic shoelaces and a rigid plastic shoe-horn are also useful
— A footstool can be useful when putting on socks and stockings
— If new clothes are being chosen, women find front fastening clothes easier to put on and for men sports shirts and cardigans with large buttons are easier
— Crease-resistant drip-dry fabrics make washing less of a chore.
— Dressing should be done in a warm room, 65–70°C, as it is such a slow process.

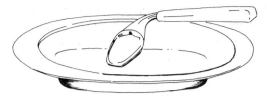

Fig. 8.1 Manoy plate and angled spoon

Eating and drinking

— Remind the patient if she has drooling and swallowing problems to close her mouth tightly before trying to swallow. This helps stimulate the swallow reflex and prevents choking
— Encourage her to take small mouthfuls to avoid the 'hamster' syndrome. Sometimes feeding with smaller spoon helps
— Plates with built-up sides (made by Manoy or Royal Doulton) (Fig. 8.1) can be used
— Plastic guards which clip onto meat plates to prevent spillage can be used
— Non-slip Dycem mats are helpful in anchoring plates when eating.
— Insulated plates (Mothercare) are useful for slow eaters — hot food is most unappetising when cold
— Double handles on a mug (Royal Doulton, Selecta heavy mug) (Fig. 8.2) instead of a cup make drinking easier
— Angled cutlery (Manoy) or gimble cutlery (Steeper) can be used
— Rocker knives (Manoy) can assist in cutting meat
— Straws can be helpful as long as swallowing co-ordination is intact
— Large towelling, plastic-backed bibs may look demeaning but they reduce the washing load considerably.

Hygiene

— WC. A raised toilet seat (heights range from 5 to 15 cm (2 to 6 in)) may help transfers

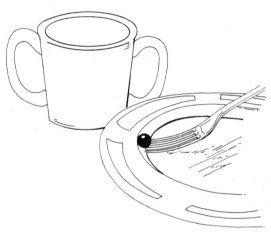

Fig. 8.2 Royal Doulton mug and plate with lip

— Or a grab rail screwed to the wall next to the WC
— Rails can be fixed to the wall behind the WC which can be hinged forward for the person with parkinsonism and back for others in the household
— A toilet frame with bilateral rails is safer with flanges screwed to the floor. Cleaning after a bowel movement is often a problem for someone with limited movement
— There are one or two bottom wipers on the market but a bidet or Clos-o-mat are the expensive answers to this problem
— Bath. Bathing should only be attempted under supervision or with someone's help — the righting reflex is reduced in people with parkinsonism
— The conventional bath seat and board with grab rail on the wall at the side of the bath are helpful
— A rubber non-slip mat to put inside the bath is an essential precaution

— It is safer to let the water run away before climbing out of the bath
— The bathroom should be heated so that bathing is a pleasant relaxing process and not a Spartan ritual
— Bubble bath is handy for cleaning people and baths effortlessly.

Shower

— The hose should be detachable from the wall and the force and temperature of the spray easily adjusted to suit individual requirements
— A non-springloaded flipdown seat in the shower (Fig. 8.3) is helpful if balance is a problem plus a non-slip rubber shower mat
— Hairwashing is best done in the shower
— If the person is able to transfer into the bath using the aids described under Bath, a rubber hose and spray can be attached to the taps and a shower taken in this fashion
— A shower cabinet or one with sliding doors instead of a curtain are the more convenient types.

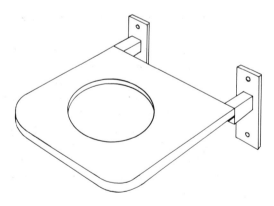

Fig. 8.3 Non-spring loaded shower seat

Washing

— A stool or chair should be kept near the wash-hand basin
— A large wash-mit or sponge is easier to handle than a facecloth/flannel.

Toothbrushing

— Diameter of the toothbrush handle can be built up
— Dentures are best rinsed after meals as well as soaked overnight in a suitable cleaning agent
— Mouthwashes are essential to keep the mouth fresh and free from food debris.

Shaving

— A battery-run shaver is the easiest type to use for a man with tremor or rigidity: attachments on the ones with flexes are very small.

Kitchen

— A kitchen stool is very helpful. There are ones with a seat which slopes forward slightly, ones with backs and others with backs and sides
— Lever taps do not require fine dexterity. Work surfaces should be continuous to avoid having to lift saucepans
— A trolley/walking aid can be useful in the kitchen for fetching and carrying
— Non-slip mats in the kitchen are useful for putting under mixing bowls, chopping boards and anything which requires to be anchored. Vegetables can be cooked in wire baskets, then the basket lifted out. The water can then be poured away when it's cold
— The kettle/saucepan can be filled by using a plastic jug
— Shelving and cupboards should be of a suitable height
— Most kitchen activities can be done when seated: for example, vegetable preparation, cooking and ironing
— Automatic washing machine plus tumble dryer are great labour savers. If clothes are folded after tumble drying there is no need to iron them.

Improve mobility

Bed

— Moving about in bed is usually a problem: brushed cotton pyjamas and sheets provide resistance and grip; nylon and silk should be avoided
— A duvet is preferable to blankets as it is light and warm
— Height of the bed should be checked for suitability and castors removed to stabilise the bed
— A divan bed aid (Renray) can help with transfers
— An orthopaedic mattress provides a firmer base from which to rise
— For night use a commode can be placed at the side of the bed. It should be of the same height as the bed.

Moving about the house

— Floor surfaces should be continuous if possible, i.e. fitted carpets not rugs
— Hesitation and propulsion problems are usually experienced when floor coverings change, i.e. from carpet to linoleum; and walking from one to the other should be practised repeatedly to reduce the incidence of 'freezing'
— Walking with a zimmerframe is sometimes successful, but not always as people with parkinsonism are often inclined to walk leaning backwards — this tendency is very hard to treat
— One should ensure that the armchair is of the correct height. Getting up can be helped if the patient rocks backwards and forwards counting at the same time '1–2–3 up' to gain momentum
— The same trick can help when the patient starts to walk if she thinks 'big' and counts at the same time. A 1–2 1–2 rhythm can often help produce the right size of step instead of the usual small shuffling ones
— Raised plug sockets are helpful and plugs with moulded strap attachments are easier to use than conventional ones (Fig. 8.4).

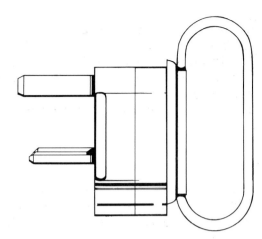

Fig. 8.4 Plug with moulded strap attachment

Communication

Spoken. The occupational therapist works in conjunction with the speech therapist and reinforces what she teaches.
— It is important to remind the patient of correct breathing techniques using the diaphragm and not the upper part of the chest. Inefficient breathing methods interrupt speech flow
— Ask her to repeat what you haven't understood
— Don't make her repeat the whole sentence — just the part you missed
— Encourage louder and slower speech.
— Wait for her answers — do not anticipate and finish her sentences for her
— Remember how frustrating speaking can be for people with parkinsonism
— Encourage her to participate in social groups so that speech comes naturally, almost reflexly.

Written

— Occasionally speech may be too difficult for others to understand and alphabet cards can be used
— Sometimes writing can be used as an alternative to speech
— To increase the size of writing, tracing over capitals and writing patterns can help.
— When writing spontaneously, ask the

patient to exaggerate the letter size and as with walking, when the person is encouraged to think big, the words may be of a reasonable size
— If writing is too small and indistinct some elderly people, especially those with previous knowledge of typewirters, find electric typewriters helpful as only light touch is required.

Timed tests pre- and post-chemotherapy

There are very few standardised hand function tests. One that is suitable for use with Parkinson's patients is the Jebsen (1969). It involves completing several fine finger dexterity tests with either hand. There are several sub-tests: writing; simulated page turning; picking up small objects; simulated feeding; stacking checkers (draughts); picking up large light objects and large heavy objects. Bilateral tests, which are not part of the Jebsen battery, highlight co-ordination and shoulder abduction problems. They are as follows:
The patient is asked to:
— take a match from the box and strike it
— fold writing paper and put in an envelope
— take three coins from a small purse
— cut plasticine with a knife and fork
— turn a newspaper inside out.
   Tests which specifically measure tremor are tracing lines, for example, mazes and circles.
   It is important that conditions and surroundings are as identical as possible to the first time a patient was tested, when she is retested after chemotherapy, so that any improvement can be accurately timed and measured.

HEAD INJURY

Head injury is usually thought of as a condition affecting young adults as the group most at risk in road traffic accidents. Conventional occupational therapy treatment described for head injuries is designed to be directed towards this very disabled group whose brain damage is extensive; recovery may be very slow and measured in months or years. Reasons for head injury in elderly people are different: most are caused by falls in the house or in the street. In a recent study (Roy et al 1985), alcohol was found to be a contributory factor in over half of the male patients in a year's study of elderly head injuries. Instead of the usual bias towards males, patient numbers were almost equal — 78 males and 68 females. Frequently, elderly people who have sustained concussion live alone and it is not possible to discharge them from hospital until their home circumstances and support systems have been ascertained. For example, home care services may have to be initiated on discharge if the person's balance is too unsteady to allow for climbing stairs and shopping. A serious complication of head injury is subdural haematoma. This is diagnosed in many older people whose conscious level fluctuates. The patient may have bouts of drowsiness, develop focal symptoms, undergo changes in personality or be in severe pain. Surgery is necessary; burr holes in the skull are made and the haematoma removed. Chronic subdural bleeding can occur in old people with friable veins or, after a slight bump on the head, in those being treated with anticoagulants.

Reasons for falls leading to head injury in elderly people

1. Stroke
2. Acute confusional states caused by sedatives/ tranquillisers or alcohol
3. Tendency to trip by:
   a. those demented people who take small steps
   b. shuffling gait of people with parkinsonism
   c. unsuitable or ill-fitting footware, e.g. slippers
4. Arthritis — because of stiff joints people are unable to regain balance if they lose it because they are unable to make quick movement adjustments
5. Postural hypotension
6. Vertebrobasilar insufficiency
7. Ménières disease.

After being admitted to a neurotrauma unit elderly people with minor head injury may not be able to be discharged as quickly as those in the younger age group. They may require treatment for other conditions. They may require a period of convalescence to recover from their trauma. They may require active rehabilitation, assessment of functional state and treatment of existing problems caused by the head injury or sustained prior to it. The following case histories demonstrate patients' physical/psychological and social conditions and how the occupational therapist was involved in planning patients' discharge.

Case history 1

Mr McP (75) had a minor head injury following a fall in the street: he was taken to a large teaching hospital. He regained consciousness quickly but was found to be confused and unsteady on his feet.

After physiotherapy treatment to help improve balance and mobility the occupational therapist was called in to assess activities of daily living, cognitive function and to take Mr McP on a home visit. When he was able to dress and move about the ward independently a home visit was arranged.

En route Mr McP became very confused and agitated, telling the therapist she was driving in the wrong direction.

At his home, a first floor flat, he was slightly disoriented, mistaking a bedroom for the kitchen, but quickly realised his mistake. He had been living with a disabled friend. She had had to move to a social services old peoples' home when he had fallen as she could not cope without his support.

The flat was sparsely furnished. The kitchen was dirty and most of the saucepans had been burnt. The couple had chosen not to have support from the home help service.

Mr McP managed to climb the twisting uneven flight of stairs but coming down he had to be saved from falling on several occasions.

In the occupational therapist's report she suggested further physiotherapy to overcome poor balance problems witnessed on the staircase. She also said that acceptance of home help support would be vital if Mr McP and his friend were to return to their home.

A second home visit was made; Mr McP was urged to slow down when climbing and coming down the stairs. This time he was not disoriented; he made a pot of tea and attempted to clean up the kitchen. He was very anxious to move home and this was arranged with support from a home help and frequent visits from his social worker. His friend was able to move home a week later, but he was unable to look after her as she was too dependent. The arrangement lasted for 3 months.

Case history 2

Mrs B (80) had been a passenger in a car driven by her husband (60) when they had had an accident and Mr B was killed. Mrs B was admitted to hospital with concussion. She had been disabled since childhood, and wore a caliper and used a stick to allow her to walk. Mrs B had been very dependent on her husband and the occupational therapist was asked to take her on as home visit to see what support services she would require on discharge from hospital.

Her home was in a sheltered housing complex (ground floor flat). The warden and other tenants were welcoming and supportive during the visit. The visit should have been traumatic for Mrs B, as the flat had not been altered since she and her husband had left it on the day of the fatal accident. Nevertheless Mrs B moved about the flat demonstrating how she could transfer on and off the WC, bed and armchair. She was at all times calm and accepting of the changed circumstances. She felt she could manage with help. It was agreed that to be able to move home she would require:
— Help with showering
— District nurse to dress her injured ankle
— Home help support
— A trolley/walking aid to help her move things about the flat.

Different agencies were contacted to supply these services when Mrs B was discharged. She continues to manage at home with this support.

Case history 3

Mr W (76), a widower, had been knocked down in the street in the dark by a hit and run driver. He was unconscious for several months and kept in the emergency hospital until he was alert. He was then moved to another hospital for active rehabilitation. He was found to have right parietal lobe damage leading to loss of proprioception and body schema. He was also confused.

After several months of occupational therapy treatment he managed to learn to look to see if he was holding things in his left hand (grip was strong); he was totally mobile, and able to wash, shave and dress unaided. He was still somewhat confused, for example he made tea with lukewarm water; when this was pointed out he willingly made another pot using boiling water. The options for Mr W's discharge were:

1. Home with maximum support from the home-help service and neighbours
2. Move to another flat in the town where his only daughter lived (with home-help support)
3. Move to a social services home in the town where his daughter lived.

The second and third options would take time to arrange, so Mr W, being anxious to move home, was discharged with daily support from the home-help and meals-on-wheels services.

HERPES ZOSTER

Herpes zoster is a viral infection which mainly affects the posterior root ganglia of the spinal cord or the sensory ganglia of the cranial nerves. This virus is the same as the one which causes chickenpox in children and younger adults. Herpes zoster may be caused by reactivation of the virus in someone with partial immunity to varicella. The affected dermatome becomes painful and red; within a few days vesicles appear. A common site is the trunk and in this case the eruption and pain occur in a unilateral band around the chest.

Involvement of the first division of the trigeminal nerve causes facial pain; scarring of the cornea cause transient and occasionally permanent damage, impairing vision, and destroying the corneal (blink) reflex. Herpes of the VIIth cranial nerve causes external ear and throat eruption and facial paralysis.

After the vesicles subside the patient is often left with pain — this is post-herpetic neuralgia and frequently affects elderly people. Many are plagued by intractable burning pain in the previously affected site for months afterwards. The pain is brought on by the slightest stimulus. Coping with persistent pain is extremely difficult at any age but the old and frail are an especially vulnerable group and adjustment does not come easily. Many become depressed, addicted to pain killers or suicidal as a consequence.

Occupational therapy treatment

The occupational therapist is asked to treat patients suffering from herpes zoster to assess functional ability in self-care and to treat depression (see Ch. 10), lower anxiety and improve self-confidence. Because of the ease in which post-herpetic neuralgia can be triggered off people recovering from shingles tend to sit very still, moving as little as possible. The occupational therapist has to try to show her patient that moving about will not make the pain worse and could in fact raise the pain threshold.

How individuals appreciate pain is relatively constant, but if someone is tense or anxious pain is felt more keenly. The therapist can encourage a person suffering from shingles to relax when carrying out activities of daily living.

REFERENCES

Draper I 1970 Lecture notes on neurology. Blackwell Scientific Publications, Oxford

Franklyn S, Perry A, Beattie A 1982 Living with Parkinson's disease. PDS, London

Godwin-Austen R B, Hildick-Smith M, Thompson M K 1982 Parkinson's disease. The general practitioner's guide. Franklin Scientific Projects, London

Hildick-Smith M 1982 Parkinsonism in the elderly Current medical research and opinion, 7

Holmes A E 1982 The many problems of head injury. Geriatric Medicine 12: 69–74

Jebsen R H et al 1969 An objective and standardized test of hand function. Archives of Physical Medicine and Rehabilitation: 311–319

Parkes J D 1982 Parkinson's disease. Update publications, London

Roy C, Pentland B, Millar J 1986 Head injury in the elderly. Age and Ageing July 193–202

Turner A 1981 The practice Occupational Therapy. Churchill Livingstone, Edinburgh

Walton J N 1977 Essentials of neurology, 4th edn. Pitman Medical, Tunbridge Wells

9

Psychiatry in old age: occupational therapy and organic conditions

S. E. E. Blair
A. H. Glen

INTRODUCTION

There are over 750 000 dementia sufferers in the United Kingdom. With demographic studies showing a continuing increase in numbers of the very old, planners have to take account of the accompanying rise in numbers of those elderly suffering from organic conditions. In recent years, a new interest has become evident. Research is considered a priority; psychologists, particularly, have spearheaded therapeutic measures and societies have emerged to promote understanding of organic illness. The challenge of treatment and management for occupational therapists centres on an understanding of the disease process and its psychological effect. Adjusting the environment to make it safer and more comprehensible also falls within our remit. In essence, our contribution is practical, as this chapter will show.

The fear in many is that old age equates with the 'sans everything' state. It is the pathetic picture of helplessness which horrifies people. In reality, the percentage of those who are ageing abnormally is small. Statistics reveal that the proportion of elderly suffering from organic disorder increases with age, and that it is higher in women than men at all ages. Those facts were reviewed by Jacques 1984 in what he describes as 'a new population of elderly women suffering from dementia and usually living alone'.

In this process of abnormal ageing, a progressive deterioration occurs. Personality is eroded, memory and intellectual functioning are impaired and disorientation is apparent. Marsden (1978) defines dementia as 'the syndrome of global disturbance of higher mental function in an alert patient'. Jacques (1984) described dementia as 'a slow death', particularly with reference to family strain where this decline is continually witnessed.

There are differing opinions on the most effective way of helping those affected by organic illness. Many advocate increases in community care and day care has emerged as a crucial resource. Residential care is described elsewhere in this book (Ch. 22) and may be private, voluntary or provided by the local authority. Ideally, the patient and her carers should have a choice. However, few have a range of services available in their area and the burden of care falls on relatives to maintain the elderly person at home.

When hospital care is deemed necessary, careful assessment is begun, and the nature of illness, degree of deterioration, and future support systems are taken into consideration. Occupational therapists are particularly involved in assessment of functional abilities as outlined by Perkins (1982) as well as designing an activity programme. A positive approach is emerging tackling this 'quiet epidemic' and is apparent in:

1. A demand to sharpen clinical acumen and determine with more accuracy the type and degree of brain damage
2. The recommendation in all reports that a multidisciplinary approach is essential
3. A realisation that services, whether health, local authority or voluntary, require co-ordination
4. Much greater recognition of the support and education required by relatives
5. The pressing need for more training for those who work with this group
6. The priority being given to research in this area.

In many respects, work with this group is a specialty within a specialty. There is so much we do not know about the process of cerebral atrophy — the pockets of deterioration and the psychological effects of multiple loss.

Occupational therapists are concerned with analysis of residual skill. When a range of opportunities is offered, it is possible to witness intact abilities. The elderly man who is disorientated for time, place and person retains the skill of bowling and approaches this with confidence. An old lady cannot remember the precise quantities of flour or margerine, but kneads and arranges pastry without hesitation. The reassurance offered by such gains instils a little confidence and raises self-esteem. The extent of activities is vast and selection according to need becomes the primary skill.

While there is undoubtedly a place for individual treatment, most activities with the confused elderly take place in small groups. An understanding of ageing and its dynamics is crucial in planning an activity programme. It is an over-simplification to regard old age as second childhood. The skill of introducing activities in meaningful and respectful ways takes time, practice and patience. A perceptive student once remarked upon the play-school type of environment in one unit, where many collages made by patients adorned the walls. Naturally, this required consideration and as a result staff decided that work of this nature required skilful mounting and more sensitive presentation. Shaw (1984) stresses an adult-to-adult approach and comments upon the necessity for purposeful and goal-directed activity with the confused elderly.

Classification of organic conditions

There are three main types of organic disorder in the elderly:

1. Alzheimer's disease was originally identified as a pre-senile dementia but it now

encompasses most cases of dementia associated with the elderly

2. Multi-infarct dementia
3. Benign dementia.

However, one of the first investigations necessary when an organic type of condition is suspected is to distinguish between acute organic reaction and one of the dementias. The former is temporary, reversible and indicates underlying physical illness. Symptoms can be less acute than in a younger person, last longer, and the causes can be more difficult to diagnose. They may be:

1. Infection, for example, chest or urinary tract
2. Malnutrition
3. Dehydration
4. Hypothermia
5. Severe pain
6. Effects of medication — over-prescribed, over-dosed or a build up of drugs in the body (see Ch. 15)
7. Psychological stress
8. Physical illness such as kidney failure, diabetes, fracture, head injury or brain tumour.

There are three factors which determine this condition:

1. Sudden confusion or marked increase in confusion
2. Fluctuating symptoms from confusion to lucidity
3. Sufferer is nearly always physically ill with rapid pulse, fever and a high temperature.

A clear comparison between the three main types of organic disorder is offered in Table 9.1 and is reprinted from Pitt (1984) by kind permission of Churchill Livingstone.

Alzheimer's disease

Symptoms are gradual, and there is a degenerative decline in intellectual abilities coupled with an associated physical deterioration. It is possible to define phases of the illness and this is outlined in Table 9.2 and is reprinted

Table 9.1 Comparison between Alzheimer's disease, multi-infarct dementia and benign senescent forgetfulness

	Alzeimer's	Multi-infarct	Benign
Age of onset	45 onwards	45 onwards	After 80
Sex	Commoner in women	Commonest in men	Commoner in women
Course	Progressive & global	'Step ladder' and focal	Slow, mainly affecting memory
Dysphasia & dyspraxia	Soon	Sooner or later	Absent
Impairment of insight, intellect and personality	Early	Late	Late
Physical symptoms	Absent	Present (headache, dizziness)	Absent
Physical signs	Few and late (e.g. grasp reflex)	Frequent (tremors, paralysis, spasticity)	Absent

with kind permission of the Alzheimer's Disease Society.

The following case history shows the downward spiral of the condition.

Case history

An unmarried woman of 58 was admitted to hospital with severe depression. She was an international bridge player. As the anti-depressants took effect the depression lifted but revealed the underlying dementia. The previous year, she had been competing in international events and writing articles on bridge for a national newspaper. Gradually she noticed signs of forgetfulness, what to bid and how to score (dyscalculia) and eventually her difficulty in dealing (dyspraxia). In time she was forced to withdraw from competitions and only played with close friends. She continued to write articles, but this too terminated with obvious difficulty in writing (dysgraphia). Losses accumulated including her job and life long interest in bridge which continued until she became totally dependent and was finally admitted to long-term care.

Multi-infarct dementia

Because of the erratic nature of this condition,

Table 9.2 Alzheimer's disease

Mild dementia	Moderate dementia	Severe dementia
Often this phase is only apparent when looking back; at the time it may be missed or put down to 'old age', 'overwork', 'laziness' etc. The start of dementia is very gradual, and it is impossible to identify the exact time it started. The person may be: — Apathetic — Less interested in hobbies, activities — Unwilling to try new things — Unable to adapt to change — Less good at making decisions or plans — Slower to grasp complex ideas — Ready to blame others for 'stealing' mislaid items — More self-centred, less concerned with others and their feelings — More forgetful of details of recent events — More likely to repeat themselves, or lose their thread — More irritable or upset if they fail at something.	Here the problems are more apparent and disabling. The person may: — Be very forgetful of recent events — memory for distant past generally seems better, but some details may be forgotten or confused — Be confused regarding time and place, and time of day — may go out shopping at night — Rapidly become lost if out of familiar surroundings — Forget names of friends or family, or confuse one family member with another — Forget saucepans, kettles; may leave gas unlit — Wander around streets, perhaps at night; sometimes becoming completely lost — Behave inappropriately, e.g. going outdoors in nightwear — See or hear things that are not there — Become very repetitive — Be neglectful of hygiene or eating (perhaps saying they have had a bath or a meal when they have not) — Become angry or upset or distressed very rapidly.	Here the person is severely disabled and needs a great deal of help. The person may: — Be unable to find their way around — Be unable to remember for even a few minutes that they have, for example, just had a meal — Constantly repeat one or more phrases or sounds — Be incontinent of urine and/or faeces — Show no recognition of friends and relatives — Need help or supervision with feeding, washing, bathing, using the toilet, dressing — Take their clothes off inappropriately — Fail to recognise everyday objects — Have difficulty understanding what is said to them, and their speech may make little sense — Be disturbed at night — Be restless, perhaps looking for a long dead relative or for a small child now grown up — Be aggressive, especially when feeling threatened or closed in — Have difficulty walking, eventually perhaps becoming confined to a wheel-chair.

decline is not so straightforward as Alzheimer's disease. Some common features are:

1. Confusion
2. Loss of judgement, reasoned thought, limited insight
3. Depression
4. Personality changes
5. Paranoia
6. Lability of mood
7. Perseveration.

Death may be caused by stroke or heart failure before the final stage of memory loss, incontinence and eventual dependency is reached.

Case history

A 75-year-old ex-fisherman's presentation is typical. On retirement, he studied electronics at night school and made wine. Suddenly he was aware of memory problems on his course and became depressed, staying in bed for most of the day. Long-term memory was good and he was very conscious of his other difficulties. Calendars, diaries and newspapers were used to retain orientation. He was referred for day care, and following assessment was found to have cerebral vascular insufficiency. He was treated for depression and continued to cope for the next six months. After a series of small strokes his personality and behaviour changed causing his wife severe concern. She also noticed black-outs, physical deterioration and that he was walking with a limp. There followed a five-year history of small strokes, increasing confusion and aggression until eventually long-term care was begun.

Summary

The main conditions of organic brain disease have been outlined. There is considerable overlap of symptoms which requires astute observation and accurate assessment.

ASSESSMENT

> All government — indeed every human benefit and enjoyment, every virtue and every prudent act — is founded on compromise and barter. *Edmund Burke*

Assessment, if viewed as 'a prudent act' is certainly founded on compromise where the elderly suffering a dementing illness are concerned. Many factors influence clinical judgement — see Figure 9.1.

Why assess?

The purpose of assessment is to determine a baseline for future action. With the elderly suffering from organic conditions, assessment covers four purposes:

1. reaching a diagnostic formulation
2. planning a treatment programme
3. outlining prognosis
4. recommending placement.

This is a complicated procedure requiring sound theoretical knowledge of the process of dementia, accurate observation and the ability to analyse information. Accurate clinical judgement is more readily achieved when it becomes a multidisciplinary exercise. Multidisciplinary assessment has been described by Jones (1980) and is a solution to the complex-

ities and variability of organic illness. Within this context, assessments are cross-validated; for example, the score on a behavioural rating scale is compared with the performance in a variety of daily living activities.

Too often, lack of precision in assessment leads to inertia in treatment. Individual care plans are possible only when the uniqueness of each person is acknowledged. Willson (1983) indicates the salient reasons for assessment in occupational therapy including the outlining of limitations, defining assets, and planning a course of action. Diagnostic dilemmas abound, not only between various types of organic illness but equally between intracerebral and extracerebral factors, which manifest themselves in similar ways. All team members have a responsibility to contribute towards a pool of information and consequently help to build a patient profile.

What is assessed?

The life situation of the elderly person is reviewed: the levels of social support required to maintain this person at home and the extent of strain on the relatives are determined. Most often, the crisis is heralded by a home help's concern or by severe distress in carers.

More specifically assessment areas are:

1. the general level of functioning in self-care, domestic and practical activities to determine residual skills
2. cognitive functioning, orientation, memory, and concentration
3. specific neurological problems of aphasia, apraxia or perceptual disorders

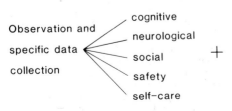
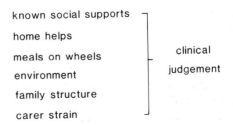

Fig. 9.1 Clinical judgement factors

4. the level of awareness and insight of the person.

Specific assessments requested from the occupational therapist tend to be in the areas of domestic, self-care or interpersonal functioning.

How to assess

The tools of assessment for each profession vary. Assessment of physical state may be reinforced by laboratory and radiological tests. The use of computerised axial tomography investigates organic changes in the brain. Psychologists have validated many cognitive and behavioural rating scales. Occupational therapists, while acknowledging the importance of rating scales (comprehensively reviewed by Brewer, (1984) attempt to reduce the anxiety of a test situation by using familiar activities as the tools of assessment. A balanced treatment programme offers the possibility for comprehensive assessment. For example, there are many ways of reviewing cognitive function in daily living. Following instructions, both written and verbal; reading the newspaper; remembering where rooms are; and handling money are a few commonplace actions which indicate memory, orientation and concentration. Points which may be covered and assessed in the course of a discussion on pensions and general money management may be:

1. recognition of coins, particularly the newer ones
2. understanding of the value of money
3. discussion of basic cost of everyday items
4. calculating costs and change

Those components could be observed in a group session using a box of groceries, in reality in the hospital shop, on an outing, or in the corner shop whilst on a home visit. Domestic assessments are ideally conducted in the home but facilities in hospital may be suitable to ascertain basic safety and nutrition. Any specific assessment, domestic, dressing, perceptual or otherwise that the occupational

therapist is invited to undertake, has to be carefully planned and sensitively executed.

1. Set the scene and explain to the patient why it is taking place
2. Reduce anxiety by having everything as normal as possible, for example, dressing is done at the right time, and place, with the patient's own clothes
3. Observe in a non-intrusive way, allowing time for completion, and only intervene when distress or danger is imminent
4. Offer appropriate encouragement without platitudes or false reassurance
5. On completion of assessment, discuss it, ask what the patient found difficult and answer her questions honestly.

Checklists are frequently preferred to assessment forms by occupational therapists, and cover essential points for consideration; a summary would then be written for the case notes.

Where to assess

The surroundings and environment are factors when considering specific assessments of the elderly person suffering from dementia. Stress and confusion may considerably increase when elderly people are out of their own surroundings. The therapist must also be aware of the patient with an excellent facade, who has all the right answers but is totally confused at home. The advantages of assessing in the home are well recognised and recorded by those specialising in psychogeriatrics. Apart from the familiarity of the person's own home, the area causing concern may dictate the surroundings. This may be the street when testing orientation or safety as a pedestrian.

There are basically three distinct places for observation and assessment.

1. Within the treatment programme

Naturally, continuous awareness of a person's level of distress, orientation or physical incapacity is assimilated within the daily contact in the ward milieu. The occupational therapist, in the design of an activity's programme, will balance a weekly timetable to cater for varying psychological needs. Within it there are rich opportunities for assessing many permutations. People can be observed in large or small groups, during physical activity, within opportunities for self-expression, in specific reality orientation groups, or in activities demanding different levels of cognitive ability.

2. Specific assessments of daily living

Most wards or occupational therapy departments are equipped with kitchen facilities for domestic assessments. The most noticeable disadvantage is that the smart chrome and formica of hospital in no way correlates with the kitchen of the average elderly person. For this reason utensils and equipment have to cover a range of sophistication. Dressing assessments and practices are most sensibly carried out in the patient's own room.

3. Home assessments

Confused people are more usefully assessed at home. Familiarity enhances performance, or highlights disorientation and progressive decline. The evidence of deterioration is often conveyed by burnt pots and kettles, fridges stacked with washing-up liquid, drawers stuffed with newspapers, scorched tea-towels, or the smell of incontinence. Those signs alert the visiting occupational therapist, whose course of action would be to discuss with relatives or carers the extent of incapacity. On such a home visit, shopkeepers and neighbours are interesting sources of verbal or non-verbal comment. The social mores of being accepted into the patient's home, shown around and often shown the treasured momentos of her life, demand sensitivity and judicious pacing of the assessment.

When to assess

The initial assessment should take place as

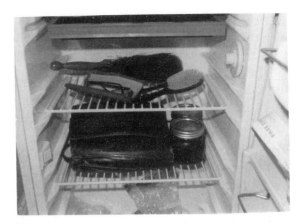

Fig. 9.2 Unusual refrigerator contents

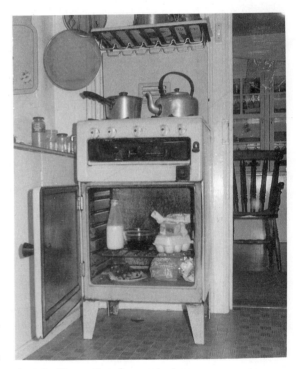

Fig. 9.3 Unusual cooker contents

soon after admission as possible but allowing the patient time to settle. Then the information gathered is presented at the first multidisciplinary meeting. At this meeting, goals are set and further specific assessments may be requested from the psychologist, occupational therapist or other staff. Further neurophysiological examinations are carried out during this period. Understanding the nature of particular dysfunctions, for example apraxia, is necessary to plan realistic treatment programmes. Holden and Woods (1982) list neurophysiological deficits together with simple assessment tests. These are particularly useful for the occupational therapist who incorporates many of the items within the context of an activities programme.

Pre-discharge assessment

Possibly the other most valuable time to assess is when the patient is due to move from in-patient status to either home, day patient, residential care or continuous care. Here,

there is a responsibility to record and equip future staff with information regarding residual skills, dependency levels and problem areas. This report is an amalgam of data collected during the admission together with recommendations. The format of the assessment report will be determined by the future placement. However, the outline would include biographical details, reason for admission, aims and summary of progress, social situation, evaluation and final recommendations.

Multidiscipline goal setting

Teamwork is of the utmost importance when working with dementia sufferers. Figure 9.4 illustrates the number of people involved in

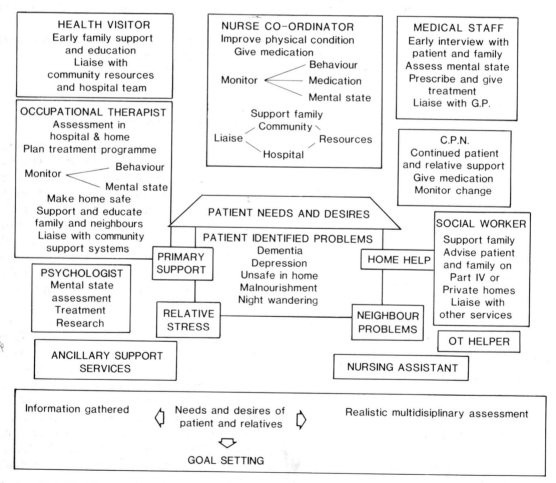

Fig. 9.4 Multidisciplinary goal setting

the necessary overlap of roles, the sharing of information, and the importance of the co-ordinator.

Most old people want to stay in their own homes for as long as possible and, if we are to respect their wishes, this should be the primary aim of each team member working with the elderly.

If eventually independence has to be surrendered, the team's aim should be to provide the quality of life that they would wish for themselves.

PRINCIPLES AND TREATMENT IN OCCUPATIONAL THERAPY

The principles around which treatment revolves are:

1. Attention to the total life-style and support systems
2. Reinforcing residual assets and skills
3. Adapting situations and the environment to minimise dysfunction
4. Acknowledging psychological needs
5. Attention to sensory deficits.

In recent years, particularly owing to the energetic influence of psychologists, reality orientation (RO) has become a fundamental base for treatment activities. Occupational therapists frequently start activity sessions by reinforcing basic orientation. It is a positive communication approach, based upon the premise that it is worthwhile explaining and talking to the elderly confused person. There are many levels of RO and it is intended as a continuous process where the environment is also adapted to include memory aids. Holden & Woods (1982) acknowledge the connections between activity, stimulation and reality orientation. Occupational therapy also bases its rationale on:

1. The use of activity to facilitate interaction with others
2. The use of structured activity to reduce confusion.

The well-known hierarchy of human needs described by Maslow (1973) is most applicable when considering the psychological needs of the elderly person suffering from a dementing illness. Basic physiological needs are readily met but more sophisticated cognitive or asthetic needs are frequently neglected. Levels of activity will be determined by the residual functional level. Flexibility in attitude and skill is essential. Components of each activity need to be analysed and modified by means of instruction or demonstration. There are many levels at which to pace activities according to the type and phase of the dementing illness. They can be broadly categorised as:

1. Activities involving sensory stimulation
2. Activities based on self-care and life skills
3. Activities designed around realistic physical exercise
4. Activities to increase social interaction and reduction of isolation.

Activities involving sensory stimulation

Everyday activities such as baking, gardening, washing and watching television stimulate the senses. When removed from the stimuli in institutions, the senses are dulled and underused. Sensory stimulation programmes are most commonly used with those in continuous care. However, a measure of this work enters RO sessions and many other activities within occupational therapy, for the mild, moderate or severe phases of organic illness. Paire and Karney (1984) completed a study to explore the effectiveness of sensory stimulation and found that this approach 'forestalled deterioration and rekindled interest in the environment'. Sessions are most effective in a group where there is a central theme, for example, winter, where snow or ice can be brought into the ward and felt, or where the ingredients of a Christmas cake can be sampled with ensuing discussion. Change in sensory input is stimulating and creates interest.

Activities based on self-care and life skills

The state of independence is relative. We are aware that dementing illness brings with it a changing body image. Therefore, deficits in basic self-care can cover shaving, grooming, bathing, eating or toileting. Dysfunction in any one of those calls for individualised programmes based on analysis of specific difficulty. When a person can no longer cope independently with personal hygiene or feeding, dignity is lost. The Alzheimer's Disease Society publishes an excellent and readable booklet offering solutions to common problems of that nature. Repetition and practice occur within treatment sessions. Familiar activities such as baking, if simplified and guided, can be successfully achieved and admiration of the shared results boosts confidence. If dressing difficulties are identified, simplified fasteners can be used and a dressing/undressing schedule worked out. Other activities associated with this stage in life — strolling, listening to music, watching television, working with money — can all be incorporated into treatment.

Activities involving realistic physical exercise

Literature describing the benefits of exercise for elderly people is plentiful. Increased well-being can be connected with cognitive improvement, although it is difficult to establish whether it is exercise or the resulting discussion that causes improvement. The sessions are best conducted in a group and carefully structured to meet concentration and fatigue levels. This is one of the simplest forms of activity for the confused elderly and can be combined with music or drama. Langley and Langley (1983) outline progressive sessions for the elderly, using drama techniques and a variety of adapted games. A comprehensive selection of 'Movement and growth programmes for the elderly and those who care for them' by Bate et al (1984) is an excellent source of reference. Adapted forms of darts, golf, football, or basketball are well accepted. Relaxation techniques with elderly patients seated in comfortable chairs can be helpful. Attention to slow and deep breathing and the use of touch and massage promote well-being.

Activities to increase social interaction and reduce isolation

The opportunity to reminisce and exercise long-term memory fosters communication. It is a social experience which satisfies many needs. There are many audio-visual aids on the market to stimulate discussion. Photographs, old fashioned utensils, pre-war music, can be used as the focus for such sessions. Music facilitates interaction, whether in clapping, tapping feet, singing or dancing. Festivals and holidays are ideal settings to involve relatives and friends in socials and parties.

Involvement with play groups or nurseries in the form of visits from children or liaison with the elderly to make puppets, dolls or toys, followed by the opportunity to hand them over, reinforces self-worth, pleasure and caring for others.

Milieu approaches, as outlined by Gottesman (1969), describe a way to counteract 'social death'. The occupational therapist, together with nursing staff, can identify tasks within the ward, for example, shopping, washing up, watering plants, which encourages the patients to have greater responsibility for each other and thus reduce custodial constraints.

Occupational therapists are challenged professionally by the multiple needs of this group. Flexibility in design of activities is essential. An understanding of the components of each activity and the balance of sessions is vital. There is scope for individual work, group approaches and attention to the wider implications or ward milieu.

SUPPORT FOR CARERS

As knowledge grows and insights deepen regarding the widespread repercussions of a dementing illness, attention is increasingly focussed on the total group, consisting of the sufferer and the carers and supporters. The amount of support and practical help varies according to:

1. How enlightened the staff are
2. Level of disability
3. The precise reason for referral — assessment, day care, prospect of residential care or continuous care in hospital.

Knowledge of resources

A knowledge of the catchment area is imperative if one is to be aware of potential resources. This can vary from an awareness of church groups interested in helping the elderly to more detailed knowledge of local support groups for carers. Relatives may require reading material designed for families of people with dementing illness. In recent years, there have been many such publications.

The occupational therapist can suggest practical aids for independent living, but in most cases she is involved in helping the relative to discover ways of adapting to problems of increasing dependence.

Relatives' meetings

This concept is widely accepted, and regular meetings with others dealing with the same problem is a most valuable part of the support system. It is an opportunity for relatives to meet with each other and a variety of staff. Relatives are interested in the occupational therapist's intervention, but it is essentially an opportunity for the therapist to learn about the patient from the carers, and for relatives to share the problems of caring with each other and the professionals. These discussions range from loneliness and loss of friendship for the carer, to how to deal with aggression and the aggravating business of being followed around every moment; from the difficulty of doing the everyday tasks of life like shopping and cooking, to the bereavement and loss felt for a loved one, while still having to physically care for someone who is totally demented. At some groups there may

be an invited speaker and various disciplines and volunteer groups have an opportunity to inform about the nature of their work.

Practical support

If the elderly person is referred for assessment or day care, it is possible for the occupational therapist to carry out a home visit to suggest memory aids and practical methods of coping with behavioural problems. A kind of diagnostic appraisal can be mutually arrived at as to how the house and environment can be made safer and simpler. This problem-solving is therapeutic for the carer, who feels actively involved in the patient's management.

Particularly in day care, diaries can be a useful method of involving relatives. Entries may be written by the patient with staff support or by the staff in discussion about the day's events. It may be a simple description about the outing, hairdresser, or what was for lunch. The rationale is linked with the aims of reality orientation, in that prompts or hints are offered to reduce confusion and encourage recall.

The great need in many carers is for more information about the disease process. However, White (1985) sensitively describes her role as an occupational therapist in helping families and carers to understand the patient's limitations and assisting them to modify their attitudes and approaches, thus achieving patterns of care which are acceptable to carers and patient.

EDUCATION

In order to meet and understand the needs of elderly people, a comprehensive education programme is required. The problem of dementia sufferers and the effect on carers is dawning on the consciousness of the public. Already, we witness an increase in media interest from television, radio and newspapers. Libraries, community centres and other local authority facilities display information regarding resources. Areas requiring further information are:

1. The general public
2. Carers
3. Staff.

The general public

Whitehead 1974 described the necessity for society to review its educational systems and to include the study of ageing. This would have two benefits:

1. To help prepare for old age
2. Attitude change

Schools do include the study of growing old within social or community studies. However, this is patchy and may be elective. Help the Aged's Education Department publishes a wide variety of teaching material for schools and colleges. Many organisations have instigated invaluable projects to inform, and attempt to revise misinformed views regarding those suffering from organic illness. The Alzheimer's Disease Society states education of the public as a clear aim of its organisation through media, press or fund raising. Age Concern has two main aims — action and campaigning for a voice for older people at all levels. Awareness of the realities faced by those enduring a dementing illness is sobering, but these organisations and others like them help to allay many of the myths and fears surrounding dementia.

Carers

Our health service relies heavily on the capacity of carers to cope and care for confused elderly people. Frequently inadequate help and resources are available which cause stress and pathology in the carers themselves. National organisations have designed informative guides on how to cope in this situation and also provide regular support meetings where carers can give each other mutual aid.

At a national conference in 1984 on Coping with Care of Ambulant Dementing Older People, Mary Marshall reminded the audience that strategies and expertise are not the prerogative of the professionals, and that relatives are rapidly adapting and discovering new ways of management. A co-ordinated sharing of care and resources between all concerned is essential.

While practical advice from professionals on management and resources is gratefully accepted, the overwhelming emotional distress surrounding this problem demands attention.

Staff

There is a pressing need for post-registration courses in this area. The majority of those working in close day-to-day contact with the elderly have very rudimentary training. Working with highly dependent people with insufficient knowledge or training taxes the most enthusiastic, and morale can slump. One solution could be the organisation of multi-disciplinary in-service training schemes.

Role-play is an active and potent teaching technique in this area. Problems enacted in this way can cover, for instance, dealing with aggression; what it is like to be confused; and how to deal with catastrophic reactions. The public are now actively campaigning for a much higher standard of care and senior staff should take the initiative in reviewing new learning methods, in the knowledge that higher morale could lead to the improved quality of care that is widely called for.

RESEARCH

The 1979 report on Services for the Elderly with Mental Disability in Scotland includes two clauses on research. One states the necessity for more information and the other makes a plea that 'such research should not delay the urgent provision of much needed services'.

As occupational therapists, our research is in its infancy and our contributions have continued to fall into the 'provision of much needed service' rather than research.

We are paying close attention to the many biological and epidemiological studies, but of more direct interest has been the dramatic growth of the contribution of the psychologist. Many new rating scales have been developed to measure cognitive ability, behavioural functioning and mood change in those with organic illness. Boyd and Robinson (1984) indicate that despite the number of available scales there remains a need to co-operate and co-ordinate the development of scales of interdisciplinary and international acceptance. This is certainly of interest to occupational therapists, considering the overlap of interest in residual functional ability.

Reality orientation has been another subject of interest and is often the co-ordinating factor in treatment programmes. Holden and Woods (1982) remains the text most in use as reference on reality orientation.

While subjective observation reveals small behavioural changes in severely deteriorated patients after activity sessions, this has not yet been scientifically researched. Other areas of interest could include the effects following early detection and intervention in dementia; the effects following sensory stimulation programmes; effects of a milieu approach in continuous care; what effect structured activity has on confused behaviour; and the most effective referrals to day-care.

CONCLUSION

This chapter has attempted to stress the need for clarity and precision in both clinical judgement and improved education of all concerned with the elderly suffering from some form of dementing illness. As occupational therapists, we know that activity can maintain functional ability and influence the quality of life. The central skill with this patient population is in the continual adaptation of activities.

Many approaches place emphasis on guiding families and carers, as in Mace and Rabins (1981), and have been an invaluable influence on occupational therapy.

Our profession is affected by the changing shape of the health service and has a strong commitment towards this challenging area.

REFERENCES

Bate R, Weir M, Parker C 1984 Movement and growth patterns for the elderly and for those who care for them. Available from Dunfermline College of Physical Education, Cramond, Edinburgh

Boyd W D, Robinson R A 1983 In: Kendall R E, Zealley A K (eds) Companion to psychiatric studies. Churchill Livingstone, Edinburgh

Brewer P 1984 Brief assessments for the elderly mentally infirm. British Journal of Occupational Therapy 47(6)

Gottesman L E 1969 Extended care for the aged: psychological aspects. Journal of Geriatric Psychiatry 2: 220–237

Holden U P, Woods R T 1982 Reality orientation. Churchill Livingstone, Edinburgh

H M S O 1979 Services for the elderly with mental disability in Scotland. Scottish Home and Health Department, Edinburgh

Jacques A J 1984 Key issues for carers. Report of Scottish National Conference, University of Strathclyde. Available from Age Concern, Scotland

Jones G 1980 Elderly confused people: a study of a multidisciplinary unit in action. Social Work Service 23: June

Langley D M, Langley G E 1983 Drama therapy and psychiatry. Croom Helm, Beckenham, Kent

Lewis S C 1979 The mature years. Charles B. Slack, Thorofare, New Jersey, USA

Lipowski Z 1981 A new look at organic brain syndromes. American Journal of Psychiatry 137:674

Mace N L, Rabins P V 1981 The 36-hour day. The John Hopkins University Press. Available from C.C.J. Ltd, Ely House, 37 Dover Street, London WIX 4HQ

Marsden C D 1978 The diagnosis of dementia. In: Issacs A D, Post F (eds) Studies in geriatric psychiatry. Wiley, Chichester

Maslow A 1973 The further reaches of human nature. Penguin, Harmondsworth

Paire J A, Karney R J 1984 The effectiveness of sensory stimulation for geropsychiatric inpatients. American Journal of Occupational Therapy 38(8)

Perkins L M 1982 Assessment and management of psychogeriatric patients. British Journal of Occupational Therapy 45(1)

Pitt B 1984 Psychogeriatrics. Churchill Livingstone, Edinburgh

Shaw M W 1984 The challenge of ageing. Churchill Livingstone, Edinburgh

White S 1985 Managing the demented patient in the community. Therapy Weekly 11(42)

Whitehead J N 1974 Psychiatric disorders in old age. John Wiley, Chichester, Sussex

Willson M 1983 Occupational therapy in long-term psychiatry. Churchill Livingstone, Edinburgh

10

Psychiatry in old age: occupational therapy and functional illness

S. E. E. Blair
R. Reynolds

INTRODUCTION

Few occupational therapists will pursue a career without encountering problems associated with ageing. Occupational therapy is characteristically suited to work with this group, as the dual training in physical and psychiatric approaches equates well with the multiple illness presentations which occur.

Mental health is severely buffeted by the cumulative effects of ageing and loss. We know that psychiatric morbidity increases with age for both organic and functional illness. Yet there are numerous instances of successful old age in literature, politics and the arts. What then predetermines some to a senescence of rich experience and others towards a sad and lonely decline? We can postulate the personality types which correlate with successful ageing but the question is largely unanswerable. However, many reassuring advances have been made in research into mental disorders of old age. There is now a realisation that the functional disorders of the aged can be treated and that of the 21% of individuals aged 65 and over with mental disorder, approximately two thirds are treatable. What is required, therefore, is careful detective work to distinguish between the similar symptoms of dementia and severe emotional disturbance; symptoms of physical illness and confusion; and the relationship of personality and behavioural disorders.

The challenge emerges in the interplay between medicine, sociology and psychology in any intervention with this age group. The complexities of later life demand an eclectic approach and creative problem-solving from a caring health service.

The World Health Organization reviewed care of the elderly in the community in 1979 and in the same year the report on Services for the Elderly with Mental Disability in Scotland was published (SHHD 1979). In the subsequent five years many recommendations from this report have been implemented. Occupational therapists were reassured in this report by the accent on the multidisciplinary team, clinical assessment and the emphasis on training and education.

The range of psychiatric disturbance arising in later life include depression, which remains the most common mental affliction of the elderly, hypomania, paranoid states, neurotic conditions, personality disorders, problems related to alcohol and the acute and chronic states of confusion.

Psychiatric morbidity amongst the elderly

The anticipated increase in the numbers of elderly patients is well known and was dealt with in the Timbury Report 1979 (SHHD 1979), the Shape Report 1980 and in the Government White Paper entitled Growing Older (DHSS 1981). To plan a psychogeriatric service at all levels and to determine priorities requires an examination of the extent of psychiatric morbidity amongst the elderly. Kay et al (1964) in Newcastle showed that 40% of the elderly living in the community suffered from a psychiatric disorder, 30% of these were considered to have a functional disorder. Surveys have continued to indicate that the elderly constitute a high proportion of psychiatric admissions. Occupational therapists are

wise to analyse surveys and review statistics at local level in order to predict staffing and ascertain priorities. This has implications for assessment, treatment and the quality of care. Early and accurate assessment is a key issue, and it is most effective when the team contributes towards a central store of information.

Assessment unit

The Psychogeriatric Assessment Unit offers consultation, investigation, assessment and diagnosis, treatment and rehabilitation. It allows a comprehensive range of services which combine to offer a profile of each patient. Lengths of stay vary, but 6–8 weeks is considered to be the optimum. A unit such as this relies heavily on the availability of alternative placements to avoid the 'blocked bed syndrome'.

The design of the assessment unit is important and efforts should be made to remove institutional features. Whenever possible, patients can contribute to the running of the unit and therefore the milieu is less hierarchical. Willson (1983) reminds us that the environment for caring depends upon co-operation and communication between disciplines, and this will contribute towards a therapeutic environment. Access to a garden not only contributes to the quality of care but can be used in an activity programme.

Significance of occupational therapy with this group

The overlap of areas of dysfunction requires the occupational therapist to be well acquainted with the complete spectrum of the ageing process. Lewis (1979) in her book entitled *The Mature Years*, comprehensively outlines theories of growth and ageing which offer a backcloth of understanding to the needs and dynamics of ageing.

In assessment units the emphasis is on prompt collection of information from all staff to build a profile of each patient. The occupational therapist can contribute specific information from home visits and domestic assessments as well as implementing an activity programme. This programme will be designed carefully. Maddox (1963) concluded, in a study of activity and morale, that there was a significant relationship between activity and morale in the elderly. As occupational therapists, our core skill is in the selection of activities. This has to marry with our knowledge of studies in gerontology regarding ageing theory, the patterns of activity throughout the lifespan indicated by Flowers and Kraiem (1983) and the readjustment to time in old age.

AGEING AND ATTITUDES

Our professional relationship with the elderly seems inextricably bound by our own experience of old age. Many believe that to feel at ease with this group, one has to have had a positive experience with grandparents or other significant people of this age group. There are identifiable barriers to effective liaison. Consider the following case:

A lady called Mrs Turnbull was transferred to a psychiatric hospital following admission to a general hospital for investigations into a transient confusional state. In the general hospital she was negative, refused food and fluids and was mute. Her daughter returned from America distressed by the knowledge of her mother's condition.

The mother was admitted to a psychogeriatric assessment ward where she had been known one year previously. On this admission investigations showed bilateral ankle oedema and a urinary tract infection for which diuretics and an antibiotic were prescribed. Confusion lessened and review of her difficulties revealed four admissions to hospital in seven months with physical problems causing confusion. A vested interest in 'illness' emerged as it ensured her daughter's stay. It was subsequently learned that the lady had complicated the clinical picture by taking her daughter's 'nerve' pills. In the ward she was a domineering woman, whose problems prevailed over the daily support group. A manipulative attitude of crying wolf was perceived by her fellow patients. Quite suddenly her physical condition deteriorated, necessitating a transfer to a general hospital where she died that evening. Despite reassurance from senior staff, the staff in the psychiatric hospital were shocked and felt guilty.

Thus behavioural features often defeat therapeutic zeal. Main (1957) eloquently conveys the frustration staff experience when they cannot make people better. Frustration and ageist prejudice are also conveyed in the attitudes of defeatism, domination and insularity described by Pitt (1982).

The necessity for supervision to allow a forum for discussion of these conflicting dilemmas is clear. Butler (1969) was the first to analyse ageism and defined the term as a 'a personal revulsion to, and a distaste for, growing old, disease, disability and the fear of powerlessness, uselessness and death'. Recently Age Concern has accummulated a wealth of information regarding prejudicial attitudes towards the elderly in a publication entitled 'Against Ageism' (1984)

The philosophy of occupational therapy revolves around attention to the whole person, and in this case the lifespan perspective is essential to establish goals. Presenting needs and difficulties cannot be understood without investigation into a lifetime's worth of adaptation.

Cicero's famous essay on old age, composed in 44 BC, is a wonderous reflection of this last developmental stage of life. It should be recommended reading for any person grappling with the intricacies of old age.

THE MULTIDISCIPLINARY TEAM

The quality of caring relies upon communication and co-operation between disciplines. However, the concept of the 'team' has elastic boundaries. There is the undisputed necessity of the primary health care team as the first line of defence. Collaborative planning is vital with this team when admission to an assessment ward is required. Upon discharge it is again imperative to liaise with community agencies as many patients fall within a high-risk category.

The assessment function of such a unit can therefore co-ordinate health services and social work services. Assessment serves as a common frame of reference for all disciplines. Contributions from relatives in understanding pre-morbid personality and significant life circumstances cannot be over-emphasised.

Team philosophy satisfies many needs and

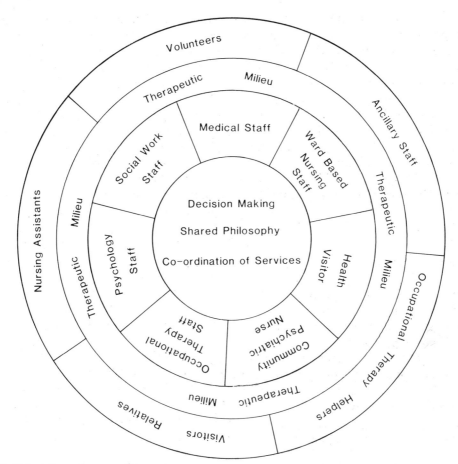

Fig. 10.1 Multidisciplinary team—milieu

has a binding effect which unites energies. Advantageous factors include a common sense of identity, enthusiastic momentum, improved organisation and management services, and the opportunity for a teaching forum. This idealism is tempered by the knowledge that any team requires co-ordination which will reflect the consensus of opinion. Everyone who has contact with the elderly person in such a ward has a contribution to make towards co-ordination of results and effort. Many therapeutic exchanges with ancillary staff exist and are considered carefully by a sensitive ward staff.

In essence, there are co-ordinators at different levels. Decision makers and day-to-day continuity staff have the patient as the main focus. It could be argued that the patient becomes the co-ordinator of effort. However, using a team approach to collect relevant information relies heavily upon a healthy therapeutic milieu. As the demands of this group are high, and decision-making is complex the team becomes a sharing and teaching vehicle.

Multidisciplinary goal setting

An example of collaborative planning is seen in a review of the progress of a 75-year-old woman referred with symptoms of depression and sporadic confusion. She had lived with her daughter for the last five years and the stress had reflected upon both herself and the family. At this time a social worker had been asked to talk to the daughter regarding the possibility of residential care. Following adjustment to the assessment unit the old lady settled with few depressive symptoms but episodes of confusion were reported by all staff including ancillary staff. Nursing staff also detected fluctuating sugar levels in urine samples which required close monitoring. A home visit was undertaken by the occupational therapist who reported that the old lady could not find the house or where things were once she was inside. Her safety when she was using electrical equipment or the cooker was unconvincing. The occupational therapist's report recommended day care in the interim until residential care could be provided. Medical staff reviewed the multifaceted nature of the problem — the diabetes, increasing confusion and the strain on the family's coping strategies — and suggested that the social worker and the occupational therapist discuss the possibility of residential care with the patient.

All recent reports indicate the value of a multidisciplinary team for comprehensive care. Boyd and Robinson (1983) also indicate the research gains inherent in combining specialised knowledge in this way.

FUNCTIONAL DISORDERS

As distinct from organic conditions, where degenerative changes in the brain produce disorders of memory, cognition and behavioural disorder, the affective disorders — psychoneurosis, schizophrenia and paranoid paraphrenia — indicate disorder of mood and thought. Elderly people experience the same range of psychiatric disorder as any other developmental group. In the Newcastle study by Kay et al (1964), looking at the prevalence of mental disorder, 30% of all people over 65 suffered from functional disorders but the neuroses and personality disorders predominated. In a psychogeriatric admission ward certain categories are prevalent; depression, hypomania, neurosis, personality disorders, paranoid states and disorders related to alcohol. Frequently, acute confusional states are referred for investigation.

Depression

The span from unhappiness to severe depression is vast, and demands careful clinical judgement. Reasons for unhappiness in the elderly are not hard to find and are normally associated with the various losses experienced. It is salutary to remember the high suicide rate in the elderly. Many old people display a 'learned helplessness' described by Seligman (1975) whereby despondency is all encompassing. It is a destructive force in those families striving to support elderly relatives, and causes resentment and frustration. Massive loss of confidence fuels this phenomenon and maintains the status quo despite therapeutic endeavour.

This is borne out in an example of Mrs Young, aged 78, who had been in an assessment unit for 9 months. There was a family history of depression in both mother and sister. Until 18 months before she had tolerated life stresses, including a stroke, and had a number of hobbies and a good circle of friends. This abruptly changed following a bad fall where she fractured her right humerus and femur. As a result of this injury she required an in-dwelling catheter which she described as the 'final straw'. Her behaviour in the general hospital was manipulative and hysterical. Upon transfer to a psychiatric hospital she was treated with antidepressants and ECT to no noticeable avail. She described herself 'a vegetable with no future'. Review of her present state revealed considerable progress in that:

1. She could manage without the in-dwelling catheter
2. She could walk with a tripod, albeit slowly
3. She was cognitively intact.

Therapeutic efforts were frustrated by Mrs Young's view of herself as a complete invalid. Clearly there were dynamic factors at work, but Mrs Young concluded that nothing could influence what she considered as irreversible change and she no longer wished to 'compete' in life again.

Reactive depression

This is extremely common as the main presenting difficulty, or secondary to physical illness, or the silent acknowledgement that life is coming to an end. Pitt (1982) defines two main features:

1. The state is justified by the subject's circumstances
2. The mood varies with changes in these circumstances.

It may be a temporary state which is resolved when the individual's coping mechanisms are resurrected, or it may require external management. The clinical picture varies, with agitation, tearfulness, loss of appetite, sleep disturbance and somatic symptoms often apparent.

Mrs Wilson has had a thirty-year history of recurrent depression with several suicide attempts. She was an only child who had nursed both parents until their death. She still lived in the large parental home which required expensive maintenance. Her work history revealed a conscientious worker, first as a secretary, and latterly as a doctor's part-time receptionist. In a recent out-patient follow-up, Mrs Wilson seemed well, apart from voicing concern about repair costs and a recent increase in rates. One week later, she was found by neighbours in a distressed, tearful and agitated condition. Following an attempted break-in she had tried to barricade windows and doors: she had not been eating in order to conserve money for repairs and she could not sleep. Clinical management included medication to alleviate anxiety and discussions with staff about the possibility of selling the parental home. Within one week symptoms subsided and with support Mrs Wilson could begin to plan her life.

Severe depression

This state is characterised by features of extreme misery, a sense of worthlessness, guilt and associated physical retardation. There is an aura of unmitigated despair. Frank psychiatric phenomena include delusions of personal responsibility, causing cancer, death of children in Ethopia, or spreading disease. The latter delusion led one 73-year-old lady to store faeces in various containers throughout the house to avoid contaminating the sewage system! She was brought to hospital as an emergency in poor physical health, uncommunicative, unkempt and with reports from neighbours that she seemed to be up throughout the night.

Auditory hallucinations frequently accompany distress: disparaging and abusive voices may be heard. 'She's a loose woman' or 'Everyone knows what she's done'. In contrast to paranoid delusions, the patient feels that these comments are true and justified. A diagnosis of endogenous or severe depression is made when there is a combination of diurnal variation, ideas of worthlessness, loss of appetite and weight, and retardation of thought and action. In extreme forms the elderly person is mute, incontinent and immobile. Cases such as this constitute psychiatric emergency and require urgent mobilisation of resources.

Although the prognosis for affective disorders is usually considered favourable, Murphy (1983) describes important findings in her study of 124 elderly depressed patients, where high-risk factors, such as poor physical health or severe life events, affected successful outcome.

Hypomania

The initial reaction of the occupational therapist to the elderly manic patient may be relief that at least one person is active, seemingly responsive and lively! Nevertheless, it rapidly becomes clear that there is a butterfly concentration span. They flit from person to person, activity to activity with impatience and expansiveness. Reactions of other patients are mixed between irritation and bemused tolerance. Schulman and Post (1980) showed that the first attack of mania, in a survey of elderly patients suffering from bi-polar affective disorder, occurred at around the age of 60. Careful investigation must be made, as this excitable state may be linked with early dementia. The numbers in any admission ward are low, no more than 4 or 6 in any year's statistics. Presenting symptoms range over a spectrum of pathological activity. Conversation is animated, often bawdy, with teasing and sexual innuendo. Heightened activity is evident in dress, make-up, many projects being attempted at once, constant demands and no completion of tasks. Energies are hurled into physical activity with frequent disinhibitions. Attempts by the therapist to monitor activity are dismissed. There is no insight or lingering reflection on inappropriate action. Extremes are evident, such as the patient wishing to buy presents for the whole ward or ordering lavish spreads on ward outings when she is financially unable to pay. Talkativeness, suspicion and irritability may also be evident.

Management requires admission to hospital where attempts are made to control activity with tranquillisers. Lithium is prescribed for the elderly with careful monitoring of side-effects. Otherwise there is full involvement in the ward programme with an accompanying firm and patient approach.

Paranoid illnesses

Paranoid symptoms may be associated with other effective illnesses or organic disorders. It is wise to investigate sources of delusion. The case of one 73-year old lady admitted with delusions of soldiers banging on her door late at night and wanting to kidnap her is interesting. On a home visit, and in discussion with neighbours in the high rise block, it was discovered that youths wearing mottled green paramilitary-style jackets did disturb the occupants, rattling letterboxes and shouting late at night. If this is magnified with extreme loneliness and fear, the 'delusions' can be understood. Paraphrenia is the term given to an illness of this type occurring for the first time in old age. The clinical picture often involves suspicion regarding relatives or neighbours. They are thought to be deriding or criticising the patient, and accompanying hostile hallucinatory voices may be present. Microphones, televisions and other electrical equipment are often the means by which the voices operate in the delusional system. Sexual delusions may become part of the picture, with allegations of rape, interference or strange sexual practices. These all-consuming fears lead to neglect of hygiene, poor nutrition and sleep disturbance. If the therapist is allowed into the house she may find evidence of attempts to hide from the voices. For example, one old lady lived in a cupboard draped with blankets; another showed evidence of attempts to exorcise the devil with open bibles and printed religious texts around the house. No insight is apparent and it is usually through providing help for other reasons that paranoia comes to light. Management is often difficult, although the condition can be relieved with tranquillisers or anti-depressant drugs. Such patients stay for lengthy periods in hospital where the delusional material seems to abate but recurs after they return home.

Neurosis

This is very common in the elderly and upon examination of the case history the patient has often had episodes earlier in life. In general practice the most common manifestation of neurosis in the elderly is physical symptoms and hypochondriasis. Anxiety, coupled with massive lack of confidence, is a very recognisable feature. There is free-floating anxiety related to dependency, social circumstance and the unknown. Neurosis is particularly evident in the socially isolated, those suffering from a physical illness and where there has been an episode earlier in life.

Careful detective work is vital to differentiate between anxiety and the early perplexity shown in dementia. Many presenting symptoms, such as loss of appetite and sleep disturbance, are characteristic of depression. Knowledge of the ageing process is essential, plus a careful study of history and present circumstances. Boyd and Robinson (1984) outline depression, obsessional neurosis, hysterical conversion and hypochondriasis under the neurosis of old age. Management revolves around psychological support and use of minor tranquillisers. Psychotherapy, behaviour therapy and occupational therapy have much to offer in resurrecting coping behaviour and raising self-esteem.

Alcohol problems

These most commonly occur in those elderly people who drink to relieve loneliness. The evidence is often hidden, and symptoms of staggering, confusion or safety problems are raised by neighbours or family. Korsakoff's psychosis is evident in the elderly who have been addicted over many years.

Personality and behavioural disorder

Personality disorder can be manifest in eccentricity, miserliness, disinhibition, uncleanliness or a combination of socially unacceptable qualities. It is not usually a new condition at this age but is accentuated by increasing dependency. Behavioural disorder is exhibited by a variety of anti-social behaviours: withdrawal to lead the life of a hermit causes others to become anxious; and sexual misbehaviour in old men causes outrage, particularly where children are involved. The anxiety of others often brings this group of people to the attention of the National Health Service. They are extremely difficult to manage and drugs have only a limited place. Acceptance and gradual adjustment is the key. Personality will not change, but the behaviour can become more appropriate to the situation and can be tempered by the reaction of fellow patients.

This briefly outlines the main categories of functional illness. The overlap of many similar symptoms necessitates careful investigation.

Differential diagnosis

Prejudicial attitudes towards the elderly have often resulted in inadequate appraisal of the psychiatric state. Haphazard descriptions of depression, dementia and personality are often based on lack of accurate observation or assessment. Most often, the differential diagnosis lies in the choice between varying states of depression, but there are diagnostic dilemmas in practically all instances where physical illness also complicates the picture. Again, members of the treatment team can challenge observation, put forward new hypotheses and provide a more comprehensive source from which to make a formulation.

ASSESSMENT

The overlap and similarities between the psychiatric illnesses of old age abound. Sleep and appetite disturbances can occur in almost all illnesses with varying intensity. Disturbances of memory occur in neurotic conditions, depressive states and dementia. Disorders of intellectual function can occur in various physical illnesses, including pernicious anaemia. Thorough collection of data and accurate observation are essential for a comprehensive assessment.

Wattis et al (1981) established the rationale for assessment prior to admission, when the psychiatrist can witness the whole life, meet the family and evaluate social circumstances. Liaison is maintained at this time with the general practitioner, health visitor or community psychiatric nurse. If admission is found necessary, a full evaluation of the psychiatric state, problem areas and existing support can then take place. An occupational therapist can contribute in a number of ways. The provision of a weekly treatment programme offers the possibility for observation in interpersonal and social settings, specific practical sessions and self-expression, as well as being a vehicle for gaugeing adjustment to the ward environment. A combination of activity groups allows a multifaceted assessment.

Initial assessment

This serves to initiate the relationship between yourself and the elderly person. It enables you to gather information and describe her possible involvement in occupational therapy. The words used have to be understandable, honest and explained with sensitivity to anxiety and loss of confidence. It is wise to conduct the assessment within the first two days of admission. Specific information to be observed would include appearance, sight, hearing, speech and physical difficulties. An appraisal of mood, orientation, memory and concentration is also necessary. It is often possible to combine this with a simple activity — making a cup of tea or strolling in the garden — where preliminary observations of safety, dexterity or recognition can be assessed. Judgement on the validity of this early interview has to be tempered with the patient's adjustment to admission.

Very frequently the occupational therapist will be specifically requested to carry out a kitchen assessment. Rationale for this hinges upon safety, basic nutrition and familiarity with fundamental living skills. Attention to nutrition is decreased in many psychiatric conditions — depression, hypomania and paranoia — for various reason. Assessment of this nature may be implemented in the patient's own home, but in the early stages of admission it would occur within the occupational therapy facilities. To ensure a standard approach, a form or checklist is helpful and would include the reason for assessment, attitude towards assessment and mental state at the time of testing. Thereafter, analysis of the kitchen assessment breaks the activity into components of:

1. *Preparation*
   — Is the patient organised?
   — Does she use appropriate quantities?
   — Does she use appropriate utensils?
   — Is she safe in the preparation of the meal?
2. *Method*
   — Is the sequence or order of the meal correct?
   — Is she aware of timing?
   — Is her concentration on the task accurate?
3. *Safety factors* — awareness and application of safety precautions
4. *Interest in nutrition* — appropriate diet — motivation and appetite
5. *Reasonable hygiene*, washing up and completion of task.

During the assessment period the occupational therapist should keep a low profile, offering encouragement when necessary and discussing aspects of nutrition and diet and subsequently gathering information from the patient. Following this, an estimation of performance would be made with various recommendations.

It is imperative that assessments of this nature do not occur in a vacuum, and that the therapist's appraisal and recommendations are shared with the patient. A natural progression would be towards assessment of this type in the familiar surroundings of the patient's own home. The participation of the elderly person within the treatment programme, and in particular her reaction to being part of a group, is outlined by Taylor (1984). There exists the potential for understanding the individual's present capabilities or deficiencies in social behaviour, intellectual ability, general level of activity and residual skills. In the course of involvement in a variety of activity groups, the therapist observes the clinical state and adjustment. When the therapist is evaluating performance, the relationship between life history and adjustment to ageing is considered.

Occupational therapists are concerned with patients ability to cope with the demands made on them and are involved in the resurrection of coping skills. As progress occurs, a home visit may be requested. This has been described by others in this book (Ch. 12) and in psychiatry the same basic format is followed. Before the visit, preliminary information is gathered with the emphasis on the patient's attitude towards this stage of rehabilitation. The procedure is divided into pre-visit components, factors during assessment and a final evaluation.

When accompanying an elderly person to her home for such an assessment, the shift in the relationship must be acknowledged. This is her home and you are a guest as well as a professional. Advice and recommendations are offered in measured and palatable amounts. You cannot impose your own standards of hygiene, tidiness and domestic skills upon others. It is a question of balance and judgement, heavily dependent upon your relationship with the patient. We are often remiss in explaining the purposes of assessment to the elderly person who can be left with mixed feelings after a home assessment. Who do the neighbours think you were? Was the home situation considered favourable? Will there be another opportunity to practise? Why did the previously familiar surroundings appear so strange? Many such fears abound and the patient should be given a chance to discuss these at a suitable opportunity. A home visit can require a lengthy investment of time, and clearly there are optimum times of the day in which to carry this out. Apart from domestic assessments in the patient's own home, shorter visits may be made to collect mail, remain in contact with the home, or to commence readjustment.

Parallel assessment procedures from nursing staff, psychologists and social work staff contribute towards a comprehensive profile from which clinical decisions can be made.

TREATMENT AND MANAGEMENT

The first principle of intervention must be to work in tandem with other approaches. Consistency and continuity are the key factors with the elderly. An understanding of drug and physical treatments is crucial to detect side-effects or a change in mental state. An holistic approach by the treatment team is favoured, examining life experiences and identifying significant problem areas. In this respect detailed formulation of the clinical state is more useful than a diagnosis. Different modes of treatment can co-exist, and indeed are preferable in dealing with multiple pathologies. Psychotherapy can offer support and the opportunity to relate to others. Although psychoanalysis with the elderly is not common in the National Health Service, the work of Hanna Segal (1981) on analysis of an old man, provides insight into the unconscious fear of death inherent in many breakdowns in this age group. Clinical psychologists have emerged as a potent force in research and treatment of the elderly. Family or marital therapy is often not employed in the belief that change takes too long. However, sensitive and far-sighted nurses are working with families and relatives, offering information and listening to their distress.

Finally, patients living in any ward or unit are affected by the living/learning experience in that milieu. A common sharing of tasks, for example a rota to collect newspapers or take messages, or baking for supper, has a binding effect on the community. Regular community meetings acknowledge the worth of comments from everyone, keep people informed of changes in staff or patients and prevent the contagious anonymity so common in institutions.

Group approaches to treatment

Treatment sessions are usually group-based. Linden (1953) was the first to outline an organised programme of group therapy for the elderly. Occupational therapists were aware of the inherent value of group work early in the profession and developed skills in the use of activity groups. Given that group work suggests talking, co-operation and sharing, the introduction of a relevant activity enhances communication, especially where confidence and spontaneity are marred by low self-esteem. The advantages of groups are outlined in a straightforward way by Priestley and Maguire (1983). Although not designed with the elderly specifically in mind, the book is a useful text for all involved in group approaches.

Treatment programmes and techniques

Occupational therapy considers the personal, social, domestic and self-care areas of the elderly person's life. Design of a treatment programme considers the selection of relevant activities and the timing of sessions. Activities offered may cater for some measure of physical activity, intellectual stimulation, social and leisure activities, and allow some opportunity for self-expression: a forum is created for activities related to personal adjustment.

Activities related to personal adjustment

Reminiscence. Reference has been made earlier to the adaptation necessary to maintain integrity in this age group. Many factors threaten adjustment, and the essential factor necessary for satisfactory adaptation is self-esteem. Activities involving reminiscence have received increasing emphasis in recent years. Evidence in support of its therapeutic qualities has been clearly outlined by Langley (1983). Audio-visual aids are commercially available from Help the Aged and are useful prompts for communication. It is also possible to centre this activity around scrap books, family photographs, music and dance, old fashioned sweets and signs or in the life review. This process is a natural instinct which may be observed in many who are approaching the end of their life. Outlining life maps, studying one's geneology or writing 'What 1 remember from childhood' are useful themes for reflection. The necessity for reflection has been described by Cicero and many others up to the present day, and it satisfies a primary need. Lewis (1979) reminds us of the necessity to listen rather than hasten activity. It is a process requiring skill and sensitivity on the part of the therapist, as unresolved conflicts are resurrected and require satisfactory reintegration.

Supportive psychotherapy

Treating the elderly in groups requires some special considerations in terms of practical aspects, and more active approaches from the staff (Blair 1979). Participation and freer exchange of communication occur when discussion revolves around an activity in the first instance. Music, pieces of relevant poetry or prose, paintings, caricatures or some techniques from remedial drama can be used successfully. Selection of members is crucial. The themes around which the group resonates reflect the group's developmental stage. Loneliness, grief, illness and family conflict are frequent themes. The goal of the sessions is growth and satisfaction through social experience.

Relaxation

Simple methods of anxiety management can be discussed in a group. This discussion covers sources of anxiety — fear of attack, burglars, physical illness, helplessness, fear of being left alone — and allows insight into symptoms. A sharing of how anxiety can be translated into physical symptoms also indicates awareness of self and response to stress. The method of relaxation is best kept simple.

Mitchell (1972) outlines a method that does not demand unrealistic feats of concentration. Time should be allowed at the end of the session for discussion of ability to control anxiety, states of relaxation and alternative methods.

Activities related to the use of leisure time

Ravetz (1984) reviews types of leisure and changes in patterns throughout the life cycle and considers the concept of leisure rehabilitation. Planning is determined by the interests of the elderly person and the resourcefulness of the staff. Leisure time represents the largest part of an elderly person's life in this country. Social contact involved with leisure is vitally important to enhance the satisfaction of life as described by Blood (1985). The range of activities available to the occupational therapist can cover review of community resources in the locality of the elderly person. Investigation with them of clubs, church-based activities, libraries, community centre groups, can engage her interest. In hospital, skittles, carpet bowls, putting, darts, crazy golf and outings offer opportunities for interaction with others. Interest in plants allows a range of activities from simple indoor procedures to gardening in a raised plot. Organisation of recreation and leisure activities is not the sole prerogative of occupational therapists. Other staff, including volunteers, have much to offer. The inclusion of such activities within the treatment programme marries with specific therapeutic goals. Factors to be considered when encouraging an elderly person's involvement in an activity of this nature are:

1. Leisure interest and activity prior to admission
2. Present ability to participate and possible constraints.

When considering readjustment once discharged, the patient's environment and financial resources will affect the choice of appropriate leisure pursuits.

Education pursuits

Within the therapeutic programme, opportunities for intellectual stimulation are considered most important. They may take the form of current affairs groups, quizzes of various types and range of difficulty, discussion of rights, retirement, or special interest discussions, documentaries or videos. Lewis (1979) expounds the importance of acknowledging the elderly person's capabilities of continued learning and achieving. Kassel (1963) strongly recommended continuing education of the elderly and resisted the view that intellectual incompetency is a natural phenonemon of later years. There may be a case for involving adult basic education volunteers, using community education centres, and investigating the possibility of evening classes as part of a rehabilitation schedule, or in some cases looking at the possibility of Open University courses.

Activities related to life skills

The inattention to basic skills of self-care and nutrition are features of the distress and preoccupation of many elderly psychiatric patients. Programmes include grooming, personal hygiene, basic laundry or use of laundry resources, menu planning and cooking. In cases of recovery from bereavement reactions, considerable readjustment to living alone is necessary and may require teaching and practice of basic nutrition. Others may have let skills lie dormant for years, and require time to re-familiarise themselves with basic coping ability. Attention to the effects of low self-esteem, dependency and lack of identity is required when designing such activities. Support, encouragement and humour are necessary to encourage and facilitate progress. Activity programmes of this kind can involve talks from dietitians about special diets, low-priced meals or the nutritional value of different foods. Domestic activities are the most readily graded. Simple beginnings, such as making tea and toast, can extend to organising lunch groups with shared

satisfaction of the end product. Attention to safety is a fundamental requisite for the therapist. Sessions devoted to analysis of hazards in the home using the ROSPA leaflets are instructive, followed up by a home visit to discover potential safety hazards. A similar outline for discussion of money management would include recognition of money, basic shopping, prices, pensions, benefits and paying bills.

Self-care in the elderly is affected by preoccupation, depression, eccentricity or delusions. The sense of personal identity is eroded by helplessness or dependency. In some cases control is held by others: by spouse, daughter or those who 'tidy up' the elderly person, much as you would a child, before she goes out. There is frequently a changed body image as physical changes or disability occur. Preoccupation with bodily functions is exacerbated by incontinence, bringing frustration and a loss of self-respect. Any activity programme designed around self-care must be undertaken with sensitivity to the biological and physical changes which occur. Sensory loss must be carefully detected and understood in terms of psychiatric phenomena, the most common being predisposition to paranoia with hearing or visual loss. It must also be remembered that gastatory and olfactory loss may affect appetite and detection of different odours. These losses impair the ability of the elderly person to adjust successfully.

EDUCATION

Learning and development of skills continues throughout our professional lives. No one is the 'fount of all knowledge' concerning the sociological, psychological or psychiatric processes in the elderly. Education is considered successful when it has its own momentum and is self-directed. Earlier components of this phenomenon were mentioned in the teaching and education which takes place in the multidisciplinary team. Attention to morale in this way acts as a spur to inform colleagues and initiate learning about new methods of assessment. treatment procedures or research. This has a most potent effect upon attitudes. While theoretical awareness may exist regarding prejudice or therapeutic frustration in working with the old, we must re-examine our own feelings and weigh up the possibilities of counter-transference.

College-based work

Most curricula in colleges of occupational therapy offer an appropriate percentage of time to the psychology and problem areas of the elderly. Students are equipped theoretically, and normally would experience clinical practice in units for the elderly. However, the translation from academic to practical application is sometimes overwhelming because of the multifaceted nature of illness. Although teaching methods in recent years have become more varied, increased time spent in analysis and differentiation of problem areas seems indicated.

Professional development

The enthusiasm and professional gains acquired in a regular in-service training programme are immeasurable. Again, it has morale as its lynch-pin. Contributions can come not only from sharing of skills within a department, but from invited speakers and specialists. Research projects, training officers from Age Concern, movement therapists, designing a guide for home visiting, or asking a relative to speak are only some of the sessions which can offer invaluable learning experiences.

Formal supervision

Occupational therapists employ psychological methods of treatment which necessitate establishing therapeutic relationships. In order to identify needs and tailor treatment, trust and rapport is crucial. This takes time, patience and considerable personal investment. Potential conflicts include a sense of helplessness,

failure and intergenerational problems. Frustration and interdisciplinary conflicts may occur, all of which require a place for ventilation and reflection. The overwhelming transference in over-protection and unwitting encouragement of dependency also often need an objective viewer to clarify the problem. These issues can be dealt with in small groups or under individual supervision. Whatever the method of choice, the educational task in dealing with them requires a supervisory alliance, careful pacing of comments and sensitivity. The resulting effects will be a better informed, more aware staff at all levels which will have a direct effect on the quality of care.

RESEARCH

Research is being undertaken at many different levels. Occupational therapists have to be cognisant of the studies which have been conducted as a baseline for evaluating priorities for staffing and for validating existing approaches. Bond and Carstairs (1982) underline the increasing interest in the elderly but stress that continuing work is required to determine effectiveness of services, support for carers and in which ways community care can be mobilised for those diagnosed with functional illnesses.

Researchers in occupational therapy have attempted to understand the relationship between activity and life satisfaction (Maguire 1984) which elicits useful information for those working with the elderly in all fields.

The variety of research of interest to us, as a problem-solving profession, can spread outwards, for instance to an interesting and humane study by Walster (1979). She investigated 'the role of the human/companion animal bond' in the mental health of the elderly. This instructive study echoes Willson's (1983) plea to abandon starchiness and rigidity in dealing with the elderly and to thoroughly promote their individuality.

Although the main body of research seems devoted to investigation of dementia, depression particularly has been the subject of a study by Murphy (1983), examining the role of a supportive relationship in determining outcome of illness. This work suggests that efforts should be made to prevent the onset of depression. In parallel with pleas from investigators into dementia, there is a need for early detection and intervention in depression.

CONCLUSION

Concluding remarks usually contain the author's recommendation for change and three main areas stand out.

1. *Education.* The evolution of services for the elderly has accelerated of late. Wattis et al (1981) conducted a national survey of resources concerning psychogeriatrics, which conveyed interesting results concerning deployment of occupational therapy staff. Occupational therapy helpers employed by nearly 80% of major services spent nearly all of their time with psychogeriatric patients. Therefore, despite the increased interest in this speciality, the day-to-day contact with the elderly is heavily dependent upon untrained staff. More education is required, particularly on a multidisciplinary teaching basis, to further a common philosophy at all levels.

2. *Prevention.* Preparation for growing old starts early. Cicero observed that 'if old age is poor it is often from the extravagance of youth'. Personality and mental hygiene are protected longer if interests are maintained and extend beyond work. However, perhaps flexible retirement, as suggested by the International Labour Organisation, could be considered. The need for hospital care may be averted if there is recognition of psychiatric problems by GPs and our community colleagues. A 'high risk' register of those recently bereaved, enduring physical illness or living alone could be compiled.

3. *Social support.* This revolves around encouraging involvement of young people to work on a voluntary basis with the old. Good neighbourhood schemes, sitting services and increased efforts to support families and relatives are urgent requirements.

It becomes abundantly clear that more is needed to contribute effectively towards the care of the psychogeriatric patient than major building or upgrading programmes. Occupational therapists, in conjunction with other health service professionals, face an immediate challenge to improve and co-ordinate psychiatric services for the elderly.

REFERENCES

Blair S 1979 Supportive psychotherapy groups with the elderly. British Journal of Occupational Therapy 42(6)

Blood H 1985 The elderly in society. Runner Up Student Award Winner. Therapy Weekly. February 7

Bond J, Carstairs V 1982 Services for the elderly. Scottish Health and Home Department, Edinburgh

Boyd W, Robinson S 1983 Psychiatry of old age. In: Kendall R F, Zealley A (eds) Companion to psychiatric studies. Churchill Livingstone, Edinburgh

Butler R 1969 Age-ism: Another form of bigotry. The Gerontologist 9: 243–246

Cicero 1903 Two essays on old age and friendship trans Shuckburgh E S. MacMillan, London

Department of Health and Social Security 1981 Growing older. HMSO, London

Flowers Y, Kraeim R 1982 Patterns of activities throughout the life span. Proceeds of the 8th International Congress of the World Federation of Occupational Therapists, Hamburg

Kay D W K, Beamish P, Roth M 1964 Old age, mental disorders in Newcastle upon Tyne. A study in prevalence. British Journal of Psychiatry 110: 146–158

Kassel V 1963 Continuing education for the elderly. Geriatrics July: 575–577

Langley D M, Langley G E 1983 Dramatherapy and psychiatry. Croom Helm, London

Lewis S C 1979 The mature years. Charles R Slack, Thorofare, N J

Linden M E 1953 Group psychotherapy with institutionalised senile women. International Journal of Group Psychotherapy 3: 150–170

Maddox G L 1963 Activity and Morale — a longitudional study of selected elderly subjects. Social Forces 43: 195–204

Main T 1957 The Ailment. British Journal of Medical Psychology 30: 129–145

Mitchell L 1972 Simple relaxation. John Murray, London

Maguire G H 1984 An exploratory study of the relationship of valued activities to the life satisfaction of elderly persons. The Occupational Therapy Journal of Research 3:3

Murphy E 1983 The prognosis of depression in old age. British Journal of Psychiatry 143: 111–119

Pitt Brice 1982 Ageing and its problems. Professional attitudes. In: Psychogeriatrics: an introduction to the psychiatry of old age. Churchill Livingstone, Edinburgh, Chs 203, pp 6–37

Priestly P, Mc Guire J 1983 Learning to help. Tavistock Publications, London

Scottish Health Authorities Priorities for the Eighties (SHAPE) 1980 A Report by the Scottish Health Service Planning Council. Scottish Home and Health Department. HMSO, Edinburgh

Scottish Home and Health Department 1979 Services for the elderly with mental disability in Scotland HMSO Edinburgh

Ravetz C 1984 Leisure. In: Willson M (ed) Churchill Occupational therapy in short-term psychiatry. Churchill Livingstone, Edinburgh

ROSPA. Publications from the Royal Society for the Prevention of Accidents, Cannon House, The Priory, Queensway, Birmingham

Schulman A D, Post F 1980 Bi-polar disorder in old age. British Journal of Psychiatry 136: 26–32

Segal H 1981 The work of Hanna Segal. Jason Aronson, New York

Seligman M 1975 Helplessness: on depression, development and death, Freeman, San Francisco

Walster D 1979 The role of the human/companion animal bond in the mental health of the elderly. Proceeds of an International Conference on Health Education. Scottish Health Education Group, Edinburgh

Wattis J, Wattis L, Arie T 1981 Psychogeriatrics — a national survey of a new branch of psychiatry, British Medical Journal 282: 1529–1534

Willson M 1983 Occupational therapy in long-term psychiatry. Churchill Livingstone, Edinburgh

WHO 1979 Psychiatric care in the community. WHO Regional Officer for Europe, Copenhagen

unable to attend. Ambulances should be exclusively allocated for day hospital use.

Elderly people prefer a set routine and it is essential to the success of day hospital treatment that patients are picked up at the same time each day to avoid anxiety.

The hub of any day hospital is an efficient and caring transport service providing close liaison between community and day hospital.

Types of service

1. *Statutory*
   National Health Service
   Social Services Department
   Hospital transport
2. *Voluntary*
   Voluntary organisations using minibuses
   Local hospital car services
   League of Friends of hospitals using private cars
3. *Private*
   Friends and relatives using
   private cars
4. *Independent*
   Use of public transport systems.

Types of vehicles

1. *Ambulance*
2. *Ambulance bus*
3. *Taxis*: can be under contract to local health authorities, and are normally only used in emergencies as a result of:
   a. industrial dispute
   b. vehicle breakdown
   c. unforseen circumstances, e.g. administrative error, emergency redeployment of ambulance service.
   Current taxi design limits their use for patients with mobility problems
4. *Local bus service*. Use of this facility is encouraged as part of a graded rehabilitation programme with psychogeriatric patients, e.g. collection by ambulance in the morning but independently return home.
   Gradually full independence may be achieved.

Associated bus travel problems:
   (i) High steps and awkwardly placed rails
   (ii) Pay on entry systems
   (iii) Destination and numeral display often too high and/or digital display can confuse the elderly.
5. *Minibus* Variety of seating: capacity 10/16 seats
6. *Private Car* Two-door cars usually have wider access for front seat passengers, but seats can be difficult for rear passengers. Four door cars are more convenient.

Escorts

Some day hospitals use escorts while others rely on a driver only. Escorts offer a valuable role in day hospital communication.
— *Duties*: vary from unit to unit
— *Liaison*: with family, carers, neighbours in communication between home situation and day hospital where appropriate.
— *Reassurance*: to patient and relative when a new patient is reluctant to attend
— *Observation*: check on medication; food; state of house; bedding etc.
— *Help*: to dress, or remind patient how to do so
— *Safety*: turn off gas and electrical appliances
— *Security*: check that the house is locked and the keys are with the patient
— *Action*: to take emergency action if the patient is unable to be contacted or when she is found in a distressed condition requiring urgent medical treatment.
In this case general practitioners are contacted as well as the day hospital.

Day hospital design

Not all day hospitals are purpose built and many have been opened in adapted premises which do not provide ideal conditions.

If a day hospital is being planned it should contain the following facilities:
— Treatment and interview rooms
— Occupational therapy, physiotherapy,

speech therapy & chiropody departments with all related facilities
— Rooms which can be used on a multi-purpose basis, for example rooms for small groups
— Well-lit areas for supportive and recreational activities
— Patients dining room
— Specialised bathrooms with aids and shower facilities
— Easily located toilets with aids and good access
— External facilities, for example a raised garden
— Support services:
  — secretarial/clerical
  — dentist; dietician; hairdresser
— Library service; shop
— Furniture of suitable design, fabric and height
— Carefully selected colours
— Good ventilation
— Clear sign-posting.

The role of the occupational therapist

In the day hospital there is much blurring of roles and overlap among various disciplines. Good communication and team work allows each discipline to contribute its specific skills.

Aims

1. Assessment
   a. Location
      (i) Home
      (ii) Hospital
      (iii) Community
   b. Aspects
      (i) Mental state
      (ii) Physical
      (iii) Socioenvironmental
2. Treatment
   a. Individual
   b. Group
3. Communication
   a. Interdisciplinary
   b. Carers

4. Reporting
   a. Oral
   b. Written
5. Remotivation
   a. Daily living tasks
   b. Hobbies; interests
   c. Social involvement
   d. Community integration.

The occupational therapist uses a holistic approach to patient care and has at her disposal a wide variety of skills and treatment media to cope with the complex problems related to care of the elderly (Fig. 11.1).

Many patients attending a medical day hospital also suffer fron dementia, especially a multi-infarct type, but it is only when their behaviour becomes socially unacceptable through aggression or wandering that they are referred to the psychogeriatric day hospital. Conversely, when a patient attending a psychogeriatric day hospital becomes physically immobile a two-man ambulance is then required to bring her to the medical day hospital. This ambulance facility is usually only available to a medical day hospital.

It is of great value to have the two types of day hospital under one roof as patients can be transferred from one to the other as their conditions and needs change.

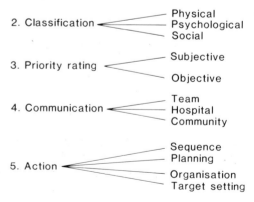

1. Identification – Collection of information

2. Classification — Physical / Psychological / Social

3. Priority rating — Subjective / Objective

4. Communication — Team / Hospital / Community

5. Action — Sequence / Planning / Organisation / Target setting

6. Re-evaluation

Fig. 11.1 Problem-solving approach to assessment and treatment

DAY HOSPITAL

Location

Treatment takes place mostly within the day hospital using the main day room area for the general daily programme. Separate rooms should be used for psychotherapeutic and other types of group work.

In addition, to reduce dependency on day hospitals, community involvement will be an integral component of the patient's programme, e.g. involvement in local library, clubs, community centres and church. Other examples are therapeutic outings to local places such as the airport, museum, swimming pool, shopping centre and cinema.

Media selection

This should reflect a 'problem oriented' approach. Careful planning and organisation is essential in the selection of the appropriate type of treatment. Appointments for speech therapy, physiotherapy, hairdressing, dentistry and chiropody have to be made in advance and accordingly fit in with the existing treatment sessions. Close team liaison is necessary as day patients' main treatment times are dependent upon transport. Most treatments have to be either late morning or early afternoon to accommodate this.

Days of attendance can be changed only after consultation with transport and community support services.

MEDICAL DAY HOSPITAL (TABLE 11.1)

Every patient referred to a medical day hospital will be seen by the occupational therapist for a detailed assessment of physical, psychological and/or social dysfunction as appropriate.

Treatment programmes will be formulated and selected media will be used (Fig. 11.2). Descriptions of assessment methods are given in Chapter 2 and specific treatment for different medical conditions are described in Chapters 3–8.

Table 11.1 Medical day hospital — reasons for attendance

Medical conditions	Possible socio-environmental problems
1. Stroke	1. Boredom
2. Cardiac disease	2. Isolation
3. Arthritis— rheumatoid osteoarthritis	3. Loneliness
4. Parkinsonism	4. Frailty
5. Orthopaedic — fractures	5. Reduced financial situation
6. PVD amputations	6. Reduced self-esteem
7. Diabetes	
8. Other reasons for referral	
a. Falls and immobility of unknown origin	
b. Thyroid disorders	
c. Gastro-intestinal disorders	
d. Respiratory disorders	
e. Obesity	
f. Anaemia	
g. Incontinence/urinary tract disorders	

Psychological conditions should be treated concurrently

PSYCHOGERIATRIC DAY HOSPITAL TREATMENT (TABLE 11.2)

Group work with organic patients (Fig. 11.3)

Generally organic patients require to be selected for groups according to their degree of dementia, e.g. mild, moderate and severe.

It is of value to include one or possibly two patients of a slightly higher level of ability. This serves to promote their self-worth, while helping the other patients by their quicker responses to orientation clues.

Organic patients require to have a more structured group programme than functional patients, giving variety of media suitably graded to meet their needs.

The duration of groups should be flexible, usually half an hour to three quarters of an hour, because of patients' short concentration span, distractability or sensory deficit. Media chosen should be graded, with emphasis on sensory stimulation and opportunity for recall and ventilation of feelings. All activities should be of short duration.

SPECIFIC GROUP AND
INDIVIDUAL PROGRAMME

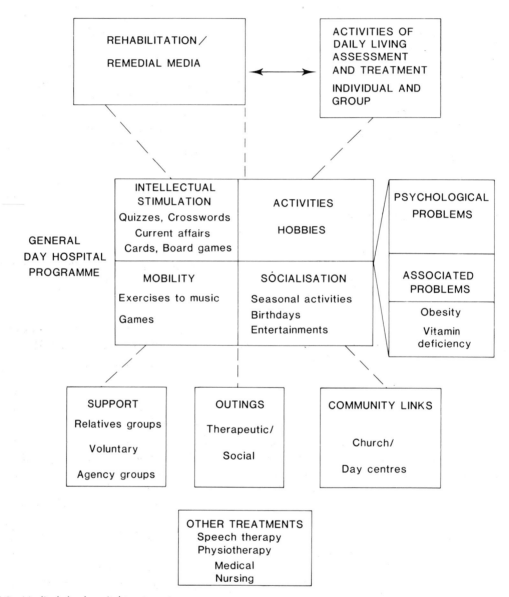

Fig. 11.2   Medical day hospital treatment

The role of the therapist is extremely important in setting a relaxed and happy atmosphere, thus lowering patients' anxiety level, reducing distractability and improving performance (see Ch. 9).

REALITY ORIENTATION

How it applies in a day hospital

Reality orientation is an important mode of management used with patients suffering

Table 11.2 Psychogeriatric day hospital — reasons for attendance

Functional disorders	Organic disorders

Affective disorders:
a. Endogenous depression
b. Mania (including hypomania)
c. Manic depressive states
 	
Reactive depression
 	
Neuroses:
a. Anxiety
b. Phobic states
c. Hysteria
d. Compulsive-obsessional states
 	
Schizophrenia/paraphrenia
 	
Personality disorders
 	
Alcoholism and drug abuse
	1. Acute confusional states
	    Causes: e.g., infection, toxicity
	2. Dementia
	    a. Multi infarct
	    b. Alzheimer's disease
	       (i) Senile dementia
	       (ii) Pre-senile dementia
	    c. Pick's disease
	    Other causes:
	       (i) Jacob-Creutzfeldt disease
	       (ii) Huntington's chorea
	3. Korsakoff's psychosis

Physical conditions should be treated concurrently	

from varying degrees of memory loss due to organic impairment. It helps them to remain independent in the community. Although mainly carried out in a psychogeriatric day hospital, it can also be used in a medical day hospital with demented or confused patients.

Carers should be educated in this approach.

Types

1. *24 hour reality orientation.* All those in contact with the patient during a 24 hour period are involved. The home environment has to be simplified, reorganised and appropriate memory aids provided (Table 11.3).
2. *Classroom reality orientation.* Daily structured group setting. This links with and reinforces the 24 hour approach (see Ch. 13).

Simplifying the home (Fig. 11.4)

Early memories and associated skills are retained longer, therefore modern household equipment may be potentially dangerous for a confused person, for example she might put an electric kettle on a lit gas burner.

Only basic household items and personal belongings should be retained in the home, for example summer clothes should be packed away during the winter.

PSYCHOTHERAPEUTIC GROUPS FOR DAY HOSPITAL PATIENTS WITH FUNCTIONAL DISORDERS (Fig. 11.5)

Day hospital attendance gives the elderly the opportunity to be introduced to a variety of groups, which is a comparatively new concept for this age group. Initially this treatment can present as extremely threatening, unless aims and methods are first carefully explained.

Elderly people suffering from incapacitating depressive illness, anxiety, phobic states or personality disorders have usually cut themselves off from social contact. They may have been neglected or avoided because of friends' ignorance of their illness and lack of knowledge and understanding in dealing with it. The benefits of treating the elderly in groups are considerable, promoting insight, building self-confidence and helping to renew those most important social contacts.

Initially this type of treatment represents a great threat to the elderly who have never previously been involved in discussing and sharing personal problems with a group. Therefore sensitivity, patience and the devel-

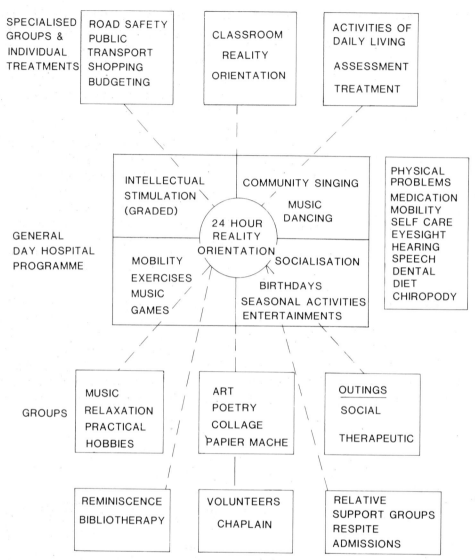

Fig. 11.3 Psychogeriatric day hospital — programme for organic patients

opment of a trusting relationship with the therapist are required before they will even consider joining a group session.

Most elderly people have been brought up to believe that it is better to keep personal problems to themselves, to keep 'a stiff upper lit' and 'to put on a brave face' in times of stress. This is especially true of men who have been taught that it shows weakness to express emotions. Bearing this in mind it can take some elderly people a long time to feel secure

and to benefit from this type of treatment. The extrovert personality can respond more readily than the introvert, being generally more gregarious. Carefully arranging where people sit in the group, while promoting an easy, caring, welcoming and friendly atmosphere, can make even the most reticent member feel involved and accepted.

When conducting groups with elderly patients, it is necessary to be more supportive and directive than with younger patients.

Table 11.3 Memory aids for confused day patients

Personal	Day hospital
Diary and pencil, notebook, photocase with pictures of family members, friends, home and pet, wallet containing name and address, watch — quartz with large numbers.	Signs to ladies and gents lavatories, large calendar, full length mirror, clock with large dial easy to see numbers, name badges for staff members, current newspapers, noticeboard, menu, timetable of activities, birthdays of patients listed.

Memory aids should be easy to read and interpret. At home, instructions regarding tablets to be taken, mealtimes, appointments, safety and security must be clearly displayed.

By using a structured approach rather than an abstract one, art, music, poetry or drama can be used as appropriate means to encourage group members to join in and to share valuable personal experiences.

Love is the most powerful emotion, capable of great healing powers. Helping to instil love of oneself and of others within the small group can be the start of recovery, replacing despair with hope. Caring for each other and sharing experiences past and present can be valuable in forming new relationships. Friendships can be developed and fostered within a small group, thus sowing the seeds of mutual help.

At a later stage these friendships can be instrumental in aiding patients' discharge from the day hospital and helping their re-establishment in the community. The therapist can contribute to these friendships by planting appropriate seeds of ideas, and allowing these to germinate, nourished by the group.

Loss is more common to the elderly than to the rest of society, i.e. loss of spouse, family, home, friends and contemporaries, role in the community, financial security, health, independence, mobility, eyesight, hearing, speech, social contact, confidence and motivation. Group work can provide a forum for discussing these often hidden feelings of loss and can be instrumental in replacing negative attitudes with positive ones (Fig. 11.6, 11.7).

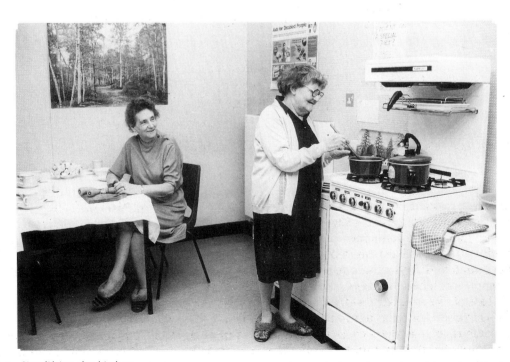

Fig. 11.4 Simplifying the kitchen

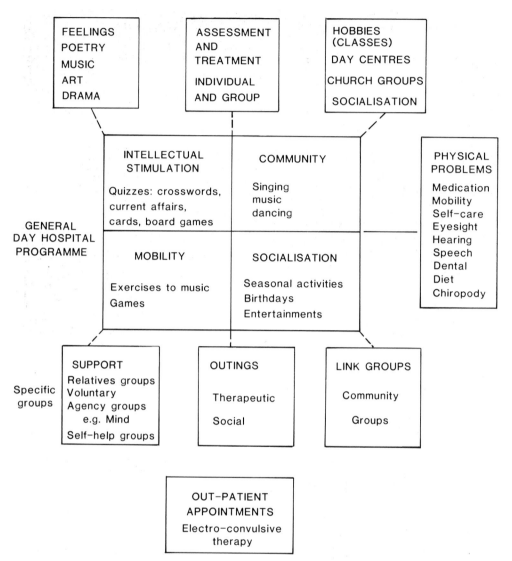

Fig. 11.5 Psychogeriatric day hospital — programme for functional patients

An important difference between younger age groups and the elderly is the loss of hearing, eyesight and sometimes speech common to the latter group. If adequate planning is carried out those with a hearing deficit, for example, need not be excluded. Sometimes it is a simple problem of wax in the ears, or a symptom of anxiety, i.e. a patient using hearing loss or low vision as a means of opting out of group involvement.

(Induction loop systems can be installed to counteract deafness by amplifying sound through a hearing aid set at the 'T' position.)

Many older people suffer needlessly through bottled up and unresolved grief reactions. It is sometimes difficult to share these feelings with close family members who may find it too painful to talk about the death of someone dear. By sharing this sorrow with others in the group who have experienced such a loss, relief can be gained. Those who have worked through the different stages of grief can be encouraged to give help to others within the caring group structure. Various

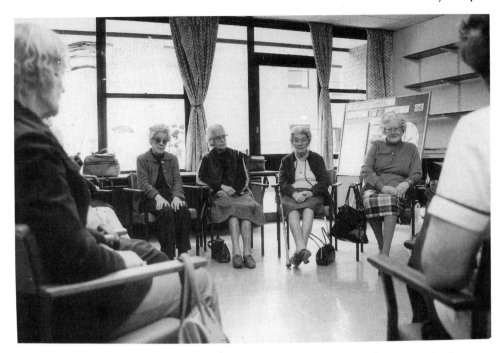

Fig. 11.6

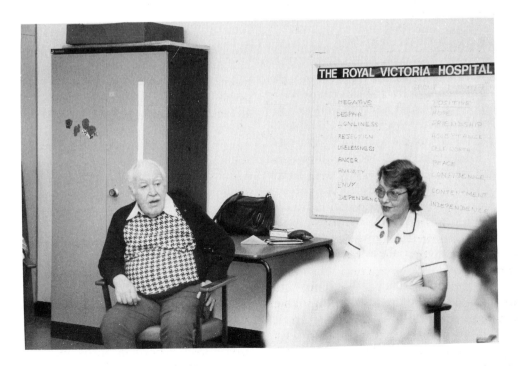

Fig. 11.7

Fig. 11.6 and **Fig. 11.7** Expressing feelings to the group

problems can be shared with the group and encouragement given by group members to find a solution.

Dependency on the day hospital can be overcome by patients being introduced to voluntary organisations and church groups, who provide education and leisure activities.

Day hospital groups where members have become used to expressing feelings can lead on to community neighbourhood link groups.

COMMUNITY NEIGHBOURHOOD LINK GROUPS (Docherty 1980)

Aims of setting up groups

— Act as a link between day hospital and community
— Maintain and improve level of function achieved by day hospital rehabilitation, in a natural setting
— Ease transition from day hospital to community
— Promote self-help concept
— Monitor progress
— Enhance quality of life
— Give support
— Help prevent hospital readmission.

In order to bridge the gap between day hospital and community these groups were developed as a natural progression of day hospital treatment for the depressed elderly, many suffering from pathological grief reactions and loneliness. Most were widows and widowers, living alone, with no family support. Within the small caring group, dependency on the day hospital structure could be reduced, behaviour modified, problems solved, targets set, insight and motivation gained, in as natural a way as possible.

By meeting initially weekly, either in each others' homes or by having outings together, relationships are strengthened and progress monitored.

Intervention can then be initiated as appropriate with support from the hospital team when necessary.

The concept of community neighbourhood link groups is now being expanded. By handing over the long-term support of these groups to specially chosen volunteers (non-practising professionals), occupational therapists are available to develop new groups as necessary.

HOME VISITS (Fig. 11.8)

The importance of assessing and treating patients in the community forms a vital part of the role of the occupational therapist. Valuable information on mental state including mood, orientation, behaviour and appearance can be observed in a true setting. Physical conditions, sensory loss, mobility, medication compliance and side-effects can also be assessed. Information collected assists in treatment planning. Problems are identified and classified in priority rating. This problem-orientated approach is used in building up a patient profile. Problems related to safety in the home can thus be identified. Home assessment can then be followed by practice in the problem areas within the occupational therapy activities of daily living area of the day hospital. Home visits are described in detail in Chapter 12. It should be stressed that the mental state and safety of the patient are priority areas to evaluate in the psychogeriatric day hospital patient at home.

COMMUNITY VISITS

Outings

Outings to re-introduce housebound patients to society are incorporated as an important treatment medium for patients attending either a medical or a psychogeriatric day hospital either on an individual or group basis.

They can be therapeutic in concept or purely social, for example:

Individual-introduction to:
    community activities
    leisure clubs
    church groups

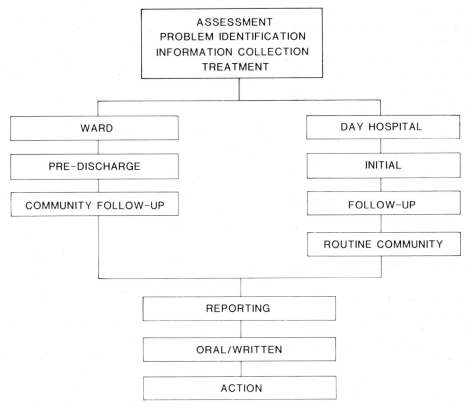

Fig. 11.8 Home visits

libraries
day centres
adult education classes
lunch clubs
Communal trips to:
museums
airport
sightseeing
seasonal scenes
picnics
theatres and cinemas
shops

Aims

— Provide stimulation: sensory, intellectual and social
— Facilitate reminiscence and recall
— Reinforce reality orientation
— Re-establish self-confidence and motivation
— Renew interest in hobbies and daily living activities
— Overcome fears and anxieties (agoraphobia and claustrophobia)

RELATIVES SUPPORT GROUPS

Purpose

Support for family plays an important part in day hospital care. Lack of understanding of the patient's illness, its management, availability of support services and prognosis, makes coping a burdensome task, greatly endangering the mental health of the caring family members.

Specific small support groups for daughters caring for parents, wives caring for husbands or vice versa can be developed on a weekly basis for a limited period, in addition to the more general monthly meeting catering for patients' relatives and carers. Representatives of the team headed by the consultant psychogeriatrician are present at the meeting.

Opportunity to express feelings (of anger, guilt, sorrow, frustration and aggression) can release pent-up emotion and help carers cope with different stages of illness and their reaction to it. Sharing similar experiences can often alleviate a feeling of isolation. Some may find that they can benefit from others' ability to cope with stress and learn from them.

Arrangements for respite admission with dates of intended holidays can be discussed with the staff.

The meeting also gives new carers the opportunity to learn about the function of the day hospital with explanations of daily programmes from staff. This information is often not relayed to carers because of patients' short-term memory deficits. The opportunity is given for carers to speak to different members of staff on specific problems.

Format

The group functions best when seated in a circle; intoductions are made, carers stating who they are, and staff describing their role within the day hospital team. Then follows an exchange of problems and a sharing of possible solutions and ways of coping.

RESPITE ADMISSIONS

Purpose

Respite admissions give relief to carers whose mental and physical state deteriorates owing to continuous stress, lack of sleep and many everyday problems. Patients suffering from chronic physical and/or severe psychological dysfunction are most in need of this very important service.

Placements

1. *Hospitals* — psychogeriatric and geriatric assessment and continuing care wards.

2. *Local authority* — Part III (England and Wales), Part IV (Scotland). Special holiday units are available in some homes.
3. *Community carers* — elderly persons looked after in a private home as part of the family under the supervision of the Social Services Department.
4. *Private nursing home* — dependent upon patient's financial state.

Advantages to carers

1. *Rest*: Relief from day to day care. Return to normal sleep patterns.
2. *Holiday*: allowing a holiday to be planned in advance.
   This sets short and medium targets for the carers.
3. *Social*: contacts to be resumed.
4. *Household*: allowing for home maintenance, household duties and other chores to be carried out.
5. *Relief*: from responsibility of elderly persons.
6. *Trial*: to see how patient reacts to various forms of care.

Disadvantages to carers

1. *Guilt*: at being parted from the patient — often reinforced by the patient saying she does not want to go for a short holiday, and would rather stay at home.
2. *Anxiety*: in case patient's personal needs are not being recognised and attended to promptly.
3. *Loneliness*: due to separation from patient.

Advantages to the patient

1. *Bridges the gap*: Between day hospital care and other forms of care on a trial basis.
2. *Severs dependence*: allows time for the carer and patient to adJust to being apart.
3. *Observation*: of mental and physical states during 24 hour regime.

Disadvantages for the patient

1. *Confusion and disorientation*: owing to unfamiliar surroundings.

Reality orientation and staff sensitivity to patient's needs can help combat these.

2. *Rejection*: separation can cause anxiety with feelings of rejection.

Summary

Respite admissions act as a lifeline enabling the carer to look after the elderly person for much longer. The advantages far outweigh the disadvantages. The system is used for patients living alone as well as for patients living with relatives. Flexibility is necessary to meet each individual's needs. Length of stay varies according to requirements. Respite admissions are especially important when continuing care beds are in short supply, and serve as an important adjunct to day hospital care.

CONCLUSION

The elderly are the largest group of people who require community services. Some of the most important challenges facing society today are to prolong elderly people's independence and enhance their quality of life.

Day hospital care, providing facilities for treatment and social integration, contributes significantly to meeting the needs of disabled elderly people living at home.

ACKNOWLEDGEMENTS

We would like to acknowledge the help of Mrs F. Mair, Miss J. Huddleston and Miss T. Fitzpatrick in writing this chapter.

REFERENCES

Bierer J 1951 The day hospital. An experiment in social psychiatry and synthoanalytic psychotherapy. Lewis, London
Brocklehurst J C and Tucker J S 1980 Progress in geriatric day care. King Edward's Hospital Fund, London.
Docherty 1980 Unpublished
Holden U P Woods R T 1982 Reality orientation. Churchill Livingstone, Edinburgh
Scottish Health Authorities Priorities of the Eighties (Shape Report) 1980 HMSO, London
Whitehead T 1978 In the service of old age. The welfare of psychogeriatric patients. H M & M Publishers, Aylesbury, Bucks

12

Home visiting
F. Meikle

Home visiting is an integral part of the assessment of many elderly patients, particularly where there is any doubt about their ability to cope at home. Most patients live at home either alone, with another elderly person such as spouse, brother or sister, or with an extended family where there may be children and grandchildren as well. The role of the occupational therapist is to try to establish an overall view of the needs of the patient; therefore it is important to consider her home and social circumstances in order to ensure a successful return.

Types of visit

A *pre-discharge visit* is the most common type of home visit, which is done to check that the patient is ready to go home after a period of rehabilitation. Information regarding difficulties which may arise due to the design of the patient's home may be available from the geriatrician who may have made an assessment visit prior to admission, or from family and friends who visit the patient. Sometimes the pre-discharge visit will show up any difficulties or areas where the patient needs further help. It can also be an opportunity to try out aids which can then be supplied before the patient is discharged, and a chance to introduce the community occupational therapist who will provide them.

A *discharge visit* may be appropriate if a patient has only been in hospital for a short time and has regained her previous level of functioning. This is also the case if the patient is well known from previous admissions.

Post-discharge or follow-up visits may be indicated after discharge if there is some concern that further problems may arise. Sometimes there are delays in the delivery of aids, or the patient may become very apprehensive after a particularly long spell in hospital and a further visit may provide reassurance all round.

Planning a visit

A variety of people may have to be invited to attend in addition to the patient and occupational therapist. These may include the physiotherapist, social worker, district nurse, community occupational therapist, home help supervisor and any relatives, friends or neighbours who provide assistance. It is, of course, not sensible to have too many people present, and it is generally best to try to arrange for additional people to call during the later part of the visit. In some instances it may be advisable to arrange for a relative or neighbour to open up the house and warm it in advance, thus avoiding extreme temperature changes. Contact with the community occupational therapist may also provide valuable information and save time where the patient is already known in the community. The patient needs to be prepared for the visit as it is important that she understands the purpose of it. It can be confusing and distressing for patients if they think they are being taken home for good, only to be taken back to hospital again. Before leaving the hospital several points should be checked:

1. The ward staff should know what time the visit is planned for and what time to expect the patient back when appropriate.
2. Ensure that either the patient or a staff member have the house keys.
3. Make sure that patients have been to the lavatory before leaving and that if necessary they are wearing a clean incontinence pad or that the catheter bag is empty.

4. Ensure that the patient has adequate footwear and clothes, particularly in bad weather, since hospital wards tend to be kept at relatively high temperatures.
5. If it is a discharge visit, check that the patient has all her belongings and essentials such as glasses, false teeth, medicines and or dressings.
6. Take any walking aids which are necessary.
7. It is helpful for the occupational therapist to take fresh milk etc. in order to make a cup of tea, and other items such as a torch (in case the electricity is turned off), matches for lighting gas and a pen and paper for writing out any messages which need to be left.

The visit

A typical assessment may well start as you leave the hospital:

1. Can the patient direct you to her home (bearing in mind, of course, that she may not be familiar with the district in which the hospital is situated)?
2. On arrival you should consider the access — main door straight off the street, garden or tenement stair; and is she able to use the keys? The access may determine how isolated or otherwise she may be. Once inside, careful consideration needs to be given to the layout of the rooms, and the accessibility of facilities such as toilet, bath and kitchen are obviously important. You should observe the patient's mobility around the house as this may differ from the ward setting where there is usually far more space available.
3. Note the patient's reaction to being home again. You have to make some judgement as to whether or not the patient actually wants to go home and whether or not she is realistic about her situation. A home visit can be stressful as patients feel that they are on trial and must perform well or they may not get home.
4. Look for any potential safety hazards, such as loose rugs, trailing wires, worn flexes

etc., access to telephone and management of medication. It is a good opportunity to point out such dangers and demonstrate how best they can be avoided.

5. Kitchen assessment should include the ability to make a hot drink and a snack if applicable. Check the food in the fridge and store cupboard. If there is anything mouldy or stale it should be removed as the elderly tend to lose their sense of smell. Ensure that the problems of shopping and money management are resolved.

6. Practise all transfers which the patient will need to do once she is home again, such as getting in and out of bed, on and off the toilet, on and off a chair or transferring from wheelchair to commode etc. This may be very tiring when done all at once, so some allowances may have to be made or tasks adjusted accordingly. It may be necessary to check on the height of all these items and note if aids will be needed. This information should be passed to the community occupational therapist will then be able to supply them.

7. Look out for any obvious signs of neglect, such as damp bedclothes, a smell of urine, bottles full of old tablets, alcohol abuse, burnt saucepans, and note the general condition of the house: if it is very cold even on a mild day, it might lead to hypothermia in winter.

8. Where possible, speak to any relatives, neighbours or other people involved in the care of the patient, as their 'story' might be different from that of the patient and how she sees the situation.

9. Before leaving after the visit, check that all the power is turned off if the house is to be left unoccupied. Remove any stale food and any old drugs where appropriate (and return to ward sister or pharmacy) — it may be important to discuss their use and value with both the patient and the ward staff. Check that the patient has any belongings that she may wish to take back to the hospital. Make sure that all doors and windows are secure if the house is to remain empty. Take the keys back to the hospital.

On returning to the hospital — where applicable

1. Inform the ward staff of the patient's return. It is useful to give a brief report to the ward staff about how the visit went.

2. Hand back any keys or valuables to be checked and locked up by the nursing staff.

3. Write up the home visit report, making any comments or recommendations at the end.

4. Refer to the community occupational therapist and any other agencies, where necessary, if they were not present on the visit.

Conclusion

It is often the case that patients who find it difficult to achieve activities in the ward or occupational therapy department, fare much better in their own well-known environment. Conversely, the security of the hospital environment may give a false impression and a failure at home may result. When dealing with elderly patients, there may be a temptation to sweep in with lots of alterations and gadgets. This should be resisted wherever possible as it may result in confusion, particularly where there is already a problem, and reluctance to use the revised situation may result in a failed discharge and readmission of the patient to hospital.

It is essential for an occupational therapist, when home visiting, to observe everything, including any behaviour or incidents which are beyond the scope of assessment.

Pre-discharge units

Pre-discharge units are often part of the discharge plan for a patient participating in a long rehabilitation programme. These units are self-contained flats attached to a ward or in a separate building within the hospital. The patient's home life-style and daily living requirements are taken into account when a plan is made of how much or how little the patient will have to do to look after herself. This ranges from carrying out all shopping, cooking, laundry and hygiene activities, to simply ordering ingredients via a nurse or occupational therapist from the hospital kitchen to make one meal or snack per day — the other meals being provided. At home, if the patients have been used to a home help or someone to help bath them, comparable forms of support are provided in the pre-discharge unit.

The efficacy of these units for elderly people is debatable. The unit can never duplicate a person's home. A different layout and, more specifically, a different cooker, equipment and utensils could add to mild confusion and lack of confidence. Conversely, a lucid elderly person recovering from an operation (e.g. joint replacement following rheumatoid arthritis) would benefit from a 7–14 day session in a pre-discharge unit to try out different aids before being discharged to use them. Stroke patients with minimal perceptual, sensory and cognitive problems can benefit from a stay in a pre-discharge unit. Managing to look after themselves unaided can boost patients' confidence and allow them to try activities of daily living at their own speed unsupervised.

A pre-discharge unit trial can also be used if there is a placement problem, and will highlight the patient's ability to function or not.

Criteria for admission to a pre-discharge unit

1. Patient should be lucid with reasonable short-term memory.
2. Patient should be independent in activities of daily living in the ward.
3. Patient should be self-medicating.
4. Premises should be used for practice and confidence boosting — any assessment should be done in the occupational therapy department.

Problems which arise

1. Often the premises are converted and not purpose-built.
2. If the pre-discharge unit is attached to the ward occupational therapists are not consulted as to equipment, and utensils and inappropriate items are ordered.
3. Selection of patients has to be done very carefully.
4. The purpose of the pre-discharge unit must be understood by all staff members.
5. Supervising patients in a pre-discharge unit is time-consuming; often they have to be visited two or three times a day. Menus have to be planned, encouragement and support given, and they may need to be accompanied when shopping.
6. Often the pre-discharge unit is not situated near the ward from which the patient was referred.
7. The nurses on the ward attached to the pre-discharge unit have to be given a full background report on the patient and on how she is to be handled.
8. There will be extra demands on the nurses if the patient is not totally independent and the occupational therapist is unable to visit very frequently.

THE AUGMENTED HOME CARE SCHEME

This research study was originally set up in 1978 by the Department of Geriatric Medicine at the University of Edinburgh and was for the benefit of elderly people over 70 years old suffering from acute and sub-acute illnesses.

Owing to the increasing number of elderly people admitted to hospital, it was felt that alternative methods of care should be investigated. A study by Currie et al (1979) suggested that 30–40% of patients admitted to acute medical wards during 1976 received the type of care that could have been provided at home. This suggested that sometimes elderly people were being unnecessarily admitted to hospital. It is widely accepted that admitting elderly people to hospital can cause more problems than it solves, often with even greater risks to those who are already frail. Some obvious problems are:

1. Confusion and disorientation resulting from the unfamiliar surroundings — this is even more likely in patients with existing difficulties in that area. Defects in sight and hearing may exacerbate the problems, resulting in agitated behaviour which may lead to the use of tranquillisers which in turn compound the dangers.
2. Elderly people may well pick up secondary and more virulent infections often resistant to the more commonly used antibiotics.
3. Incontinence may become a problem, particularly where bladder control is precarious. Simple factors such as lengthy distances to the bathroom or insufficient opportunities for regular toileting may result in a wet bed and thus loss of dignity and morale. This situation is often extremely difficult to reverse.
4. Falls, fractures and pressure sores are all well-known hazards.
5. Less obviously, perhaps, is the loss of an existing support system within the community, varying from the loss of a trusted home help to the withdrawal of support from family and neighbours.

All this reinforces the view that the frailer the patient, the greater the risks attached to hospital admissions.

For many years the medical profession has held the belief that hospital was the best solution to the care of the elderly. This is not surprising since most of their education would have almost exclusively been in hospital. Family and carers often have the same view. However, many elderly patients themselves often have a realistic appreciation of the hazards and are aware that whilst admission to hospital is very simple, the return to the community on discharge is much more difficult.

It was therefore felt that many of these potential problems could be avoided by providing a system of augmented home care.

The scheme entailed close co-operation between general practitioners geriatricians, the home help service and the community nursing service. In the pilot study, the research team consisted of a nurse who monitored the input of services by the home help and district nurse, an occupational therapist who measured the functional level of independence over the period of each patient's inclusion in the scheme (6 weeks), and a secretary who manned the contact number.

Potential patients were referred by the general practitioner visited soon thereafter by a geriatrician. If the person was suitable then the necessary support was arranged and took effect as soon as those involved had been alerted. The main conditions thought suitable for the scheme were respiratory infections, urinary tract infections, cardiac failure, uncomplicated myocardial infarctions, viral illnesses and falls with soft tissue injuries.

Assessment

A new functional assessment had to be designed to evaluate change in functional status, and after considerable work, 41 questions were collated as follows:

Feeding

1. Cut food
2. Feed self
3. Drink from cup/glass

Continence

4. Continent

Transfer

5. Transfer to and from toilet/commode/use bed pan
6. Transfer to/from bed
7. Transfer to/from chair
8. Transfer to/from bath

Indoor mobility

9. Stay up $\frac{1}{2}$ hour or more
10. Move from room to room, same floor
11. Move freely about the house
12. Go up and down stairs

Outdoor mobility

13. Go up and down stairs
14. Go in and out of the house
15. Be mobile outside
16. Transfer to/from car
17. Use public transport
18. Shopping
19. Visit others

Dressing and Hygiene

20. Get dressed
21. Underwear/nightwear on/off
22. Upper extremities dressing on/off
23. Lower extremities dressing on/off
24. Wash upper body
25. Wash lower body
26. Clean teeth, shave, brush, manage hearing aid

Work duties

27. Prepare snack
28. Cook for self
29. Cook for family
30. Do light household tasks
31. Do heavy household tasks

Communication and social contact

32. Hold normal conversation
33. Use telephone indoors
34. Have visitors
35. Hobbies and interests

Safety

36. Be left alone
37. Raise alarm
38. Balance
39. Let people in/out

40. Take medicine
41. Manage plugs and switches.

A baseline for the comparison of functional change during and after the illness was constructed by establishing the patient's pre-morbid activities of daily living status by asking the relevant people involved with the patient. The questionnaire was designed to measure what the patient actually does rather than what she is capable of doing. The patients were visited 9 times over the six week period on days 1, 3, 5, 7, 10, 14, 21, and 42. Scoring was on a simple yes/no basis:

Yes = can do independently or using an aid which is always available.

No = cannot do; or needs help which is not always available; or not applicable such as no telephone.

There were only 61 patients involved altogether in the pilot study which is a low number from which to draw any significant conclusions. However, in general, the time taken to recover the pre-morbid functional levels was within 10 days, whereas a comparable group of hospital patients took 17 days.

This pilot study showed that assessment and appropriate help could be provided almost immediately — the home help service appeared to be the most important single factor in the success of the scheme — and patients particularly appreciated being in their own surroundings with familiar faces to help them.

Second study

A second study was completed in May 1985 which was specifically designed to determine whether augmented home care, as provided in the pilot study, could be effectively carried out by general practitioners on their own, without the considerable support provided by the professorial medical staff in the diagnosis and management of patients in the pilot study. 56 patients were admitted to this second study. 88% of the patients referred were women, and of the whole group 86% were either single or no longer married. 77%

of the group lived alone but in spite of this, communication with others was potentially good as 80% of them had a telephone.

The types of ailments were similar to those in the pilot study but there was very little evidence of mental impairment such as might be expected in that proportion of the population. This suggests that general practitioners avoided referring such patients for home care.

Before the illness began, 18% made use of the district nursing service, 32% received meals-on-wheels and 25% were visited by the health visitor. By contrast 66% used the home help service, the commonest number of hours being 6 per week. The study showed, however, that help from relatives or friends was received before the illness by as many as 64%. The home help service was used by 70% of those living alone and by 54% of those living with another person. The relatives helping were offspring, apart from two spouses.

The presence of acute illness was naturally a stimulus to an increase in support. The main burden fell on the home help service which attended 95% of the patients. The district nursing service increased attendance to cover 59% of the patients. The additional burden on general practitioners and district nurses was not large and on other services was very small. The work of the home help service in hours was 30 or less for each of 47% of the patients attended and 40 or less for each of 58%. The general practitioner made 4 visits or less to each of 61% of patients and 6 visits or less to 86%. The modal value of 3 visits was made to 23% of patients.

The speed with which patients obtained the necessary service is shown by the fact that 46% of those attended by the district nurse and 68% of those receiving extra home help were visited within 24 hours of entering the study.

Non-statutory helpers (relatives or friends) were significantly important and attended a similar proportion of patients for household activities and patient care as the home help and the district nurse. A slight increase in pressure sores and incontinence was revealed

but this had returned to the previous situation by the end of the six weeks. Only two out of 56 patients in this second study developed new respiratory infections.

Of more concern was the number of patients who fell during the study. 36% of patients had fallen at home before entering the study. 13 of the 56 (23%) fell after admission, but only 9 of the 13 had fallen before admission. Considering the high proportion who lived alone, falling in 23% might need some special provision if home care was to be more generally used for acute illness in the elderly.

The study showed an increase in the use of aids during the illness. Almost the same number used walking aids at the end of the illness compared with before, but three more than formerly were using a zimmer rather than a stick. For other aids, except bath aids, a greater number were using them at day 42 than before the illness.

By day 42 the functional level had returned to that before the illness in feeding, communication, staying up half an hour, moving from room to room, putting on and off underwear and nightwear and most problems related to safety. This suggested that there was a need to allow access from outside to the patient's home by another person for a week or so at the start of the illness. It also seemed necessary to provide specially for unsteadiness in patients for about 3 weeks. Otherwise, safety considerations did not form a bar to augmented home care.

For other functional disability, in respect of ability to transfer, outdoor mobility, dressing, work duties, moving freely all over the house, using public transport and shopping, a proportion of the group failed to return to the level of competence present before the illness. This study cannot compare this proportion of incomplete recovery with that which is present in acutely ill elderly patients treated in hospital. The clinical impression certainly is that such patients at home fare no worse than in hospital.

In most patients, adequate arrangements were made during the illness in respect of keeping warm, summoning help, controlling the environment and letting people in and out. These items are, however, so important that if home care of acute illness were in general use, it would be necessary to ensure adequate arrangements for all patients.

The outcome of treating 56 acutely ill elderly patients at home was that 47 (84%) were at home after 6 weeks, but during the illness 15 (27%) were sent to hospital. Of the 15, 8 came home, 5 died and 2 went to long-term care. Total deaths were 5 (9%), of which 2 occurred at home.

It is disappointing that so few patients were referred to the Augmented Home Care Scheme but there have been difficulties in other home care schemes in securing the interest of the general practitioner. Wade et al (1985), in their study of a home care service for acute stroke, in Bristol found that while many agreed with the need for the service, when it came to actually referring patients, few were committed to using it. They thought this resistance might be the most important factor in determining success or failure in developing any new service.

One factor which reduced the numbers entering the study was that only one patient at any one time could receive extra home help in any one social work area. This resulted in 6 patients being turned away from the study.

The Augmented Home Care Scheme reported here was reasonably popular with practitioners in the pilot study but in this the geriatrician played a major role. Once decisions in the scheme were handed over to the general practitioners as in the second part of the study, and the department of geriatric medicine supplied research observers only, the interest and enthusiasm of the general practitioners appeared to wane. The inevitable conclusion is that the scheme as offered is not wanted on a significant scale by practitioners at the present time. The general practitioner retains responsibility for the proper care of patients at home (Ashworth 1959). If present arrangements eventually fail to cope with the increasing numbers of elderly persons in the population and with the treatment of relatively simple acute or sub-acute illnesses, then new systems may have to be developed to link general practice, community nursing. social work departments and hospital departments of geriatric medicine (Opit et al 1976).

The methods used to collect and analyse data were satisfactory. If two groups of patients had been included, randomly assigned to care in hospital or at home, it would have been simple to arrange the further analysis required.

REFERENCES

Ashworth H W 1959 The care of old people in general practice. Medical World 91: 314–315

Currie C T, Smith R G, Williamson J 1979 Medical and nursing needs of elderly patients admitted to acute medical beds. Age and Aging 8: 149–151

Opit L J, Shaw S M 1976 Care of the elderly sick at home; whose responsibility is it? Lancet 2: 1127–1129

Wade D T, Hewer R L, Skilbeck C E, Bainton D, Cox C B 1985. Controlled trial of a home-care service for acute stroke patients. Lancet i: 323–326

13

Continuing care units

N. Munro

This chapter covers reality orientation techniques and occupational therapy activities used in a practical way with the following patients:
— Confused
— Severely physically handicapped
— Long-term psychiatric.

INTRODUCTION

The National Health Service has had to provide extra facilities to allow for the growth in the elderly population, including additional continuing care units. The role of the occupational therapist in working with these chronically disabled people is to improve their social and personal skills as well as cognitive function and motor ability (Trevan-Hawks 1985).

CRITERIA FOR ADMISSION TO CONTINUING CARE UNITS

Patients in the United Kingdom are admitted on the basis of the following criteria:
— They must be 65 years or over and live within the catchment area of the unit.
— They are no longer able to look after themselves at home or be supported by their family or any other agency.
— Loss of independence is caused by a disabling physical and/or psychiatric condition

requiring specialist nursing care and drug monitoring.

Referral for continuing care is made by a patient's general practioner, or consultant if she is already in hospital. A geriatrician assesses the patient to see whether she requires immediate permanent care or if she might benefit from assessment in a geriatric unit.

PHILOSOPHY OF CONTINUING CARE

Staff must be aware of, and have a good understanding of peoples' basic needs in order to offer them long-term care at a socially acceptable standard (Shaw 1984). Everyone has the right to 'be herself', to be treated with dignity, and to be given freedom of choice and privacy. Care and help should be offered to, not foisted upon, patients in continuing care.

The ward is a new home for its residents and the decoration, furnishing and atmosphere should reflect this. Patients are able to get up later and get ready for the day at a leisurely pace. There are no doctors' 'rounds' to prepare for as in acute wards.

The role of continuing care ward staff is to enable, encourage, befriend and occasionally cajole, as much as it is to give physical help and care.

OCCUPATIONAL THERAPIST'S ROLE

When a new patient is referred to a continuing care unit, she will bring her medical notes which should include a functional assessment from the last occupational therapist who treated her. The therapist will carry out a new assessment for comparison, looking for improvement or deterioration in mobility, mood, cognition and daily living activities. She carries out the assessment in a small quiet room with no visual distractions, in order to try to gain the patient's total concentration. She also uses this opportunity to spend time in getting to know her new patient. It is diffi-

cult for most to adjust to life in an institution and support must be available during this settling in period. When working with patients in any institution, it is important to remember what they have left behind in the outside world and to try to compensate for this lack — in other words, to try to enhance their 'quality of life' (Harris 1971).

The occupational therapist offers a balanced programme combining social, intellectual, domestic, physical and personal activities. These will be fully described later in the chapter.

STAFFING

When organising activities for continuing care patients, occupational therapists must call upon other staff to help with their programmes. Trained occupational therapists are in short supply and especially so in wards for chronically disabled people. Occupational therapy helpers are invaluable in working with this group of patients (see Ch. 2).

Occupational therapists work in co-operation with nurses, physiotherapists and speech therapists to give patients the treatment they may require. Volunteers are often very helpful if using them is accepted practice by the local hospital management group.

Much interest is created by young people visiting wards for the elderly. They might be school children undergoing job experience, youth training scheme trainees or apprentices; all are valuable sources of interest for the elderly and vice versa. Because of the constantly repetitive nature of treatment and the degree of commitment required by staff working with highly dependent patients, morale can be poor and patients and staff can become adversely affected. Often staff working on these units have the highest record of sickness and absenteeism.

To boost staff and patient morale the following points have to be implemented:

1. Appropriate staffing levels should be maintained.

2. Good communication amongst occupational therapy staff and with other disciplines should be established.
3. Careful consideration should be given in order to plan varied and interesting programme of activities. Innovation is all important as a morale booster.
4. Staff members should be deployed to treat as many patients as possible who might benefit from occupational therapy.
5. Another reason for careful assessment is to gauge who will or will not benefit from individual and/or group therapy. Groups are unsuccessful if they contain noisy, confused members.
6. Regular meetings with patients' relatives are important to encourage their help within the ward. Many want to help but, without reassurance from the staff, think they might be encroaching, be unwelcome and feel out of place.
7. People working with high dependency patients require more praise and encouragement than other staff. They have to give so much of themselves to achieve even a small improvement.

Space for occupational therapy activities

Groups for 6 or 7 people take place in a simulated sitting room. This provides a quiet, friendly atmosphere for discussion.

Cooking groups for 4 people take place in the small simply furnished occupational therapy kitchen. This encourages exchange of cooking ideas, general conversation and a concerted effort to produce a meal or make some cakes for teatime.

If activity areas do not resemble home settings they do not give the opportunity for normal social and role performance; there is then the danger of 'social death' (Sheppard 1984). Larger group activities take place in the ward sitting room; in most continuing care units space is limited and public rooms have to be at least dual purpose.

Not all residents are fit enough to participate in groups, but may benefit from seeing and hearing what is happening within the group. (When patients suffer from severe senile dementia they are unable to relate to more than one person at a time.)

Treatment

If choice and preference are not offered, the patient who is already dependent and passive may become institutionalised (Willson 1983).

Group therapy is usually given to continuing care patients, but there are times when a programme for individual treatment has to be drawn up. When patients are being treated in a group their personal identity must never be forgotten. Their names must always be used and each patient's personal qualities and interests must be appealed to and brought out during group activities.

Newcomers

Some patients may have difficulty in settling into the ward routine, and can become aggressive and disruptive. The following is an example of such a patient who was referred to occupational therapy for behaviour modification.

The patient was unsociable, unkempt, unwilling to make decisions, unco-operative and hostile to the ward staff. She had been ostracised by the other patients.

The occupational therapist's aims of treatment were to make the patient more sociable and manageable, improve her self-esteem, integrate her with patients of a similar intellectual level and try to make her less dependent on tranquilisers. This patient's programme lasted from Monday at 10.30 to Friday at 4.00 (occupational therapists and physiotherapists do not work at weekends on these wards and the shortage of nurses prevented the programme from being continuous.)

Programme

A contract was made. Therapists offered to make her life more rewarding if she agreed to control her behaviour and try to be more independent.

Rewards for acceptable behaviour were offered as follows:
— A bus outing was offered in return for an end of aggression to staff.
— An outing with one other patient and a therapist was offered if the antisocial behaviour stopped.

Improvement of self-esteem was helped by a visit to the hairdresser. She was encouraged to choose what to wear and subsequently took more interest in her appearance.

Mixing with other patients was initiated to give her mental and social stimulation. This renewed her self-identity as well as demonstrating ward policies.

Conclusion. After three weeks of behaviour modification, the patient was able to make eye contact, initiate conversation, participate in ward activities and behave well on outings. After seven months this patient is respected by staff and other patients and fulfils a useful role in the ward.

It is important that behaviour modification be carried out objectively and that all ward staff know the reward system for each patient being treated in this way.

Sandra Cutler Lewis (1981) said that 'since occupational therapists are trained in the restoration of an individual's cognitive, emotional and physical functioning it is our obligation and mandate to provide treatment that is responsive to each consumer, client, patient problem'.

Reality orientation

Reality orientation (Fig. 13.1) is a technique to treat confused patients or to stimulate a mixed group of continuing care residents so that the alert ones continue to use their memories and minds to remain lucid, while those with failing memories are encouraged to grasp the 'here and now'. There are two variations: classroom and 24-hour. Both are used in continuing care wards.

Classroom reality orientation

The classroom version of reality orientation involves one occupational therapist working with a small group of patients. This session starts the therapist's daily programme. Normally she uses a board with the name of the hospital, the day, date, month, year, the season and the weather outside printed boldly and legibly on it. (Magnetic boards and letters are useful but not essential.) It is important that this session takes place near a window so that patients can look outside for visual clues as the therapist asks them about the month and season. She will often have clues inside the room as well: spring or summer flowers, autumn leaves, bare branches or dried fir cones.

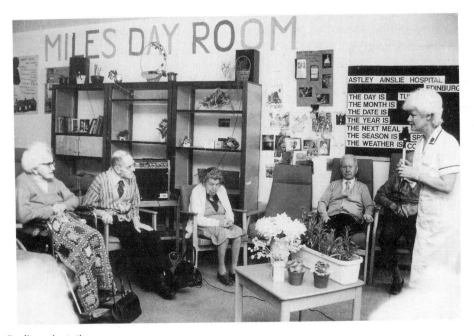

Fig. 13.1 Reality orientation

24-hour reality orientation

This involves all staff working with confused patients, reassuring them about where they are, the time of day, the date, names of other patients and staff and sometimes reminding the patient who she is. In fact staff fill the gaps in patients' memories, as well as tactfully modifying their inaccurate recall. When the patient makes a mistake, she can be gently reminded of the correct answer; for example 'Remember you had fish for lunch, it's the afternoon now'.

Other tactics when working with delusional patients are to distract them by changing the subject from the delusion or to ignore the content of what has been said and react to how they are feeling.

Ward reality orientation clues are clocks, calendars, and signs. They should be large, clear, simple, accurate and legible from a distance. Patients feel more secure if they can see the signpost to the lavatory or dining room from the sitting room, and are more likely to remain mobile and independent.

When the therapist uses treatment activities she must always try to use reality orientation techniques which combine use of all senses. Some examples are:

— *Olfactory*: smelling flowers, perfumes, onions, oranges, coffee
— *Visual: looking at photographs, cuttings from magazines, collages, colours*
— *Auditory*: hearing tape recordings, music, records
— *Tactile*: touching sand, soil, leaves, flour, clothes, wood, coal
— *Gastatory*: tasting food they have cooked, distinguishing between different tastes, sweet, sour, salt and so forth
— *Kinesthetic/vestibular*: throwing, catching, bending, stretching, leaning in different directions.

Using reality orientation techniques stimulates patients to think and makes them more cheerful and co-operative, better oriented and motivated. Willson (1984) reports 'from the evidence and experience of using this form of treatment it appears to work best in behav- ioural retraining and combatting depressive withdrawals'.

Suggested occupational therapy timetable for continuing care patients

9–10	Washing and dressing practice for those patients who still wish to attempt these personal activities, most require some physical help or prompting.
11.00–11.15	Reality orientation
11.15–12.00	Intellectual activity
2.00– 3.00	Social and/or physical activity
3.00– 4.00	Domestic activity

ACTIVITIES

These are chosen to stimulate patients' inter- ests. They offer patients the chance to make decisions, to maintain previous skills or to talk about them; they answer peoples' needs to make friends, to be competitive, to communi- cate, to remember, to maintain self-esteem. Most equipment is inexpensive and usually modified by the occupational therapist and helpers to suit their patients' needs. Some expensive items are required, for example a microphone and amplifier to reach deaf group members.

Activities are generally divided into intellec- tual, physical, social, domestic and personal, but most combine two or three of these descriptions.

Intellectual activities

These tend to be for smaller quieter groups to help improve concentration.

Discussion groups. Topics are chosen by the patients. The occupational therapist acts as chairman, to encourage the quieter people to air their views and keep the noisy ones from monopolising the discussion.

Newspaper and news awareness (Fig. 13.2) The therapist or one of the patients will read out a news item which stimulates discussion about things past or present.

Quizzes can be organised with patients in ward teams for competition, and so that those who have difficulty in replying can refer to

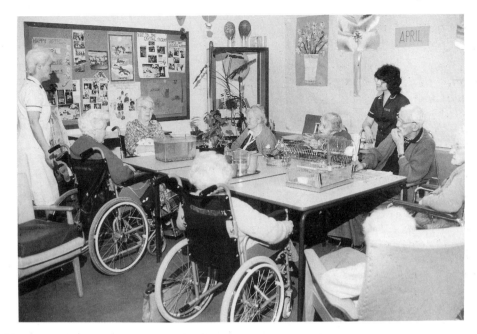

Fig. 13.2 Newspaper and news awareness group

their team for the answer. Alternatively the occupational therapist can pitch her questions to suit patients' various levels of intellect, in order to obtain a response.

Crosswords (Fig. 13.3) are drawn on a large grid and as clues are guessed, the words are filled in by the therapist. This also acts as a discussion group as each response must be

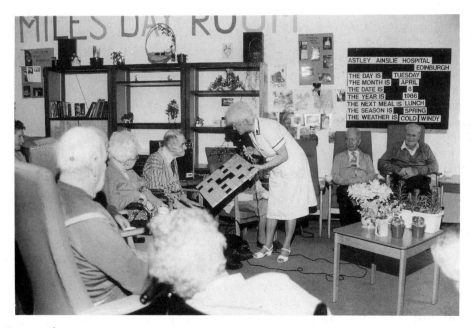

Fig. 13.3 Crossword group

commented upon and positive feedback given to patients for attempting to provide the correct answer.

Physical activities

These are usually carried out with large groups of patients and plenty of helpers.

Skittles are played with plastic skittles and beanbags. The patients are seated in a circle and have to knock over as many of the 9 skittles as possible — they are given three throws. They have to try and remember their scores but there should be an official scorer to avoid arguments.

The games of beetle, Aunt Sally and quoits can be adapted in a similar way for exercise, competition and numerical capability.

Music and movement is a lively activity requiring many helpers to remind patients what the current movement is. This exercises all muscles and patients have to concentrate in order to keep up with therapists and helpers showing them what to do.

Simon says is another way of exercising and getting patients to concentrate on which movement should be performed.

Dancing is an excellent exercise for mobile elderly patients.

Unihock is a two team hockey game using plastic sticks; alternatively rolled up newspapers can be used. Two teams sit opposite each other and try to hit the ball to one end or the other to score goals. This is very stimulating and an excellent way to work off excess energy.

Walks with a purpose are popular but only active patients or a few in wheelchairs can be taken. To give the walk a purpose, flowers for pressing can be gathered. These can be used in a reality orientation group or as part of a collage.

Social activities for large groups

Bingo is one of the most popular board games in continuing care wards. Bingo cards are made of firm white card, with numbers and grid drawn in indelible pen (black shows up best for the partially sighted). Small squares of paper are used to cover the numbers so that the cards can be reused frequently.

Parties, seasonal or birthday, are enjoyed by the whole ward, as are film shows and concerts organised by local entertainers. A good example of a party which alerts all patients' special senses is a Burns supper to commemorate the birth of the poet Robert Burns, born on 25th January. Singing and percussion bands are enjoyed by most elderly people. Dysphasics often gain great relief when banging a tambourine or shaking a maraca! It is best to use a record in the background to provide the beat and melody.

Social activities for small groups

Collage making (Figs. 13.4 & 13.5) can use current themes such as St Valentine, Easter, Christmas, royal event, gardens, historical event.

Charades, play reading and poetry recitals can be organised for those with a special interest in drama.

Bus outings to concerts, museums, parks, shops and exhibitions can be arranged. Often these visits can be commemorated by making a montage from photographs and programmes or a collage from Polystyrene. card, paper, paint, cartons, egg boxes and so forth.

Domestic activities for small groups

Well-known previous skills can be practised by two or three patients together:

1. Washing a few personal items
2. Baking for friends
3. Making marmalade, jam or chutney
4. Home-made wine or beer
5. Polishing shoes
6. Mending clothes
7. Watering plants
8. Planting cuttings or gardening using window boxes or waist high borders to avoid stooping. In summer this is a good outside activity.

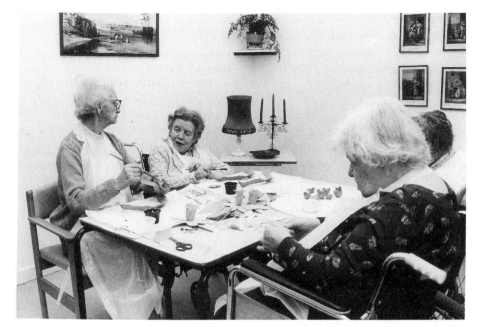

Fig. 13.4 Making a collage

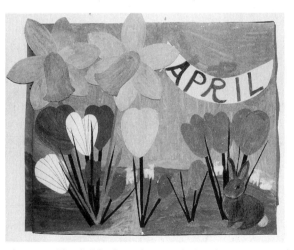

Fig. 13.5 The finished product ready for display

A person's spiritual side should also be fostered. Sunday services are very important to many people in continuing care wards. The opportunity to discuss death and the after-life should be freely given, and not just with a clergyman. This could be one of the subjects chosen for a discussion group.

The help of patients' relatives and of volunteers is most welcome when planning fund-raising events or ward entertainments. They are also a boon if they offer to push wheelchairs when taking patients for walks or accompany them on bus outings with therapists. There are relatives who enjoy helping out with several activities in the full treatment programme organised for continuing care patients. Relatives are often pleased to supply any extra materials, books and scrap items for collages.

Personal activities for small groups

Ladies have more scope for this but men can join in a few:

1. Trimming nails and/or manicuring them
2. Skin care, and make up sessions
3. Hairdressing/barber.

CONCLUSION

Occupational therapists working with chronically disabled patients have to be realistic about treatment limitations. Progress is not immediately apparent but with daily stimulation, gradual small improvements can be noted, the end result is a happier, livelier and more contented group of patients.

REFERENCES

Cornish P M 1983 Activitiies of the frail aged. Winslow Press, Winslow

Cutler Lewis S 1981 The mature years. Chas B Black, Thorofare, NJ, USA

Harris A 1971 Handicapped and impaired in Great Britain. HMSO, London

Holden V P, Woode R T 1984 Reality orientation. Churchill Livingstone, Edinburgh

Paire J A, Karney R J 1984 The effectiveness of sensory stimulation for geropsychiatric in patients. American Journal of Occupational Therapy 38:(8)

Shaw M W 1984 the challenge of ageing. Churchill Livingstone, Edinburgh

Shepperd G 1984 Institutional care and rehabilitation. Longmans, London

Trevan–Hawks J 1985 Occupational therapy and the role of leisure. British Journal of Occupational Therapy 48(10)

Willson M 1983 Occupational therapy in long-term psychiatry. Churchill Livingstone, Edinburgh

14

Urinary incontinence

N. Hood

INTRODUCTION

Incontinence of urine is not a life-threatening condition. Its emergencies and disasters do not involve ambulance dashes through the night or admission to intensive care units. It brings no drama — only shame and embarrassment. Its consequences to the well-being and independence of the sufferer are none the less calamitous and its demands on health care resources enormous (over £36 million was spent by the NHS on equipment for incontinence in 1981).

Perhaps the lack of glamour surrounding the management of uncertain urinary control explains the general reluctance among all types of caring professionals to come to grips with the problem. Little formal teaching on the subject is given to occupational therapists, physiotherapists, nurses or doctors in training. Thus many doctors feel that it is not a problem with which they should involve themselves. There still exist therapy departments where the strongest conviction felt about incontinence is that its presence is an automatic bar to attendance in the department.

At any age the onset of incontinence is a personal disaster. In the school child the fear of ridicule is ever present. She is often unable to join in games or to stay overnight with friends. The teenager finds the prospect of joining in active sports which take her into communal changing rooms daunting. School camps and later university halls of residence create obvious problems. The young adult may find it difficult to form relationships with the opposite sex, to hold down a job or to keep lodgings. A study of homeless young adults found that urinary incontinence was a frequent factor in forcing them onto the streets. The middle-aged individual with a problem of incontinence becomes more and more isolated, and to the elderly the onset of incontinence may herald the final loss of independence.

INCONTINENCE AND OCCUPATIONAL THERAPY

It is surprising that the discipline of occupational therapy has not become more involved in dealing with incontinence, since it can be argued that, in theory, retraining towards continence most appropriately lies with this discipline.

Continence depends on two distinct abilities of the lower urinary tract. Firstly the bladder is required to hold large volumes of urine without discomfort, and secondly it is required to void all or part of that volume at will. This is at its most developed in territorial mammals where urine is held and voided in small quantities to mark boundaries. With the development of social integration among higher mammals, territorial disputes receded and the need to conserve urine for marking diminished. As a consequence they have become indiscriminate in their voiding and are in effect incontinent. Thus the higher primates which build rudimentary shelters, move on and build afresh when soiling makes their home uninhabitable.

In the human the restraints of clothing and permanent housing have made continence advantageous once again. So the human infant is forced to learn a physiological trick which has been rejected by its immediate evolutionary predecessors. Continence then can be regarded as an activity of daily living of the same degree of sophistication as dressing or cooking. It is thus in the sphere of concern of the occupational therapist. By the same token, because it is a newly acquired art and dependent on very high levels of cerebral function, it is vulnerable to damage from a wide variety of aetiological factors, many of a seemingly trivial nature.

THE SIZE OF THE PROBLEM

Incontinence is a hidden problem. It is no more talked about in polite society today than it was in Victorian days. Few people boast of their bladder problems at cocktail parties. Even when a patient brings herself to speak about the problem, her doctor may be less than willing to listen because of embarrassment and a sense of therapeutic impotence. The public has a very low expectation of medical intervention in incontinence and this means that there is little incentive to report the problem. With particular regard to the elderly, all too often incontinence is viewed as an expected concomitant of ageing and quietly accepted. These factors combine to make incontinence a problem associated with low levels of self-reporting at all ages.

Two studies, one on each side of the Atlantic, have been carried out amongst nulliparous female college students between 18 and 30 years of age with almost identical results. 52% admitted to a urinary leak at some time in their lives. Almost 17% claimed it happened at least once per day. Although it is likely that many of these girls had very slight problems, it is significant that the percentage of them with daily problems is extremely close to the known incidence of stress incontinence in middle aged and elderly woman.

Several studies have suggested a high incidence of incontinence in late middle aged and elderly people living at home (Table 14.1). Over 30% of patients admitted to geriatric hospitals are incontinent at the time of admission (compared with 8% of over 65-year olds admitted to general medical wards).

Two facts are certain. Firsty, there is a high incidence of unrecognised incontinence in

Table 14.1 Incontinence in the elderly living in the community (All figures %)

	Sheldon (1984)	Brocklehurst (1968)	Milne (1972)	Thomas (1980)
Male	7	17	25	7
Female	13	23	42	12

the ageing population of our country. Secondly, if all cases were identified we do not have the resources to meet their needs.

ANATOMY AND PHYSIOLOGY

Although it is customary to consider the bladder and urethra separately, they are, in fact, one muscular organ and in health act as a co-ordinated unity.

Bladder

The bladder (detrusor) has three muscular coats. They are closely intertwined throughout most of its substance, but around the bladder neck separate into an inner longitudinal, a middle circular, and an outer longitudinal coat. The longitudinal coats continue downwards to form the urethra while the middle forms the internal closure mechanism.

The triangular area bounded by the two ureteric orifices and the urethra is called the trigone and is the most sensitive part of the bladder.

Urethra

Female

In the female the urethra is a canal 3–5 cm in length. It is closely related to the vagina, especially towards the external meatus.

Male

The male urethra is an 'S' shaped tube 20 cm in length, passing through the substance of

the prostate, the urogenital diaphragm and the erectile tissue of the penis.

Structural supports

Like all pelvic organs the bladder rests on the levator ani muscles which are comprised of two main muscle groups, the pubococcygens and iliococcygens. In the female the bladder neck and proximal urethra are supported by two strong ligaments attached to the pelvic bone, the anterior and posterior pubovesical ligaments. The bladder neck in the male is more firmly fixed by its attachment to the prostate gland, and the puboprostatic ligaments.

Urethral closure mechanisms

Early anatomists described an internal urethral sphincter near the bladder and this has given rise to much confused thinking. There is no evidence of any intrinsic urethral structure more adapted to closure than the rest of the organ. The circular fibres holding the bladder neck closed have already been mentioned but they do not pass down into the urethra.

Three components are thought to play some part in the inherent closure properties of the urethra:

1. Intrinsic smooth muscle tone
2. The turgor of the abundant blood vessel network within the substance
3. The exuberance and sponginess of the folds of mucosa and submucosa.

The resting tone of the muscle fibres is, of course, under autonomic neurological control. It is of interest to note that all three components are in varying degree affected by the circulating levels of oestrogen and this in part is responsible for the increased incidence of micturition problems in women of post-menopausal years.

The external urethral sphincter consists of striated muscle under voluntary control. It surrounds the middle third of the female urethra and the membranous part of the male urethra. It is normally relaxed, and acts as a secondary defence mechanism brought into play only during emergencies. It is the muscle group which allows the small boy to cross his 'Ts' and dot his 'Is' when writing his name in the snow and allows the adult to interrupt the flow midstream.

Innervation

The main motor supply to the bladder is parasympathetic, and leaves the spinal cord from segments S2–4.

The two important sensory modalities in the bladder are proprioception and pain. Proprioception consists mainly as an appreciation of stretch. Pain is a reflection of extreme stretch or inflammation.

CAUSES OF INCONTINENCE

Neurological

The various levels at which neurological control of micturition may be affected are shown Figure 14.1.

a. Frontal lobe

The deterioration in social habits and self-care resulting from high neurological damage will produce loss of urinary control.

b. Cerebral cortex

The stroke patient may be wet because although she has reasonable urinary control she cannot rise and go to the toilet unaided. She may be concerned that a request to be taken will only increase the work-load of the already busy nurses. She may, on the other hand, be desperate to tell the nurse that she wants to go but because of dysphasia or dysarthria is unable to convey her needs. All staff in the ward must be alert to both situations.

It is also likely that her bladder control has been affected and that she will have detrusor contractions with little warning. With regular toileting and active rehabilitation, incontinence should settle within three months in

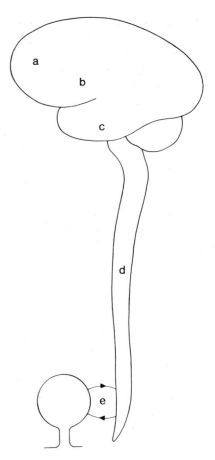

Fig. 14.1 Neurological levels of incontinence: (a) frontal lobe, (b) cerebral cortex, (c) basal ganglion, (d) cord damage, (e) peripheral nerves

almost all stroke patients who are intellectually preserved. Indeed, return to continence may be a sensitive indicator of the efficiency of the early stages of stroke rehabilitation. It should not need to be said that the careless insertion of an indwelling catheter in the early days of rehabilitation may ensure incontinence for the rest of the patient's life.

c. Basal ganglion

There can be few conditions more calculated to produce incontinence than parkinsonism. The sufferer takes an age to reach the toilet and, when there is poor manual dexterity, she is very slow to arrange her clothes to allow micturition. A normal bladder would be hard pushed to cope. Very few parkinsonian patients have normal bladders. An almost invariable component of the autonomic neuropathy associated with the disease is detrusor involvement. The most common manifestation is a hyperactive bladder. No more certain recipe for disaster can be imagined than an urgent bladder in a pathologically slow body. However, in around 10% of parkinsonian patients, at cystometry an atonic bladder is found. Incontinence is caused by overspill from an overfull bladder but the symptoms may be indistinguishable from urgency. Only proper investigation will give the clue to appropriate management.

d. Cord damage

Trauma to the cord, although all too common in young adults, is a rare cause of bladder dysfunction in the elderly where multiple sclerosis and cord tumour (often benign) are commoner problems. The pattern of incontinence is one of involuntary emptying around a set volume of bladder filling. In some cases of multiple sclerosis, other micturition mechanisms are involved and voiding is also problematic.

e. Peripheral nerves

Involvement of the nervous connections between the bladder and the sacral micturition centre will produce a poorly reactive large capacity bladder which fails to empty efficiently and will eventually lead to overflow incontinence. The classic textbook cause of syphilitic tabes dorsalis is now rarely if ever seen. A much commoner cause is the autonomic neuropathy of diabetes mellitus. Around 25% of established diabetics have a measurable tendency to bladder atonicity. They are already compromised with regard to continence because of the increased urine production associated with hyperglycaemia, and any disturbance of micturition mechanisms will quickly lead to incontinence.

General

a. Excess urine production

In a normal individual this will not lead to incontinence, but where continence is precarious it may be enough to tip the balance. While organic causes such as diabetes mellitus and insipidus should not be forgotten, by far the most common reason for problematic polyuria is prescribed diuretics. Most elderly individuals on diuretics have frequency. Many have learned not to take them on days when they have engagements. Although most are incapacitated only during morning hours it should be appreciated that in the presence of moderate renal impairment the effect of a so-called short-acting diuretic may last throughout the whole day and night.

Most prescriptions of diuretics given to the elderly are unnecessary and carry considerable risks. Each individual case should be scrutinised to see if a better alternative exists. For example, dependent oedema of ankles and calves is most appropriately managed with the use of support stockings and increased activity.

b. Mental state

There are two alterations in mental state which predispose to incontinence:

1. Clouding of consciousness
2. Confusion.

1. Clouding of consciousness. Many medical conditions can produce clouding of consciousness and in that state the patient is likely to be incontinent Obviously the correct management of the underlying problem will tend to bring a return of continence. In the elderly, inappropriate drug therapy is a common cause of drowsiness. The problems associated with sedative drugs are readily apparent but it must be realised that drugs which seem to have no direct effect on the central nervous system are at times implicated as a cause of drowsiness or confusion.

2. Confusion. The causes and implications of acute confusional states and irreversible mental deterioration are dealt with elsewhere. It is clear that if an old person is too disorientated or forgetful to manage other basic activities of daily living, she is unlikely to keep herself dry. At that level the widely conceived correlation between mental deterioration and incontinence is observed. Some further thought, however, must be given to this relationship. It is too easy to lump dementia and incontinence together, adopting a circular argument. 'If she is demented she will be incontinent If she is incontinent she must be demented'. Looking at every new referral to a geriatric service no correlation was found between incontinence and mental state. There is a small group who are incontinent because they are confused and forgetful. The majority of elderly incontinent patients are, like their younger counterparts, ordinary people who are wet. Their incontinence is as embarrassing and as incapacitating at 80 as it would have been at 40. The last thing they need is to have their incontinence paraded as the first sign of decrepitude.

c. Physical state

In any disabled population there will be a group who are regularly wet, not because of any urinary problem but because their disability prevents them reaching the toilet or arranging their clothes in time. Both in hospital and at home they depend on good occupational therapy to ensure that the environment is conducive to continence and that their garments suit their disability.

d. Psychological state

There are three accepted psychodynamic pathways to secondary enuresis (i.e. loss of established bladder control):

1. Regression
2. Sensory deprivation
3. Rebellion.

1. Regression to an earlier stage of development is a response which is accepted as important in enuresis among school children

subjected to stress. It has been suggested that regression as a reaction to the physical and emotional stresses of old age may explain some cases of incontinence. Everyone involved in the care of the elderly, for every example of 'spontaneous' regression can identify several whose regression is a response to 'mothering' by family or ward staff. It is a maxim of rehabilitation that the level gained must be maintained. The individual who today struggled to the toilet and was dry will be wet tomorrow if a commode is brought to her bedside.

2. Sensory deprivation. Healthy teenage volunteers kept in a sound-proof grey room with no extrinsic stimulation become incontinent within a few days. Prisoners of war in solitary confinement became incontinent. Too many of our old folks live in their own 'grey rooms' at home or in hospital and surrender to apathy. One of the most fundamental observations in the literature of long-stay care is that the level of incontinence in an institution fell in whichever ward the painters were working at the time.

3. Rebellion. Political prisoners with few mechanisms of protest available to them have been known to use their excreta to further their cause. It has been suggested that the elderly do likewise on occasions, using incontinence, in a manipulative way. To suggest that this is a common situation would be to underestimate the inventiveness of the human mind and the opportunities for devious behaviour open to the elderly. Few need to sit uncomfortably in cold wet clothes to get their own way. Incontinencc should only very rarely be regarded as volitional.

e. Local causes

Urethra and bladder neck

(i) Outlet obstruction. In the elderly male, benign prostatic enlargement frequently leads to outlet obstruction and secondary detrusor instability which produces urge incontinence. Occasionally in women, outlet obstruction leads to similar problems. In both cases

surgery to relieve the obstruction may cure the incontinence, but of course the rare complication of bladder neck incompetence leading to stress leakage must be borne in mind.

(ii) Stress incontinence.

Involuntary urinary leak of a stress type occurs to some degree in every woman from early adulthood onwards. Although there is some increase in incidence among multiparous women, pelvic floor weakness is not always related to childbirth. Indeed the incidence is the same in nulliparous women and those of modest parity. The stimulus required to produce the leak may vary from a slight change in the sitting position to violent exercise or prolonged coughing. The increased popularity of exercise programmes such as aerobic dancing has increased the referral rates to incontinence clinics in women of all ages. The majority of these women have no problem at any other time but are right to present early since at that stage the weakness is liable to be easily reversible.

Bladder

Anything which irritates the sensory receptors in the bladder will tend to increase detrusor excitability and will lead to urinary urgency and eventually to urge incontinence. Perhaps the most striking example is the bladder stone which is in regular traumatic contact with the trigone. A commoner cause is bacterial inflammation of the bladder wall or of the tissues beyond the vesico-ureteric junction. The acute cystitis or pyelonephritis thus caused is associated with urgency which may produce incontinence.

This does not mean that every patient with a positive urine culture will be incontinent or that, conversely, treating asymptomatic bacteriuria in an incontinent patient will change the incontinence in any way. About 25% of elderly women admitted to hospital will have a positive MSSU. The majority will have no urinary symptoms. By no means all with bacteriuria will be incontinent and some of those with sterile urine will be. There is no certainty that in those who have bacteriuria and are wet, rendering the urine sterile will improve continence. Indeed the only conclusion that can be drawn is that, if there are no symptoms of cystitis or pyelitis, treatment of bacteriuria is irrational, unlikely to produce benefit and needlessly introduces the not inconsiderable problems of antibiotic side-effects.

MANAGEMENT OF INCONTINENCE

Assessment

The first essential of successful management is a comprehensive assessment. A clear picture of the extent of the problem and its pattern will be gained from a clear and detailed history. The following twelve questions may serve as guidelines:

1. How long have you had this problem?
2. Was the onset sudden?
3. When does the leak occur? Day/night/both.
4. Do you have pain or discomfort when passing urine?
5. Do you wet yourself without being aware of your bladder being full?
6. Is the leak a little or a lot?
7. Do you have a leak when you cough, sneeze or on exertion?
8. Do you have difficulty starting the stream?
9. Do you dribble after passing urine?
10. Do you have a feeling of urgency?
11. How much warning do you get?
12. What wakens you at night? Desire/wet bed.

An attempt should be made to quantify the problem objectively by charting the events of a few days. The most successful way to do this is to keep accurate charts (Fig.14.2). Only in this way will a true picture emerge. This detailed display of the day's events will in some cases be enough to enable the patient to deal with the problem herself. It will also serve as the ground plan on which rational management is built.

For those whose problem is mainly nocturnal a clock and pad trial may be of use. This is a

LONGMORE HOSPITAL

CONTINENCE ASSESSMENT

Name._____

TOILETING REGIME

— NO

✓ YES

Date	Time	Pad Wet	Clothing / Bed Wet	Did Patient ask or for Toilet	Routine Toileting	Did Patient pass urine	Signature

Fig. 14.2 Continence assessment

variation of the bell and pad system so beloved of paediatricians. Rather than have the patient subjected to the noxious stimulus of the ringing bell, the device uses the voiding episode to stop the clock. After a few nights the pattern will be discernible and the patient or carer may be trained to anticipate the event. Rising at a particular hour may be enough to maintain continence.

In most instances the problems will have been elucidated by this stage, but if they have not, referral should be made to a specialist unit for further investigations of which the most useful is cystometry — the measurement of the bladder's pressure responses to filling and voiding.

Design toward continence

Most hospitals could have been designed to produce incontinence. On the day of admission the patient, confused and frightened, has been subjected to some of the most embarrassing hours of her life. The young doctor has gone at last and she would like to visit the toilet. Where is it? In public places toilets are clearly signposted. In hotels and restaurants they are marked with simple symbols on the doors. Not so in hospitals. Victorian reticence is the order of the day. Modern hospitals are particularly difficult. The toilet is behind one of perhaps six identical doors with no identifying marker. It should be a simple matter to identify routes to toilets in a clear fashion.

It has been arbitrarily decided that the maximum accepted distance an old person can be expected to walk to a toilet is 30 feet (over three times the greatest distance in a sheltered house). Two thirds of geriatric units have beds more than 40 feet from a toilet. We need more readily accessible toilets, also chairs and beds from which the elderly can rise quickly to respond to a call of nature.

An old person with urge incontinence will regularly be wet in the toilet if she has to struggle with several layers of under-garments. She should be encouraged to wear as few lower garments as possible and those worn should be able to be easily and quickly arranged. Some general statements may be made. Loose garments are easier to manage than tight fitting ones. Buttons should be as large as possible. For some, toggles will be more manageable. Zips, if essential, should be long with an adequate tab to pull. Velcro is extremely useful and is better in short rather than in long strips.

Men may find 'Edgeware' trousers useful. They have an extended fly. Some may prefer trousers with Velcro fastenings at the front. If shirt tails are shortened they are less likely to become wet. For women, wrap-round skirts and night-dresses with French knickers or suspender belts and stockings make a combination that can be managed quickly. Suggestions for further reading are given on page 158.

Working with the patient

Many of the causes of incontinence discussed earlier will require specific intervention which may be surgical or based on drug therapy. The details are outwith the scope of this book and will not be considered further. However, the general principles of approach to the problem are important to all.

First, a word about the newly admitted hospital patient: she is embarrassed about her problem and may feel that her difficulties are unique. All geriatricians see patients who are reluctant to come to hospital because they have always coped with incontinence by themselves and are reluctant to have others involved. She must be set at ease by considerate staff who do not appear to underestimate the enormity of the problem in the patient's mind but who calmly accept it and can promise practical help. She should be shown where the toilets are and should find out how long it takes to reach them. It should be made clear that not asking to be toileted is liable to result in more rather than less work for the nurses, who will not mind as long as the request is made when the need is first felt. If a patient has used a bedside commode for years she should have a commode in the same situation beside her bed. Bed and commode should be at the height of her bed at home. Lastly, it is an unforgivable insult to human dignity to expect voiding in anything but complete visual, auditory or olefactory privacy.

Bladder retraining

Although frequent toileting is regarded as important in the management of incontinence, it must be realised that while this may maintain dryness it will do nothing to restore normal bladder function. We must not be surprised when an old woman who has been dry in hospital where the nurses have taken her to the toilet every hour, is wet when she returns to live on her own. At any age the problem of urge incontinence is worsened by the tendency to go to the toilet as soon as urge presents. The patient ends up a slave to the urges of her bladder. Fortunately, as soon as she has emptied her bladder she begins again to feel the urge to go. At this point the appropriate intervention is bladder retraining.

Bladder retraining (sometimes referred to as bladder drill) is often done under hospital supervision but may just as easily be done at home by a co-operative patient. In the first instance she empties her bladder at short regular intervals (usually every hour) but not between times. A safe garment is worn to deal with any involuntary voiding. Once this interval is mastered, i.e. when she can empty by the clock every hour and is dry in between, the intervals are gradually lengthened until two hours is reached. At this point reasonable bladder control will have returned and she is encouraged to forget about her bladder and resume normal living. This procedure is designed to bring detrusor function under volitional control and is akin to infantile toilet training. It has been shown to be at least as effective as drug therapy in dealing with detrusor instability.

Pelvic floor exercises

In the early stages of stress incontinence the type of exercises taught at antenatal classes may be enough to restore sphincteric control and should be tried in all cases. The following instructions should be give to the patient:

1. Sit, stand or lie comfortably, without tensing the muscles of the seat, abdomen or legs, and pretend you are trying to control diarrhoea by tightening the ring muscle round the back passage. Do this several times until you feel certain that you have identified the area and are making the correct movement.

2. Sit on the lavatory or commode and begin to pass water and while doing so make an attempt to stop the flow in mid-stream by contracting the muscles round the front passage. Do this several times until you feel sure of the movement, and of the sensation of applying conscious control.

3. Exercise as follows: sitting, standing, or lying, tighten first the back passage muscles and then the front, and then both together. Count four slowly, and then release the muscles. Do this four times, repeating the whole sequence once every hour if possible. With practice the movements should be quite easy to master and the exercises can be carried out at any time — while waiting for a bus, standing at the sink, watching television or lying comfortably in bed.

Remember that these must be carried out daily for at least two or three months as frequently as possible.

AIDS

While hospital-based services have access to an acceptably wide range of aids for incontinence, the availability of aids and services in the community varies from area to area. There is a statutory requirement placed on all local authorities to provide a removal service for soiled disposables, but only permissive legislation applies to the provision of a disposables delivery service or community laundry service. The occupational therapist should be familiar with the services available in her own area.

Commodes

In many areas the supply of commodes in the community is undertaken by the NHS and voluntary organisations. Occasionally those supplied by local voluntary groups are old fashioned and quite unsuitable for disabled patients. The occupational therapist should be involved in selecting the most suitable model for the individual patient. A commode which is rigidly fixed to the bed is often of considerable advantage to the patient who needs a hand-hold when rising. If a commode is necessary in the living room it need not be the focal point in the room but should rather be screened. The task of emptying the commode can often be left to a relative. It is not an agreed duty of a home help. When no one is available to perform this task on a daily basis a chemical lavatory will enable the district nurse to cope on twice weekly visits.

Many men will manage with a bottle type of urinal which should be fitted with a non-return valve. A considerable amount of apparent incontinence at home and in hospital will be prevented by this inexpensive non-spill adaptation. Soft polythene, flat-fold versions are now available and are invaluable for car or train journeys.

At present the available female equivalents are varients of the narrow St Peters Boat receptacle or the Feminal which consists of a rigid close fitting vulval mould with disposable collecting bags. Both types of devices can be used in the sitting or supine position.

ROLE OF THE OCCUPATIONAL THERAPIST

Continence is as important as all the other activities of daily living and because of its embarrassing nature is one that has to be handled in a sensitive manner. The patient should never be made to feel inferior or disgusting, and cleaning up following an accident should be carried out in an efficient, matter-of-fact way — a normal part of an occupational therapist's work with elderly people.

Hospital occupational therapist

Nurses are normally the first to be aware that a new patient has an incontinence problem. When patients are referred for occupational therapy, medical and psychological symptoms are normally listed on the referral card from the doctor, but sensory deficits and incontinence are not necessarily mentioned unless very obvious, e.g. blind, stone deaf.

In hospital, provision of incontinence aids and charting of incontinence episodes are the nurse's main concern. Nevertheless, the occupational therapist must be aware of any continence programme instigated by nurses; for example, if the policy is to take a patient to the WC every two hours and that time scale falls when the patient is in the occupational therapy department the policy must be implemented. During dressing practice it is essential for the occupational therapist to check that the patient is able to use her incontinence aids efficiently. Very often a patient with limited hand function is supposed to be able to fit a Kangapad into the tight pouch of the pants and this is found to be impossible. The occupational therapist should mention the problem to the ward sister so that an alternative, e.g. Maxi pads and pants, can be prescribed. Another common dressing problem which arises is a patient's inability to put on the small stretchy pants normally supplied with Maxi pads. She may have a recent fractured neck of femur, osteoarthritis or simply be too obese to reach her feet. A helping hand to get the pants over the feet sometimes works or a suggestion that the patient wear more voluminous pants. The knicker leg elastic of these should be loose or absent for added efficiency in dressing. Men with similar problems should be advised to wear boxer shorts/underpants instead or jockey or long john variety.

As has been mentioned, urodoms and leg drainage bags are efficient and discrete urinary incontinence aids for men. Very often it is the occupational therapist who has to show the wearer how to apply the aid and how to use the valve for periodic emptying of urine.

Community occupational therapy

As it is the hospital nurses's preserve, advice on incontinence at home is the district nurse or health visitor's task. Occasionally an occupational therapist will be referred a client who is unknown to community nurses. In this case she should refer her to the general practitioner who will ask the appropriate nurse to call. The general practitioner after careful assessment will prescribe pads for the type of incontinence described, i.e. stress, or dribbling. If the old lady is not being treated by a community physiotherapist and if home physiotherapy treatment is too hard to come by, the community occupational therapist should suggest pelvic floor exercises, as described in this chapter, and give a written hand-out so that regular practice can be started.

Bedside commodes for women and bottle type urinals with spill-proof non-return valves are useful incontinence aids at home. They also lessen the chance of old people falling on the way to the WC during the night.

Continual urinary incontinence at home is usually the last straw that breaks a carer's back. The community occupational therapist must be aware of local incontinence laundry facilities and of the most efficient aids to incontinence and who supplies them, and instigate these services as soon as possible.

Mobility is sometimes the cause of incontinence, therefore the community occupational therapist should check height of chair, height of bed etc., in case the old person has difficulty getting up to go to toilet. Assess for mobility aids, toilet aids, commode (for daytime use, bedside chair). For information on suitable clothing and clothing adaptations, see Chapter 19.

SOURCES OF FURTHER INFORMATION

1. Association of Continence Advisors (ACA)

This is a comparatively recently formed association whose members are drawn from various disciplines involved in the management of incontinence. It exists to provide a forum for discussion and information, sharing all aspects of the practical management.

It has two extremely useful and comprehensive directories of aids and equipment for incontinence. These can be obtained from:

> A.C.A. Secretary
> c/o Disabled for Living Foundation
> 380–384 Harrow Road
> LONDON W9 2HU

2. Aid centres

— Disabled Living Foundation, 380-384 Harrow Road, London.
— Newcastle Upon Tyne Council for the Disabled, Mea House, Ellison Place, Newcastle Upon Tyne, NE 1 8XS.
— Disabled Living Centre, 84 Suffolk Street, Birmingham B1.
— Merseyside Aids Centre, Youens Way, East Brescott Road, Liverpool 14.
— Scottish Information Service for the Disabled, Claremont House, 18–19 Claremont Crescent, Edinburgh, EH7 4RD.
— Aid Centre, Astley Ainslie Hospital, Grange Loan, Edinburgh, EH9 2HL

3. Useful reading

Mandelstam D 1977 Incontinence. Heinemann Health Books, London
Ruston R 1977 Dressing for disabled people. Disabled Living Foundation, London

15

Drug problems

R. G. Smith

INTRODUCTION

The annual bill for drugs prescribed in the United Kingdom is now in excess of £500 million. Over 60% of the total population receive at least one prescription per year, but over 75% of the over-75-year-olds are prescribed drugs (Skegg et al 1977) — two thirds of them are taking between one and three drugs and one third four or more.

Repeat prescriptions are commonly given to the elderly and this often causes problems. General practitioners are under considerable pressure to prescribe for the elderly for various reasons — the increasing number of elderly people in the population, a tendency for old people to present with a multiplicity of complaints and symptoms, and families demanding that 'something has to be done'. Because of the social and psychological stresses on the elderly they may consult their general practitioner with ill-defined recurring symptoms.

There is a tendency amongst doctors to expect the patient to want a prescription, but often the patient, and particularly the elderly patient, would more appropriately be 'treated' by a sympathetic or reassuring word or by being allowed to talk through her problem. Various studies have shown that approximately 85% of the over-65-year-olds are taking medicines regularly, but about 15% had had no contact with their general practitioner for the past six months, i.e. they were having repeat prescriptions (Shaw & Opit 1976). 20% of patients discharged from hospital had not contacted their general practitioner by the end of the first month and many had returned to the drugs they were taking before their admission to hospital (Deacon et al 1978).

The common types of drug being consumed by elderly patients are diuretics, digoxin, analgesics and psychotropics which include the benzodiazepines such as diazepam. Sleeping tablets and laxatives are often taken by the elderly although many of them do not consider them as drugs but more a way of life.

Although prescribing is carried out by medical staff, the occupational therapist will almost certainly be involved in the compliance of prescribed drugs in the community. On home visits, questions may be asked of the occupational therapist about the drugs being taken, or difficulties of packaging and usage may come to light.

PHARMACOKINETICS

Any drug is absorbed into the blood stream, distributed around the body, metabolised and excreted. The effect of any drug is dependent on (i) the amount of 'free' drug in the blood and (ii) the sensitivity of the tissues or organs on which the drug is to act. There is evidence that elderly cells are more sensitive to the effects of drugs than those of younger patients. For example, morphine and barbiturates have a greater effect, dose for dose, on the elderly brain. The hypnotic nitrazepam has been shown to have a much longer effect on psychomotor function in the elderly patient than in the young when the same dose of 10 mg is given, despite plasma levels being the same (Castleden et al 1977). Therefore, when prescribing certain drugs a lower dose should be prescribed and the dosage increased slowly and in small increments until the desired effect is obtained.

Absorption

Most drugs taken orally are absorbed from the stomach or small bowel. With ageing there is a reduction in the blood flow to the cells, a reduction in the total number of cells, a reduction of the absorptive surface of the small bowel and a reduction in gastric acid; but despite these changes there is probably little change in absorption with age. More importantly, concomitant treatment may affect absorption. By giving a drug such as propantheline, which slows down gastric emptying, the absorption of digoxin, which is mainly absorbed in the stomach, is increased, thereby increasing the amount of free or bio-available drug in the plasma. This in turn may cause side-effects of nausea, vomiting and confusion even though a 'normal' dose of digoxin has been given. Conversely, by prescribing metoclopramide which speeds up gastric emptying, less digoxin is absorbed and the therapeutic effect is substantially less. Other examples of drug interaction affecting absorption are giving tetracycline with metal compounds such as iron or aluminium (in antacids) which form insoluble compounds with the tetracycline.

Distribution

With ageing there is an alteration in the main constituents of the body, which can affect the distribution of a drug. There is a reduction in the proportion of body water, which may lead to higher plasma concentrations of a drug. There is an increase in body fat, which may lead to a more protracted action of a lipid-soluble substance stored in fatty tissues. The decrease in the lean body mass in an elderly person leads to higher plasma levels, following similar doses, than in the younger person.

Many drugs, when they are absorbed into the plasma, are bound to albumen and are thus non-bioavailable. In any condition in which the plasma albumen falls, there is an increase in the proportion of drug which is free or bioavailable. It was previously thought that albumen levels fell with age, but we now know that it is only in ill elderly people that albumen levels are low. If two or more drugs are given, there may be competition for these albumen sites and more of one drug becomes bioavailable. For example, salicylate, which is highly bound, will free more of the anticoagulant warfarin, which is less highly bound. This has serious implications as an elderly patient may be stabilised on warfarin in hospital; she is then discharged and subsequently takes an aspirin for her headache or other pain. This frees more warfarin in the plasma, resulting in an increased likelihood of bleeding. Other patients who are at risk of the effects of albumen competition are diabetics stabilised on oral hypoglycaemic agents such as a sulphonamide.

Metabolism

Most drugs are metabolised in the liver. With age the liver mass is reduced as is its blood flow. The microsomal enzymes involved in drug metabolism become less efficient with an increase in plasma levels of certain drugs. Drug interaction occurs at this level and drugs such as phenothiazines, alcohol, barbiturates and phenytoin are powerful microsomal enzyme inducers, leading to increased metabolism of themselves and of other drugs being given concomitantly. For example, the combination of a phenothiazine with warfarin reduces the anticoagulant effect because of the increased metabolism of the warfarin. Similarly, phenothiazines with tricyclic antidepressants reduce the therapeutic effect of the tricyclic antidepressant for a standard dose. It may be thought that the drug is not working or that the diagnosis is wrong. Another danger occurs when an enzyme inducer substance is stopped and there is a rebound rise in the plasma level of the other drug, leading to possible adverse effects. Other drugs tend to inhibit hepatic metabolism, causing higher plasma levels of drugs being prescribed with them. Aspirin, for example, can increase the activity of other drugs such as tolbutamide and phenytoin, making the control of diabetes mellitus and epilepsy respectively more difficult. It is important to remember that aspirin is contained in many 'over-the-counter' preparations and

the patient's general practitioner may not be aware of this potential hazard. All of these effects are commoner in elderly patients because of poly-pharmacy.

Excretion

The kidney is involved in the excretion of most drugs and is subject to changes with increasing age. The glomerular filtration rate falls by 46% between youth and very old age and the renal blood flow by over 50% (Dawes & Shock 1950). The decline in renal function is due to loss of nephrons and not to loss of efficiency. As a result, the half-life of many drugs is increased in the elderly, causing increased plasma levels which may cause adverse effects. Digoxin has been shown to have a half-life of 51 hours in young adults and 73 hours in the over-80-year-olds (Ewy et al 1969). Plasma digoxin levels can be measured. The aminoglycoside antibiotics, lithium and chlorpropamide may lead to adverse effects in the elderly due to their capability of causing renal damage in standard doses. Renal excretion may vary from individual to individual and change suddenly when renal reserves are reduced. For example, after a myocardial infarction the renal clearance may be greatly reduced and a patient previously stable on a drug may suddenly experience toxic adverse effects.

ADVERSE EFFECTS

Almost every drug has the potential to cause adverse effects, but these effects are much more common in the elderly, especially in the very elderly. The incidence of adverse effects increases with age. In a multicentre study of elderly people admitted to geriatric departments in the UK, 15% of those taking prescribed drugs suffered adverse effects (Williamson & Chopin 1980). The commonest drugs prescribed were diuretics and analgesics. Diuretics were found to be the commonest cause of adverse effects, followed by psychotropic drugs, digoxin, hypnotics, analgesics, hypotensive agents and rigidity and tremor controllers. However, the risk associated with each drug is highest for hypotensive agents and rigidity and tremor controllers, and lowest for diuretics, hypnotics and analgesics. Adverse effects were commoner when an increasing number of drugs was taken. In 10.5% of the sample, adverse effects of drugs were the sole or contributing factors in the need for admission of the elderly person to hospital. Full recovery occurred in 68% of patients with adverse effects, but this varied depending on which drug was causing the effects. Digoxin had the highest recovery rate (80%) and rigidity and tremor controllers the lowest (46%). Extrapolating this study to the whole of the United Kingdom, about 4000 admissions to geriatric departments are solely due to adverse effects of drugs, and for another 11 000 patients drugs are a contributory factor. About 4500 will not make a full recovery from the adverse effects of drugs prescribed to them.

SPECIAL PROBLEMS

Certain drugs are commonly associated with problems in the elderly.

Digoxin

Digitalis preparations are often prescribed to elderly patients for heart conditions. It has been shown that 75% of elderly patients on digoxin on a long-term basis suffered no deterioration in their condition when it was withdrawn (Dall 1970). Digoxin used to be prescribed routinely in cases of cardiac failure but now is only recommended in cases of rapid atrial fibrillation with failure, or in paroxysmal supraventricular tachycardia. Lower dosages are recommended in the elderly but as has already been stated the effective dose depends on renal function in particular. Plasma digoxin levels can be measured and are helpful in finding the correct dose. The common adverse effects are nausea, vomiting and confusion.

Case history

Mrs C. F. was an 86-year-old widow living alone and looked after by a 5-day home help. She recently had become confused and paranoid, accusing her home help of poisoning her. She was on digoxin 0.25 mg twice daily. She was, in fact, being poisoned — by her GP, not her home help. Her mental state returned to normal on stopping the digoxin.

Diuretics

The speed of action of diuretic drugs is important in the elderly patient. Loop diuretics, such as frusemide, have a short half-life and cause a brisk diuresis within four hours. This is an effective way of reducing the fluid overload in cardiac failure, but in a frail elderly patient with mobility problems from osteoarthritis or stroke, urinary incontinence may occur before the toilet is reached. Males with prostatic hypertrophy may be precipitated into acute retention of urine, especially if an anticholinergic drug is being prescribed concomitantly. Potassium loss and postural hypotension leading to falls are other possible adverse effects of diuretics.

Case history

Mr R. T. was an 85-year-old, living on his own. He presented with recurrent falls and dizziness on getting out of bed. He was supposed to take frusemide, one tablet daily, and Slow K, three tablets per day. Due to his forgetfulness and the label on both bottles saying. 'Take as directed' he knew he had to take three of one but could not remember which one. He took three of each 'to be safe', and his symptoms of postural hypotension were relieved when he was taking only one frusemide tablet per day.

Psychotropic agents

These are widely and often unneccessarily prescribed.

a. Hypnotics

Hypnotics are grossly overprescribed in the elderly, with an increased demand with increasing age. Nearly 20% of the over-70-year-olds in the USA take a regular hypnotic. They tend to cause an exaggerated sedative effect which in turn impairs orientation, stability, mobility and continence. With age, the body requires less sleep and there is a loss of deeper sleep. Observed wakings increase from two in young people to over seven per night in the 75-year-old. There is an increased tendency to sleep during the day, which affects the length of sleep at night. Going to bed earlier means waking up earlier. It often helps to explain to an elderly person why she needs less sleep, and this may stop her taking sleeping tablets. Hypnotics suppress natural sleep and withdrawal of the hypnotic leads to rebound wakefulness and possible night-mares. Rather than prescribe hypnotics for difficulty in sleeping, it is much more appro-priate to investigate the cause of insomnia — pain, breathlessness, depression — and to treat the cause. Barbiturates are no longer recommended for elderly patients. Problems with addiction and difficulties in withdrawing the drug are two good reasons for this view. Falls and confusion were common adverse effects. Benzodiazepines are widely used in the elderly as hypnotics. The short-acting ones are recommended for use such as nitrazepam and temazepam. Nitrazepam is the common-est in use in Europe, but in some elderly patients there is a prolonged effect on psychomotor performance. The general guidelines for the use of a hypnotic agent are shown in Table 15.1.

Table 15.1 Guidelines for use of hypnotics

Limit use to exceptional times
Prescribe a specific dose
Begin with a small dose and increase slowly if necessary
Stop drug if day-time alertness is impaired
Avoid long-term dependence

Case history

Mrs C. McA. complained of waking at 2 am, and not being able to get back to sleep. She asked her doctor for a sleeping tablet. Closer inquiry revealed that she in fact went to bed at 6 pm and slept well. Explanation of normal sleep patterns and advice on changing her daily routine prevented the prescribing of a hypnotic.

b. Antidepressants

The most commonly used antidepressants are tricyclics such as imipramine and amitripty-line, which are still as effective as many of the newer preparations and a lot cheaper. Unfor-tunately they have anticholinergic adverse effects — dry mouth, confusion, constipation and bladder atony. Postural hypotension is the most important adverse effect and is poten-tially dangerous to an old person. Erect and supine blood pressure measurements must be taken regularly if patients are receiving tricyclics. The main problem in using tricyclics is that the therapeutic plasma levels are very close to the levels likely to cause adverse effects. Low doses should be used when initiating treatment and small increments added slowly until the beneficial effect is seen. Depression may be difficult to diagnose in the elderly but is worthwhile treating.

Case history

Mr T. L. was not coping at home following the death of his wife. He was thought to be demented, as he scored poorly on formal mental testing. However, on more careful assessment, it was noted that he could not be bothered trying to answer the questions, and he was, in fact, suffering from pseudodementia associated with an underlying depression.

c. Tranquillisers

Agitation, anxiety and restlessness are symp-toms that respond well to tranquillisers. Any underlying cause for these symptoms should be sought before embarking on treatment. The common mild tranquillisers prescribed are diazepam and chlordiazepoxide. Treat-ment should be started with small doses and slowly increased to avoid the adverse effects of falls, unsteadiness and postural hypoten-sion. Paradoxically, some tranquillizers may occasionally induce a period of increased rest-lessness. The phenothiazines and butyrophen-ones are the common major tranquillisers prescribed. They should only be given for short periods, otherwise drowsiness, consti-pation, postural hypotension, confusion and parkinsonian features will develop.

Case history

Mrs A. H. lived alone, and as she was not managing despite considerable community support, arrangements were being made for her admission to residential care. She had been troubled with dizziness for two years and had been prescribed prochlorperazine (which is a phenothiazine). On examination she was found to have classical signs of parkinsonism — bradykinesia and rigidity. The offending drug was stopped, her parkinsonian symptoms were relieved and she was able to live an independent existence at home with her community support.

Anti-parkinsonian drugs

Parkinson's disease is commoner in elderly patients and therefore it is important to understand the drugs used to treat it. Sometimes the diagnosis is difficult to make as a 'senile' or 'essential' tremor may be misdiagnosed as Parkinson's disease, and the bradykinesia and shuffling gait of cerebrovascular disease mimics Parkinson's disease. L-dopa therapy has transformed the treatment of Parkinson's disease over the last twenty years and between 80 and 90% of sufferers will benefit from this treatment, especially if bradykinesia and hypokinesia are the main features. The common side effects of nausea and vomiting have been reduced by combining the L-dopa with a decarboxylase inhibitor which inhibits the conversion of L-dopa to dopamine (the active ingredient) outside the brain. A low starting dose is again important as nausea, confusion, postural hypotension and oro-facial dyskinesia may occur. The use of anticholinergics should only be used for tremor which is severe enough to interfere with daily function or where there is embarrassing excessive salivation.

COMPLIANCE

The majority of elderly patients in the community are responsible for taking their own medicines, but as many as 75% make mistakes, a quarter of which are potentially serious (Report of the Royal College of Physicians, 1984). Much of the reported noncompliance is accidental, secondary to complex drug regimes. The greater the number of doses, the more likely it is that mistakes will be made (Wandless & Davie 1977). Inadequate instructions are often given or the patient is too confused to understand. Bad labelling with 'as before' or 'as directed' is one cause, and recently the introduction of child proof containers has led to problems (70% of the elderly were found to be unable to open these containers). The very elderly person who lives alone not coping very well, whose memory is poor and is confused, is most likely to make errors in compliance. Hoarding of medicines by the elderly is common as a result of poor compliance, and a recent campaign against hoarding in Glasgow produced two and a quarter tons of medicines (Pharmaceutical Journal 1978). Tablet counts and checking the frequency of prescriptions can help to identify those at risk of poor compliance. Methods of improving compliance include reducing both the number of drugs and doses per day (preferably to not more than four per day), relating doses to meal times, giving simple clear legible instructions, and arranging supervision of medication by relatives, carers etc. The containers should be made of clear glass or plastic with a screw top or wing-nut lid. Labels should be large and typewritten with clear instructions. Patient prescription cards for use both by the general practitioner and hospital departments and specially designed dispensers-containers, such as Dosett boxes, have been suggested and tried with varying success. Regular review by the general practitioner and the limited use of repeat prescriptions are important, but the problem patient will continue to be the one with poor vision, poor hearing, poor memory and confusion.

ROLE OF THE OCCUPATIONAL THERAPIST

It is important for occupational therapists to be aware of the problems of the possible adverse effects of drugs and of compliance in elderly patients. In hospital, the assessment of the activities of daily living should include patients' ability to take their prescribed medicines. Ability to open drug containers and knowledge of drugs being taken and their frequency, should be assessed. When a pre-discharge home assessment visit is carried out, relatives or carers may ask about drugs. A check should be made on drug bottles already in the home, and the presence of over-the-counter drugs noted. A trial of self-medication before discharge may be helpful in assessing a patient's ability to cope with drugs at home. The community occupational therapist also should check on the elderly person's capabilities of taking her drugs, and report any problems to the person's general practitioner. Any suspicion of adverse effects should also be reported. Good liaison between hospital and community occupational therapist should include awareness of potential problems with drugs and their possible adverse effects.

TOWARDS SAFER PRESCRIBING

Prescribing any drug to an elderly person is potentially hazardous, but the elderly have the most to gain from good prescribing. Following certain guidelines (see Table 15.2) will reduce the hazards and increase the benefits. It is essential that the diagnosis is accurate and that a drug is necessary for treatment. The use of a placebo may be helpful as long as it is an inert substance. As already stated, reduce the number of drugs and doses to a minimum and commence treatment with a lower dose (sometimes a quarter or a third of that recommended for younger patients) and build up the dosage slowly, always watching for adverse effects. Suitable containers should be used and clear instructions given. If there is any doubt about compliance, arrangements should be made for suitable supervision. Finally, over-the-counter preparations may interact with prescribed drugs, and specific questions about their use should be asked when taking a drug history. Stewart and Cluff

Table 15.2 Guidelines for safer prescribing

Accurate diagnosis—treat the cause, not the symp...
Is drug treatment really indicated?
Reduce number of drugs and doses to minimum
Always start with low dose and increase slowly
Give clear instructions
Package in suitable containers
Enlist help where compliance is poor
Watch for adverse effects

(1972) summed it up when they wrote 'In our society better instructions are provided when purchasing a new camera or automobile than when patients receive a life-saving antibiotic or cardiac drug'.

REFERENCES

Castleden C M, George C F, Marcer D A et al 1977 Increased sensitivity to nitrazepam in old age. British Medical Journal 1: 10–2

Dall J L C 1970 Maintenance digoxin in elderly patients. British Medical Journal 2: 705–6

Dawes D F, Shock N W 1950 Age changes in glomerular filtration rate, effective renal plasma flow and tubular excretory capacity in adult males. Journal of Clinical Investigation 29: 496–507

Deacon S P, Hammond L, Thompson B 1978 Drug supply requirement for patients discharged from hospital. British Medical Journal 2:555

Ewy G A, Kapadia G G, Yao L et al 1969 Digoxin metabolism in the elderly. Circulation 39: 449–53

Journal of the Royal College of Physicians, London 1984 Medication for the elderly: A report of the Royal College of Physicians 18: 1–10

Pharmaceutical Journal 1978 Report on 'Dump' campaign 220:417

Shaw S M, Opit L J 1976 Need for supervision in the elderly receiving long-term prescribed medication. British Medical Journal 1: 505–7

Skegg D C G, Doll R, Perry J 1977 Use of medicines in general practice. British Medical Journal 1: 1561–3

Stewart R B, Cluff L E 1972 A review of medication errors and compliance in ambulant patients. Clinical Pharmacology and Therapeutics 13: 463–468

Wandless I, Davie J W 1977 Can drug compliance be improved? British Medical Journal 1: 359–61

Williamson J, Chopin J M 1980 Adverse reactions to prescribed drugs in the elderly: A multicentre investigation. Age and Ageing 9: 73–80

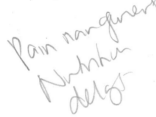

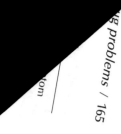

16

Eating and nutrition

E. Henery

INTRODUCTION

The purpose of this chapter is to give occupational therapists a basic understanding of what good nutrition is and how an elderly person can eat healthily.

What is good nutrition?

The science of nutrition is the study of all processes of growth, maintenance and repair of the living body that depend upon the intake of food. It is necessary to understand something of the basic nutrients in order to apply the principles of good nutrition to everyday practice. Food is anything solid or liquid which, when swallowed, can do one of three things:

— give the body material from which heat, work or energy forms can be obtained
— give the body materials to enable growth, repair or reproduction to occur
— give the body materials which are needed in the regulation of energy production, or for growth or repair.

The diet may be chosen from a large variety of foods, all of which contain essential nutrients. A balanced diet is therefore one which contains all the nutrients in the required amounts.

GENERAL GUIDELINES FOR A BALANCED DIET

There are three golden rules to be followed for a balanced diet:

1. Use a wide variety of foods, i.e. lean meat, fish, fruit, vegetables, wholegrain cereals, and not too much of any one food.
2. Most foods are good for you but some are not as good as others i.e. cakes, baked products and fried foods. This is well illustrated in Figure 16.1.
3. No food is essential; foods disliked should be substituted with foods liked, e.g. eggs, fish or other red meat for liver.

In the following section we shall see exactly what is meant by a balanced diet and how the 5 food group is involved.

A balanced diet and the 5 food group

The 5 food group is just another way of cate-

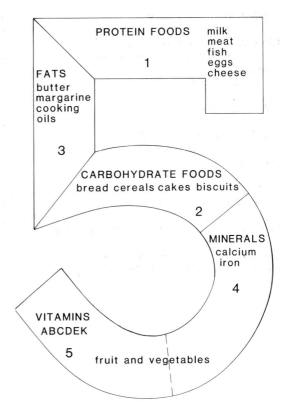

Fig. 16.2 Eat a variety of foods from each group every day

gorising the nutrients from which food is made up.

Protein

This substance is the basis of all life and is the main constituent of all the body's cells. There are many types of protein, each made up of a number of amino acids which are grouped together in different ways. There are 22 amino acids in all, 8 of which are essential to adults and 10 essential to children: these cannot be manufactured in the body. The protein we need comes mainly from:
— animal sources such as meat, fish, eggs, cheese and milk
— cereal foods, such as bread, flour, rice and pasta

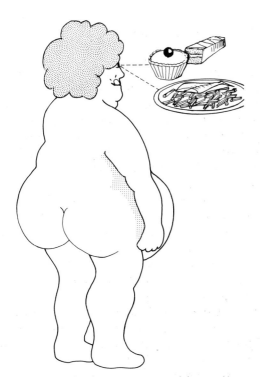

Fig. 16.1 Some foods are not so good for you!!

Table 16.1 Nutrients and their main functions

Group	Nutrient	Function
1	Protein	Provides building material for repair of body tissue and for growth. It can also be used for energy but this is not a main function
2	Carbohydrate	Provides the body with energy and has the capacity to act as a protein-sparing nutrient. This means that the protein may be used for growth and repair. It may also be converted to body fat
3	Fat	Provides a concentrated source of energy and it may also be stored as body fat
4 and 5	Vitamins and minerals	Vitamins are essential to life and are needed to regulate body processes. They also ensure the proper use of other nutrients. Minerals regulate many of the body's processes and provide material for growth and repair

NB. Fibre is discussed on page 173

— vegetables such as beans, lentils, peas and nuts.

The diet should contain a mixture of protein foods from each of the animal, cereal and vegetable groups. The protein obtained from animal sources contains almost all of the essential amino acids and is therefore known as a high biological value protein or first class protein. The protein obtained from cereals and vegetables does not contain all of the essential amino acids and is therefore known as a low biological protein or second class protein. Protein also provides the body with minerals and vitamins which are essential for a healthy diet.

Carbohydrates

These provide heat and energy for the body and are essential for the efficient metabolism of protein and fat. Some carbohydrates also provide a good source of fibre as well as containing vitamins and minerals. Carbohydrate provides the biggest proportion of calories in the British diet, usually somewhere between a half to two-thirds of the total calorie intake. The body cannot manufacture carbohydrate — we need to take it in as part of the daily diet. Carbohydrate can be subdivided into starches, fruits and vegetables and sugars:

Starches

Bread, potatoes and cereals, including breakfast cereals and biscuits, are all important to the diet. They provide heat and energy in addition to being a good supply of protein, minerals, vitamins and fibre, especially the wholegrain varieties.

Fruits and vegetables

Apples, pears, oranges, all berries and bananas should be included in the diet, either fresh, frozen, or tinned in natural juice form. Fruit also provides us with a good supply of vitamin C and fibre.

Carrots, beetroot, swede, turnip, sweetcorn and other pulse vegetables help to provide us with carbohydrate, minerals, vitamins and fibre in the diet. They can be fresh, frozen, canned or dried.

Sugars

These include sugar, glucose, jam, marmalade, syrup, sweets, confectionery, baked goods and soft drinks. They are not an essential part of the daily diet because, generally, they only contribute energy and no other nutrients.

Fats

These are needed to provide the body with an insulating layer and protective covering for vital internal organs. They provide the body with fat soluble vitamins and essential fatty acids. They enhance the palatability of foods, and because they are more slowly digested they provide the body with a greater satiety value. They are also the most highly concentrated sources of calories taken in our diet. Fats can be subdivided into animal and vegetable origin:

— *Animal* — beef and mutton fat, pork, bacon, lard, dripping, herring, mackerel, sardines, milk, dairy produce, eggs. These fats contain high levels of cholesterol which has been linked with heart disease.
— *Vegetable* — polyunsaturated margarines, polyunsaturated cooking oils: sunflower seed, ground nut, maize oil.

Minerals and vitamins

Minerals

Although protein is the basic cell-building material, minerals also play a large part in body processes. They help to form the main constituents of bones and teeth. They are contained in all body cells such as muscle, vital organs and blood corpuscles.

They form soluble salts needed to maintain a constant balance in body fluids. Minerals are found in a wide variety of foods and a good balanced diet should cover the body's needs. Table 16.2 summarizes some of the functions and the best sources of the main minerals.

Vitamins

These are present in very small amounts in foods and are essential for life. They can be divided into fat soluble vitamins and water soluble vitamins, and each vitamin has one or more specific functions. Fat soluble vitamins A,D,E,K, can be stored in the body and are not destroyed by cooking or storing processes. Water soluble vitamins B complex and C are

Table 16.2 The minerals: their functions and sources

Mineral	Function	Sources
Calcium	Needed for the development of healthy bones and teeth. Important for blood clotting mechanism. Needed for normal muscle function	Milk and dairy products, white bread, fish, eggs, dark green vegetables
Iron	Needed for the formation of haemoglobin. A deficiency of iron can cause anaemia	Liver and kidney, red meats, pulses, dried fruit, bread and wholegrain cereals, leafy green vegetables
Sodium	Present in all body fluids for fluid balance	Present in most foods and also added to foods being cooked or at the table: cooking salt, tinned soups, sauces, savoury dishes, bacon, ham, tinned meats and fish, smoked fish, pickles
Potassium	Is essential for blood cells and muscles action and it is also found in body fluids.	Instant coffee, natural fruit juice, malted drinks, e.g. Horlicks, bananas, dried fruit, potatoes, oranges, tomatoes.

not stored in the body and they are less stable than fat soluble vitamins. They are readily destroyed by exposure to air, soaking and the cooking process. Table 16.3 summarises some of the main vitamins, their functions and sources.

NUTRITIONAL PROBLEMS OF THE ELDERLY

There is an ever increasing number of elderly people in the population today. People now live longer due to better living conditions, medical and social cover, and sanitation. One would think that in an affluent western society, malnutrition would be a thing of the

Table 16.3 The vitamins: their functions and sources

Vitamin	Function	Sources
Fat soluble vitamin A	Is essential for healthy protective epithelial tissue. It is also essential to prevent night blindness	Milk, butter, margarine, egg yolk, liver, oily fish. The precursor of vitamin A (carotene) is found in leafy green vegetables and coloured fruits, e.g. carrots, apricots, tomatoes, oranges
Fat soluble vitamin D	Needed for healthy bone and teeth formation along with calcium and phosphorus	Eggs, margarine, fortified yoghurt and evaporated milk, oily fish and liver. It can also be synthesised from ultraviolet light by pigmentation in the skin
Water soluble vitamin B1 Thiamine	Needed for the release of energy from carbohydrate	Wholewheat cereals, bran and marmite, meat, milk, eggs and potatoes
Water soluble vitamin B2 riboflavine	Needed for energy release. Lack of B2 in the diet can cause sore mouth and tongue thus leading to a greater dietary problem	Milk, liver, eggs, marmite, bovril, yeast, green vegetables, beer, wholemeal products
Water soluble vitamins B12 cyancobalamin and folic acid	Needed for new blood cell formation and to prevent anaemia	Liver, kidney, red meats, fish, eggs, milk and green vegetables
Water soluble vitamin C ascorbic acid	It is very easily lost in the preparation and cooking process. It is needed for the absorption of iron in the gastrointestinal tract. Vitamin C is needed for tissue repair and to aid the healing process	Citrus fruits, e.g. grapefruit, oranges, blackcurrants, lemons. Leafy green vegetables e.g. lettuce, watercress, sprouts, spinach, potatoes, tomatoes

past. This is not so as more and more malnourished and nutritionally deficient elderly people are being seen in clinics and hospitals every day. Malnutrition in the elderly is brought about by changes in economic circumstances and way of life which often occur in the elderly and retired, and by the increasing incidence of disease and disabilities which leads to a change in dietary intake, absorption and metabolism of nutrients. 7% of subjects studied in the DHSS Survey of the Elderly in 1972 (DHSS 1979) were suffering from clinical malnutrition. This should give us cause for concern because it shows probably only a tiny part of the real problem. Exton-Smith (1978) showed that there is a long latent period before a low dietary intake leads to clinical problems. For every diagnosis of malnutrition, there are many cases where people exist on sub-standard diets, their chronic nutritional status may only become apparent and critical at a time of stress, such as after a fall or during an illness

Causes of malnutrition

Physiological changes take place in the elderly person's body about which they can do nothing. With increased age there is a reduction in the basic metabolic rate (BMR is the rate of consumption of oxygen by the patient after an overnight fast and at least an hour's complete rest), which is mainly due to a reduction in metabolic tissue and physical activity. The differences in energy expenditure observed in the elderly can often be accounted for by complicating factors such as disability and disease which have an increasing prevalence in the age group above 75. In many cases the energy expended by someone with a disability is much greater than by a non-disabled person. When someone is physically capable and has a well-balanced diet the energy and nutritional requirements are met. However, when she is physically disabled and housebound the intake of many nutrients may be insufficient. Exton-Smith (1978) drew up a list of factors which lead to dietary deficiency in the elderly.

Primary factors

Ignorance

The elderly of today were brought up in times of hardship when financial stringency dictated their dietary habits and moulded their knowledge of nutrition. Ignorance about basic nutrition and meal planning is most common amongst elderly men, who have to fend for themselves when widowed. Women who have been used to a lifetime of cooking for a family, lose the incentive to cook for one.

Social isolation

Eating is very much a social event which loses its value in solitude. Dietary intakes were found to be higher in those people who ate at luncheon clubs in the company of other people. In contrast, those people living alone in social isolation seemed to lose interest in food and consequently ate less and had less variety of food in their diet. In these circumstances meals tend to be made up of snack products and are eaten more quickly than if eaten in the presence of others.

Physical disabilities

Many elderly people have physical disabilities such as Parkinson's disease, poor eyesight, arthritis and hemiplegia which can complicate such activities as shopping, preparation and cooking of food. This is a particular problem of the isolated, housebound person with little or no outside support.

Mental disabilities

Confusion, senile dementia and depression affect many elderly people. These mental disabilities often lead to loss of appetite and forgetfulness in preparing and eating food. The number of malnourished, mentally disabled elderly people is very high and they are very difficult to treat.

Iatrogenic

Special diets continued for longer than necessary can lead to malnutrition. For example, 'gastric' diets which are low in citrus fruits (vitamin C) may lead to scurvy if continued indefinitely. Low fat diets followed for longer than necessary may lead to a lack of energy and fat soluble vitamins (ADEK). Restrictions in diet due to advice from friends, information obtained from advertising, articles in magazines and television, can have a detrimental effect on nutritional intakes.

Poverty

Making ends meet on a pension is very difficult and food eaten by pensioners is often dull, tasteless and monotonous. Existing on a pension demands individual skills in budgeting, and the motivation to shop around for bargains to vary the diet. It has been shown that those elderly people who have a supplementary income have a better diet than those who rely solely on their pension. In winter many elderly people have to choose between spending money on fuel or food. Commercial concerns should show more consideration to elderly shoppers and provide food packaged in smaller quantities to meet their needs and their pocket and enable them to vary and enjoy their diet.

Secondary factors

Impaired appetite

The time needed for an elderly person to regain her appetite following an illness is longer than in a young person. Malnutrition can occur easily in a person whose diet was previously only marginally adequate.

Masticatory inefficiency

An elderly person may select a soft diet which is poorly balanced if she has bad teeth or ill-fitting dentures. Poor oral hygiene can cause taste and smell distortion, and in the elderly this can lead to unpalatability of food and a loss of appetite.

Malabsorption

Mild degrees of malabsorption are not uncommon in the elderly. There are a number of causes and the main nutrients affected are fat and fat soluble vitamins (ADEK), folic acid and vitamin Bl2.

Alcohol and drugs

When alcohol intake is excessive, calorie needs will come mainly from alcohol and the intake of other nutrients will be negligible. Drugs can have a harmful effect on nutrition. They can cause nausea and loss of appetite; they can deplete the body's mineral stores, cause internal bleeding which can lead to anaemia and they can interfere with vitamin metabolism.

The new NACNE guidelines and their relevance to the elderly.

NACNE stands for the National Advisory Committee on Nutrition Education. This committee was set up early in the 1980s to look at the nation's diet and to see how it could be improved. Britons in the 1980s are suffering from conditions caused by poorly balanced diets and over-nutrition: the opposite situation existed before the war. Dietitians now have the NACNE guidelines and the (1979) DHSS 'Recommended Daily Amounts' to use together, as a guide to better nutrition for the nation. Special considerations should be made for 'at risk' and 'special' groups such as the elderly and children.

At a meeting in December 1984 held by the Nutritional Advisory Group for the Elderly (NAGE), a sub-group of The British Dietetic Association, the NACNE guidelines in relation to the elderly were discussed.

It was felt that imposing these guidelines on an elderly person very much depended upon the individual, her age, activities, health and normal eating habits. Table 16.4 gives the results of the meeting in relation to NACNE; and Table 16.5 is an example of a week's menu using NACNE recommendations. Special diets have to be prescribed for elderly people with specific problems — they are as follows: reducing, diabetic, high protein, liquid/soft, dietary fibre, sodium restriction, low fat, low cholesterol, gluten free, low protein. Details of these diets can be obtained in Davidson et al (1979) and Goode et al (1985).

GUIDELINES FOR EMERGENCY STORE-CUPBOARD

There are a number of reasons why people may not be able to go shopping for themselves, e.g. bad weather, or physical or psychological illness. Many housebound people therefore rely on neighbours and friends to do their shopping for them. With this restriction it is very easy for an elderly person to slip into a routine of snacks instead of proper meals and thus lose the enjoyment of meals. It is essential to have a stock of food for a store-cupboard and also a supply of fresh food bought more regularly, e.g. milk, eggs, cheese, meat, bread, fruit and vegetables. Elderly people should be encouraged to check for 'sell-by' and 'use-by-dates' because even dried and tinned foods do not last for ever. A freezer can be useful for storing individually prepared meals, bread, fruit and vegetables etc., particularly for someone living on her own. Table 16.6 includes a comprehensive list of foods suitable for a store-cupboard.

Table 16.4 NACNE and Nutritional Advisory Group for the Elderly (NAGE) guidelines

NACNE guidelines	Nutrients	NAGE
The energy intake should be sufficient to maintain ideal body weight as defined in Royal College of Physicians Report on Obesity 1983. An increase in exercise should be encouraged to increase energy expenditure	Energy intake	It was felt that the weight tables were not relevant for the whole elderly population. The importance of exercise and good eating habits should be emphasised to retirement groups
For dental reasons sucrose should be halved to an average of 20 kg per person per year. Sugary snacks and drinks between meals should be discouraged, remembering underweight and normal weighted people are free to eat from this group	a. Sugar-sucrose	Many older people eat sugary snacks and sweets between meals; as sucrose is a known appetite suppressant, decreasing sugar in the diet may increase the appetite for other foods. If the patient is not overweight it may not be appropriate to decrease sugar intake, so long as the remainder of the diet is balanced
There is much evidence now of a link between total fat in the diet and coronary heart disease (CHD). Approximately 38% of the total calories in the diet come from fat. A reduction in fat intake will help to reduce serum cholesterol levels. A reduction of total fat levels is recommended in the diet, 34% in the short term and dropping to 30% of total calorie intake in the long term	b. Fat	A reduction of the fat levels to 30% of the total calorie intake was thought to be inappropriate for the elderly. It would cause a reduction in the fat-soluble vitamins A and D and essential fatty-acids. Menus would have to be changed drastically in most cases and unfamiliar foods would have to be eaten, e.g. cottage cheese. This could result in meals not being eaten and a poorly balanced diet. It was felt that the choice of butter or margarine and whole or semi-skimmed milk should be given to this group
Because of the link between low fibre and disease of the bowel, an increase in dietary fibre is recommended. An increase in fibre from all sources, unrefined cereals, fruit and vegetables should be gradually introduced, aiming for a final level of 30 g per day	Fibre	An increase in dietary fibre is difficult to achieve with some elderly people, due to their reduced appetite. An increase in dietary fibre would be beneficial for this group due to the high incidence of constipation and the amount of laxatives taken. There is some question over the connection between an increase in fibre and a reduction of some minerals and their absorption; this is especially significant to the elderly who are more at risk to develop mineral deficiencies through poor diet and reduced gastrointestinal function
Salt is said to be a major risk factor in the development of ischaemic heart disease and hypertension. Evidence suggests a general reduction in the level of salt in the diet: the present intake of 12 g per day is well in excess of the daily requirements and comes mainly from processed and convenience foods. A reduction to 9 g per day would give an adequate intake. This can be done by reducing the intake of processed and convenience foods, reducing salt used in cooking and at the table and by using more fresh foods.	Salt	A general reduction of salt should be advised, remembering, however, that a large part of the elderly person's diet is made up of convenience foods for ease and quickness

Table 16.5 Sample of a week's menu for a varied, healthy diet using NACNE guidelines for the elderly

Meal	Monday	Tuesday	Wednesday	Thursday	Friday	Saturday	Sunday
B'Fast	Small glass fresh orange jce (unsweet) Porridge + little milk sl. toast + little butter & jam	Small helping of grapefruit/segments Weetabix + little milk wholemeal roll + little butter	Small glass fresh orange jce (unsweet) Branflakes + little milk toasted bran scone + little butter & Jam	Small glass fresh orange jce (unsweet) boiled/poached egg sl toast + little butter	Small helping grapefruit/segments Weetabix + little milk sl. wholemeal bread + little butter & m'lade	Small glass fresh orange jce (unsweet) porridge + little milk roll + little butter	Small glass fresh grapefruit jce (unsweet) scrambled egg + sl. toast + little butter
	tea + milk	tea + milk	tea + milk	tea + milk	tea + milk	tea + milk	tea + milk
Mid-morning	tea/coffee + milk	tea/coffee + milk Digestive (if desired)	tea/coffee + milk	tea/coffee + milk Digestive (if desired)	tea/coffee + milk	tea/coffee + milk	tea/coffee + milk Digestive (if desired)
Lunch	Soup (homemade or tinned) mince & vegs (carrots, onion, turnip) + 1 potato boiled/mashed banana tea + milk	Glass fresh fruit jce (unsweet) Scrmb. egg & tomato sl. toast + little butter ice crm & jelly tea + milk	Baked haddock & tomato + boiled potato sl. fresh melon tea + milk	Chicken casser. with carrot, turnip, m'rooms + brussel sprts + boiled potato sml help Jelly tea + milk	Brsd liver & onion cabbage & mashed potato fresh fruit salad tea + milk	Small grilled bacon & poached egg sl. toast + butter ice cream & jelly tea + milk	Rst chicken & peas & carrots small roast potato sml std fruit & cus tea + milk
Mid-afternoon	tea + milk Digestive (if desired)	tea + milk apple	tea + milk Digestive	tea + milk orange	tea + milk Digestive	tea + milk Digestive	tea + milk banana
Evening meal or mid-day snack	Sliced lean gammon + tomato + beetroot, lettuce + cucumber slice wholemeal bread + little butter low cal/low fat yoghurt tea + milk	Shepherd's pie + peas + carrots little stewed fruit + little custard tea + milk	Small grapefruit segs small macaroni cheese + carrots small helping ice cream tea + milk	Soup (small helping) corned beef + lettuce, tomato cucumber slice bread + butter stewed fruit tea + milk	Soup (small helping) grilled haddock + tomato, peas Little Oven chips slice bread + little butter tea + milk	Gigot chop + cabbage boiled pot. slice bread + little butter fresh fruit salad tea + milk	Soup (small helping) tuna or salmon sandwich + tomato small helping ice-cream tea + milk
Bedtime (if desired)	Tea + milk slice toast + little butter	Tea + milk Digestive biscuit	Tea + milk slice toast + little butter	Tea + milk Digestive biscuit	Tea + milk 2 oatcakes + little butter	Tea + milk Digestive biscuit	Tea + milk Digestive biscuit

Table 16.6 List of foods suitable for a store-cupboard

Beverages	Cereals	Fats	Protein foods	Fruit & vegetables	Misc.
Tea, coffee, squash, dried skimmed milk powder, evaporated and condensed milks, tinned or cartoned fresh fruit juice tinned or packet soups, malted drinks	Oatmeal, breakfast cereals, pudding cereals, flour, pasta, rice, tinned spaghetti and macaroni	Butter, margarine, low fat spreads, spreading cheese, cooking oils	Canned fish, canned meat, pre-packed cheese, pre-packed cooked meats, canned stews and mince, tinned or packet puddings e.g. rice, semolina, instant desert	Canned fruit, dried fruit, canned vegetables, dried vegetables, dried potato	Salt, pepper, herbs, spices, sauces, stock cubes, sugar, jam, biscuits, packet jellies

CONCLUSION

Future prospects for occupational therapists, dietitians and the elderly patient

The principle aim of this chapter is to give a basic understanding of nutrition, problems related to the elderly, and to show how easily poor eating habits can all too often lead to malnutrition. The aim of the dietitian is to make sure that people know how to keep healthy by eating a well-balanced diet. The future prospects for the dietitian and occupational therapist working together, both in hospital and in the community, look very interesting and challenging and will give greater insight into each other's professional roles.

REFERENCES

British Dietetic Association 1985 Dietary advice for diabetics on insulin, diet alone, or diet and tablets

Dietetic Department, Brighton Health Authority 1984 Dietary leaflets: How to slim sensibly; Healthy eating as you grow older; Dietary fibre

Brown S 1984 Vegetarian kitchen. BBC Continuing Education Advisory Council, London

Burket D 1981 Don't forget fibre in your diet, Martin Dunity, London

Davidson S, Passmore R, Brook J F, Truswell A S 1979 Human nutrition and dietetics, 7th edn, Churchill Livingstone, Edinburgh, pp 3–14, 62

Davies L 1981 Three score years. . . . . and then? Heinemann Medical Books, London

Davies L 1977 Easy cooking for one or two. Penguin, Middlesex

Davies L 1974 Notes on: What is a balanced diet; The food store-cupboard; Keeping food fresh without a refrigerator. Geriatric Nutrition Unit. Queen Elizabeh College, University of London

DHSS 1972 A nutritional survey of the elderly. HMSO, London

DHSS 1979 Recommended daily amounts of food energy and nutrients for groups of people in the United Kingdom, HMSO, London

DHSS 1975 Health service catering manual, vol I. Alexander House, London

Exton-Smith A N 1978 Nutrition in the elderly. In: Dickerson, J W T, Lee H A (eds) Nutrition in the clinical management of disease. Edward Arnold, London, pp 72–105

Goode A W, Howard J P, Woods S 1985 Clinical nutrition and dietetics for nurses. Hodder and and Stoughton, London, pp 2–4

Health Education Council leaflet, Look after yourself 1982 Fat–who needs it? London

Mathews W, Wells D 1972 Second book and Nutrition, 1973. Home Economics in Association with Flour Advisory Bureau, London, pp 1–6

National Advisory Commitee on Nutrition Education (NACNE), 1983 Paper on proposals for nutritional guidelines for health education in Britain Health Education Council, London

Nilson B 1971 Cooking for special diets. Penguin, Middlesex, pp 1–4

Nutrition Education Service 1979 Malnutrition and disease in the elderly. Elmutt Clifton, for Van den Bergh & Jurgen, Sussex

Pyke M 1973 Teach yourself nutrition. English Universities Press, London, pp 1–8

Thomas S J 1980 A study of the nutritional status of long-stay patients in Springfield Hospital. Unpublished. Copies available from Geriatric Teaching and Research Unit, Clare House, St George's Hospital, Blackshow Road, London SW17

Thomas S J 1982 Getting the most out of food 1982 Nutrition Awards, Prize Papers, The elderly — A forgotten nutrition problem? Van den Berghs & Jurgens, Sussex

Walshe M, Smith I, Black A E 1985 Nutrition guidelines. Heinemann Education Books, London

17
Wheelchairs
M. Rainey

INTRODUCTION

Occupational therapists are often responsible for assessing elderly people for wheelchairs, either in hospital or at home. It is essential that there is sound knowledge of the person's disabilities, needs and environment as well as knowledge of the range of wheelchairs available.

MANUAL WHEELCHAIRS

Provision

There are three main ways of obtaining a manual wheelchair: permanent loan, short-term loan and private purchase.

Permanent loan

Anyone elderly or disabled in need of a wheelchair is entitled to one on permanent loan through the Department of Health and Social Security. The *Handbook of Wheelchairs* is a book published by the DHSS (1982) which lists, describes and illustrates the range of wheelchairs available through this service. It can be obtained by anyone involved in wheelchair prescription from local authority offices.

   For a wheelchair to be supplied, the doctor in charge of the patient has to send an application form (AOF 5G) to the nearest Artificial Limb and Appliance Centre (ALAC), describing the patient's clinical condition and recommending the appropriate wheelchair model. This recommendation may be based on information given by an occupational therapist or physiotherapist. If required, advice can be sought from the medical officer or technical officer in the centre, especially where special adaptations may be necessary.

A large range of standard wheelchairs are stored locally by the ALAC and can therefore be supplied reasonably quickly once the application has been approved by the medical officer in the centre. Following supply it is the responsibility of the patient to contact the centre if the chair is no longer suitable or is in need of repair. This contact is not always made for a number of reasons, e.g. ignorance of the procedure, and the community occupational therapist should routinely check the condition of a patient's wheelchair.

Short-term loan

Many Health Authorities have a temporary loan service, where the chair is only required for a short period of time. This can be organised through the GP.

A wheelchair may also be borrowed from organisations related to the person's disability or from the local branch of the British Red Cross Society.

Private purchase

Wheelchairs can be bought privately by individuals. However, this involves considerable expense with the risk of money being wasted on an unsuitable chair. Most old peoples needs can be adequately met through the DHSS service, as long as a proper assessment is carried out. Professional ignorance is often the cause of poor wheelchair prescription, and in many cases chairs are bought privately as a result of lack of awareness of the existence and extent of the service available. If, however, private purchase is desired, it is important that advice is received from someone with knowledge of wheelchair types in relation to the person's disability. There are a number of Aid Centres throughout Britain

where trained occupational therapists and others can demonstrate a wide range of commercially available chairs.

Considerations

How long the chair will be needed for

This will determine the source of provision. If, for example, a wheelchair is required for two weeks to enable a family to take their elderly relative on holiday, then short-term loan may be the answer. Similarly, if the old person has a fall leaving her immobile for a short period of time the chair should be borrowed on a short-term basis so as not to encourage dependency. If, however, the person is capable of walking around at home, but requires a wheelchair to go on outings with her family, then permanent loan should be sought.

Attitude to the use of a wheelchair

Many old people are aware of and fear increasing infirmity and the loss of independence that it will lead to. As a result they may become stubborn, resenting any kind of help offered, whether it be from another person or an aid. They may become depressed and withdrawn. A wheelchair for many people is seen as the ultimate in disability, and to accept it may mean admitting defeat. These feelings must be respected and the person should be given as much encouragement as possible to remain 'on her feet'. However, there may come a point where safety becomes a priority and time must be spent gently helping the person adjust to the change. Reasons for using the chair should be pointed out in a positive manner. Many people do not want to be seen in a wheelchair by friends and neighbours, yet social isolation as a result of reduced mobility can have a devastating effect on an old person's well-being.

On the other hand, there are those who become too dependent on a wheelchair too soon. A wheelchair may be necessary in a large hospital ward, but may not be at all practicable at home. Dependency should not be encouraged in this type of case.

A multidisciplinary decision must be made where there is conflict between attitude and need.

The person's size and weight

(i) Seat width — this will depend on the person's hip measurement when sitting. If the chair is going to be used outside, room must be allowed for the person to wear a heavy coat. Seat width should be looked at in conjunction with the overall width of the chair where narrow doorways are going to have to be negotiated (Fig. 17.1).

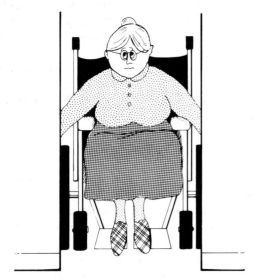

Fig. 17.1 Check width of doorways

(ii) Seat depth — there should be a space of about 2.5 cm (1 in) between the front of the seat and the back of the knee. Poor posture causing the person to slide down the seat will alter this and should be corrected if possible.

(iii) Seat height — the footplates should be adjusted so that the thighs are lying horizontally on the seat without any pressure from the seat edge. If the footplates are too high, excess weight will be put on the ischial tuberosities which will result in discomfort

and possibly pressure sores. There should be a minimum clearance of 5 cm (2 in) from ground to footplate.

(iv) Arm-rests — these should be high enough to support the forearms comfortably to prevent slouching, but not so high as to cause elevation of the scapulae. If the arm-rests are too low, there may be inadequate lateral support for those with poor sitting balance.

(v) Weight of person — a light chair is easier to propel and transport, but it will be less robust, and a heavier tubular steel chair may be necessary for the large overweight person.

The person's disability

(i) Method of propulsion.

a. Attendant propelled — many old people retain the ability to walk around the house either independently or using a walking aid. However, they may have difficulty walking for any distance out of doors and will depend on others to push them in a wheelchair. An old person has seldom the strength to propel a wheelchair herself for any distance. Attendant wheelchairs usually have smaller rear wheels which are pneumatic so as to provide a more comfortable ride over rough surfaces. Some people find large rear wheels easier to negotiate kerbs.

b. Self-propelled — chairs with large rear wheels are most commonly used for self-propulsion. Wheel size varies but, generally speaking, the larger the rear wheel, the easier it is to propel. However, sideways transfers may be made more difficult and the turning circle greater. Chairs with large front wheels are seldom suitable as they are difficult for an attendant to steer: they encourage poor posture, impede sideways transfers and are difficult to position close to work surfaces. They are occasionally prescribed where there is a limited range of movement in the shoulders. They may be prescribed for a person with a double amputation of the lower limbs to provide adequate stability; chairs with rear wheels set back 7.6 cm (3 in) are generally preferred for such conditions. One-arm drive chairs have two hand-rims on one of the rear wheels to enable someone with the use of only one hand to propel the chair. These are often found to be heavy, difficult to transport and difficult to manoeuvre in confined spaces. They require good co-ordination, strength and comprehension. It may be more appropriate to use the good arm and leg for propulsion, remembering that the footplate should be swung back out of the way and the seat should be low enough for the person to comfortably place her foot flat on the ground. Some people may have difficulty using their hands, e.g. due to rheumatoid arthritis, and foot propulsion may be recommended. Again, the seat should be low enough to facilitate this. It may be easier to propel the chair backwards.

(ii) Posture. Good posture can usually be obtained if the person is properly measured for her chair. Accessories such as trays, head-rest extensions and extra side padding may be used to improve posture. A reclining back may help someone with weak truncal muscles, although this increases the overall length of the chair and may be unsuitable for use within the home. Padded wheelchair inserts are available commercially and, in addition to comfort, can give extra lateral support. Special adaptations may be necessary to maintain a good sitting position, e.g. moulded seating, and advice from the technical officer in the ALAC may be necessary. A square of non-slip netting between the person's bottom and cushion may be all that is needed to prevent someone from slipping down the chair. Alternatively, a wedge cushion positioned with the thickest part at the front of the seat may have the same effect. Waist straps can provide extra security. The Buxton Chair (McLaughlin Ltd) can be prescribed for the person who cannot be supported in a standard wheelchair. It is a large hospital-type chair which has a tilting mechanism which can be locked in the required angle. This gives limited lateral support, however, and can encourage poor posture.

(iii) Cognitive ability. Insight, perceptual ability, memory and general intelligence must be considered. Some people may have difficulty judging distance or working out right from left. Some may forget to take their feet off the footplates before standing up or may forget to put on the brakes. One-arm drive and powered wheelchairs are particularly difficult to become accustomed to by the elderly if there are learning and perceptual problems.

(iv) Ability to transfer. If a person uses a standing transfer, the seat and arm-rests must be high enough to facilitate this. The foot-rests may have to be detachable to allow the person to position the chair properly. If a sideways transfer is used, the size and position of the propelling wheels will be important, and also the provision of detachable arm-rests. Most elderly people carry out standing transfers, and time should be taken to teach them the correct procedure, i.e. position the chair, put the brakes on, lift the foot-rests, move forward on the seat, push up from the arm-rests, stand. Equally important is the need to teach carers transfer techniques.

Environment

Is the chair going to be used indoors, outdoors or both?

(i) Indoors considerations include the width of doorways, manoeuvring space, type of flooring, and obstacles such as door sills, steps, loose mats and furniture. The home environment may have to be adapted to accommodate wheelchair use. Solid tyres are easier to propel indoors, especially on carpets. Small front castors allow the chair to turn more easily in confined spaces. The length of the chair will affect the turning circle.

(ii) Outdoors pneumatic tyres make journeys over rough, uneven surfaces more comfortable. They must be kept well pumped up, as soft tyres make steering and propelling difficult. Small front castors tend to stick in cracks, and small stones can halt the chair suddenly, sometimes even tipping the occupant out (Fig. 17.2). If the area in which the

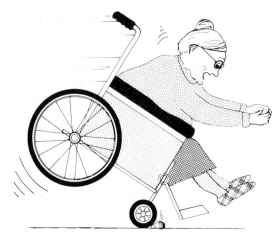

Fig. 17.2 Small front castors are less suitable for use outdoors

person lives is hilly, the attendant may have difficulty pushing the chair, especially if he himself is elderly, and an electric wheelchair may be required.

(iii) Indoors and outdoors. It is impossible to find a chair that will meet all requirements and it will be necessary to find a compromise by working out the various priorities. Access in and out of the home must be assessed and steps ramped, paths widened etc.

What the the chair will be used for

This has already been partly covered under 'Transfers' and 'Environment'. Consider also:

(i) The provision of accessories which will make everyday tasks easier, e.g. trays, desk arms. Wheelchair capes are available for protection against the weather, although most people find that a warm rug wrapped around the legs and a thick coat suffice. Care must be taken not to allow any garments to get caught in the wheels.

(ii) The provision of a second chair may be necessary and, indeed, can be supplied by the DHSS. For example, many need a heavy robust chair for use within the home or hospital, as well as a lightweight collapsible chair for transporting purposes. A second chair will not be supplied merely as a stand-by, should the one in use breakdown.

Transport of the chair

Most chairs supplied by the DHSS can be folded to fit into the back of a car. Folding back-rests and detachable leg-rests make the chair more compact for storage in a car boot. Difficulties may arise when the chair is too heavy to lift in and out of the car, especially where the helper is also infirm through age. In such cases it may be appropriate to prescribe the Baratt 7 or 10 (see Types of wheelchairs) as these are only 16.8 kg (37 lb) in weight and fold in such a way as to facilitate lifting. Folding does tend to be tricky, however, with these and some other light-weight chairs are available.

Handling a wheelchair

Carers should be given careful instructions on how to use the wheelchair, e.g. opening and closing the chair, checking tyre pressure, negotiating kerbs and steps, lifting the chair for transportation. They should be shown how to work the foot-rests, arm-rests and brakes. What may be obvious to the professional may not be to the layman.

Coping with kerbs is often a worry. The best way to go up a kerb is frontways: tilt the chair back on its rear wheels using the tipper lever, push it forward until the rear wheels touch the kerb, lower the front wheels and lift and push the chair onto the path. To go down a kerb, the chair should again be tipped back onto its rear wheels and gently lowered down the kerb frontways (Cochrane & Wilshere 1982) (Fig. 17.3).

DHSS range of wheelchairs

The needs of most elderly people can be met by the range of wheelchairs available through the DHSS. For the purpose of this book, therefore, mention will be made of those chairs most commonly issued to this category of people through the DHSS. Further details of these and the other chairs supplied can be obtained from the 'Manual of Wheelchairs' (DHSS, 1982) Up-to-date information on

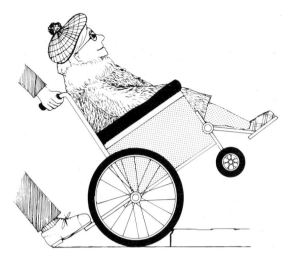

Fig. 17.3 Climbing kerbs

commercially available wheelchairs can be obtained from the Disabled Living Foundation, 380/384 Harrow Road, London W9 2HU, tel: (01) 289 6111; and the Scottish Council on Disability, Princes House, 5 Shandwick Place, Edinburgh, tel: (031) 229 8632.

1. Self-propelling

Barratt Model 7. This chair is usually supplied where other chairs in the DHSS range do not fit into the person's car for transporting. It fits into the boot of a Mini, when folded, and is one of the lightest chairs to lift. The propelling wheels are smaller than those of other chairs, making it more manoeuvrable though possibly slightly more difficult to propel. The low seat height is advantageous for foot propulsion.

Model 8LJ. The seat width of this chair makes it suitable for the smaller person, with a smaller overall width for narrow doorways. It is quite long, however, which may affect manoeuvrability. Its castors are larger than the 8BL which make it better for outdoor use.

Model 8BL. This is a frequently supplied chair to the elderly. It is light, compact, manoeuvrable and good for use in confined spaces. It is shorter than the 8L and 8LJ. Its small front castors make it less suitable for use over rough, uneven surfaces outside.

Model 8L. The seat widths accommodate the larger person although its overall length and width make it less manoeuvrable in confined spaces. It is sometimes preferred to its attendant propelled counterpart, Model 9L, for use outside, as the larger wheels cope well with kerb climbing.

Everest and Jennings/Carters. A chair made by either of these two companies will only be supplied where there is a proven clinical need which can only be met by this type of chair. Special requests will be met by whichever make is most readily available at the time unless specific reason is given for a particular make. It may take longer for such chairs to be supplied.

Standard chairs. Recommendations for these wheelchairs will only be accepted from the Consultant or Medical Officer in the ALAC (DHSS, 1982). They are attractive, robust wheelchairs. They are heavier than those in the 8L range and can be difficult to lift for transporting.

Fully or semi-reclining. These may be prescribed where the person has weak truncal muscles, poor head control, breathing or swallowing difficulties. The wheels are set back to keep the chair stable when the back is reclined; the chair is therefore long with a large turning circle and is not suitable in confined spaces. Elevating leg-rests are usually prescribed in conjunction with the reclining back and this will increase the overall length. The high back makes it difficult to lift the patient into the back of the chair from behind. The chair is large and heavy to transport.

One-arm drive. Two hand-rims are fitted to one propelling wheel and can be for right- or left-handed use. To go backwards and forwards, both rims have to be moved together; to turn, one rim is moved. They require strength, co-ordination and good comprehension. They are wide and may not be suitable for some households. They are large and heavy for transporting. They are found to be suitable for only a small number of elderly people, and more suitable for hospital than home use.

Carters guideabout/commode chair. These

are highly manoeuvrable where space is limited. The 5HC (mobile commode) is particularly suitable where there is insufficient space in the toilet area for positioning a standard wheelchair beside the toilet for transferring. The person can transfer onto the 5HC outside the toilet area and can then be wheeled directly over the top of the toilet. The commode chair can greatly reduce the number of transfers that have to be carried out. These are not standard issue, however, and recommendation will only be accepted from the consultant or medical officer in the ALAC.

2. Attendant-propelled chairs

Model 9LJ. This chair is suitable for small adults. It is designed for outdoor use with longer pushing handles to make the negotiation of kerbs easier. The standard chair has solid front castors. Balloon tyred castors give a smoother, more comfortable ride. It is possible to get 32 cm (12.5 in) pneumatic tyres but the chair loses its manoeuvrability and has to be tilted back on its rear wheels for turning. It is light, compact and easy to fold for transporting.

Model 9L. This chair has similar features to those of the 9LJ, except that it has larger seat widths. It is the most commonly prescribed attendant-propelled wheelchair.

Barratt Model 10. This chair has similar features to the Model 7 except for its small rear wheels. It will only be supplied where the chairs in the Model 9 range are not suitable for transporting.

Variations on all of the above models may be possible and the DHSS 'Manual of Wheelchairs' should always be referred to when prescribing a wheelchair.

Accessories. Readily available accessories include elevating leg-rests, head-rest extensions, safety straps and trays. Capstan hand-rims may help the person to secure a grip on the propelling wheels but care must be taken with arthritic hand joints as overworking them can have destructive long-term effects. A powered wheelchair with joystick control may be more appropriate. Extended brake levers and single brake levers are available, as are attendant controlled brake levers which are valuable in helping the pusher control the chair in hilly areas, especially if the occupant is heavy.

Cushions available include:

1. PVC-covered foam cushions. These come in 5 cm, 7.6 cm or 10 cm (2 in, 3 in or 4 in) thickness. The height of the cushion will affect the overall sitting position and may affect the person's ability to transfer. PVC can become hot and sticky but the cushion can be turned over to reveal a cotton covered base. This surface is less slippery and may improve posture. Hard-based cushions prevent sagging. Wedge cushions can be used in many different ways, e.g. at the back of the chair or on the seat. If toileting is a problem, cushions with a U-shape cut-out for a urinal can make life easier. Sheepskins often improve overall comfort.

2. Where the person is at risk of getting pressure sores, special cushions can be issued through the DHSS, e.g. gel or air. There are many special cushions available commercially. If possible, the person should be able to try out various cushions for a period of time in order to ascertain which is the most effective.

ELECTRICALLY-POWERED WHEELCHAIRS

Some elderly people are too weak to propel a manual wheelchair independently. In many cases, upper limb joints are so badly affected by rheumatoid arthritis, that it would be impossible and destructive to attempt self-propulsion. A powered chair may be the answer if the person can responsibly operate the controls. It involves good co-ordination perceptual awareness and general comprehension; careful assessment is required.

An electric wheelchair may be required for indoor use, outdoor use or both.

Indoor chairs

Indoor electric wheelchairs can be issued

through the DHSS to elderly people who can neither walk nor propel a manual wheelchair. They are for indoor use only and must not be taken outside the home environment. The DHSS models include:

Model 102. This chair has been described as being indestructable and, though no longer manufactured, is still available through the DHSS. It is very compact and manoeuvrable with its three small wheels, although this feature means it is not stable enough for use in the garden. It has a comfortable, supportive seat with an adjustable back-rest. The main disadvantages are that it cannot be disengaged for free-wheeling, it cannot be folded and the arm-rest with the control cannot be removed (Harpin, 1981).

Model 103. This chair is lightweight, folds easily and is compact for indoor use. It has frontwheel drive, giving it a sharp turning circle but making it a little more difficult to steer. It has a 2-speed standard control or a proportional control.

Model 109. This has similar dimensions and controls to the 103 but has rear wheel drive, which makes it easier to steer, and it has a stronger frame.

Power drive (Carters). Although this chair is for indoor use only, it has a longer travelling range and is robust and stable for the heavier person. It is heavy to transport, however, does not fold easily and its length gives it a larger turning circle than the other DHSS models. The reclining chair in particular is often found to be unpractical for use within the home.

Outdoor chairs

Many old people become housebound because their spouse can no longer push them outdoors as a result of their own infirmity, particularly where the district is hilly or the occupant heavy. If this is the case, an application can be made for an outdoor attendant-operated power chair (Model 28B) through the DHSS; alternatively an occupant-controlled chair can be bought privately.

Model 28B. This chair is attendant operated

and requires a certain amount of skill to control. It has a 2 speed fixed control box with forward and reverse, with a range of $3\frac{1}{2}$ miles. It has a fairly large turning circle and is unfortunately often found to be cumbersome, difficult to manoeuvre and inadequate in climbing kerbs. Storage space may be a problem for many people.

Outdoor powered chairs controlled by the occupant are not issued through the DHSS. Motability is an organisation set up by the government to help disabled people use their mobility allowance to purchase an electric wheelchair. However, you have to be under 65 years old to receive mobility allowance which ironically deprives the age group most in need of power chairs of assistance. This is a sad fact, and the only possibility of assistance may be from some form of charity or voluntary organisation. In such a case, it is important that the person is still assessed for the most appropriate chair and not given a surprise present of the cheapest chair available. Money can be wasted this way (Fig. 17.4).

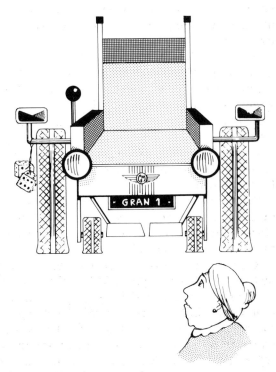

Fig. 17.4 Unwelcome surprise

Maintenance money and insurance costs must be considered. If the person cannot cope with the running costs herself, the extra money must be put aside by the donor for this purpose. Only a minority of elderly people can afford to buy a chair, but some companies have hire purchase schemes and a bank loan may be arranged. Second-hand chairs are available and can be found advertised in various newspapers and journals. They have no guarantee, however, and may require new batteries, tyres and a general service. A free home demonstration of new chairs can be arranged with suppliers. If possible, an Aid Centre should be visited. There are three main categories of outdoor power chairs.

1. Wheelchairs — there are many variations of powered wheelchairs, with different types of kerb climbing devices. Most can climb kerbs of 10–13 cm (4–5 in) and cope with 1:4 gradients with a range of anything between 15 and 30 miles. A certain amount of skill and co-ordination is required to climb kerbs and many elderly people would prefer to find a route avoiding such obstacles. Climbing and descending kerbs gives a jolt and can be painful to arthritic joints. Powered wheel-chairs come in various seat widths. Many are compact enough for indoor use as well as for outdoors and some can be controlled by an attendant.

2. *Scooters* — these are compact 3-wheeled vehicles which can be dismantled fairly easily for transporting in a car. Few can climb kerbs and 3 wheels are obviously less stable than 4. They are not suitable for people who are very heavy or who have poor sitting balance. Steering is usually similar to that of a bike, which many elderly prefer to joystick control as it is easier to become accustomed to. Many elderly people find scooters appealing in that they do not have the 'institutional' look of a wheelchair. They cope with 1:12 gradients and have an average range of 10 miles. They can be used indoors and out.

3. *Buggies* — these are larger vehicles for outdoor use only, with a travelling range of about 22 miles. They cope with 10–13 cm (4–5 in) and kerbs 1:4 gradients. Steering is by a tiller column which some elderly people may find heavy, especially where upper limbs are arthritic. One major advantage is their hoods for protection against the weather. They are stable vehicles and can climb kerbs fairly easily, but they may require a storage area outside the house and cannot be trans-ported in a car.

All powered vehicles are meant for use on pavements with a speed limit of 4 mph. No licence is needed but it is advisable to take out insurance for breakdown, injury to 3rd parties and accidental damage, fire or theft. Batteries should be charged regularly so there must be an easily accessible power point. This operation is simple and the batteries do not have to be removed from the chair. They should never be allowed to go flat and the level of electrolyte should be checked once a week, and more distilled water added if necessary. Lead acid batteries have a life span of about two years, depending on how well they are cared for. Standard accessories can be fitted to most wheelchairs, e.g. elevating leg-rests, head-rests, safety belts, shopping bags.

Assessment

The following points should be considered when assessing the suitability of an electri-cally-powered wheelchair for an elderly person:

(i) *Steering*
   a. Joystick power steering allows the user to control both the direction and speed of the chair with a small single movement. The chair will move in the direction that the joystick has been pushed. It can be positioned for left- or right-handed use; chin control and similar adaptations made.
   b. Manual steering involves the movement of a steering column or tiller which acts directly on the wheels and therefore requires more strength and movement.

(ii) *Speed control*
   a. Proportional control gives a gradual increase and decrease of speed, similar to that

of a car accelerator. The further the joystick is pushed, the faster the chair will go. This gives a smooth movement. It is sometimes possible to get an accelerator limiter which delays the build up of speed: this is useful for someone with poor co-ordination.

b. Standard/fixed control gives a fixed speed when the joystick is pushed forward—again, useful for someone with poor co-ordination or a tremor. However, take-off tends to be jerkier.

In all cases it takes a while to get used to the different controls and it takes a while to build up confidence. Unfortunately, there are many elderly people who will never be able to master the controls and, for their safety and the safety of others, must be advised against doing so. For example, those who lack mobility as a result of a stroke may have additional perceptual and comprehension problems. Vascular diseases can result in intellectual and confusion. Eyesight may be too poor to control a powered chair, safely. Careful assessment is required.

(iii) *Posture* and method of transfers have to be considered when choosing the most appropriate chair, as with manual wheelchairs.

(iv) *Prognosis*—progressive disorders may result in sitting balance becoming worse: arm strength may lessen etc. A scooter may be the answer initially, but with time a chair with sensitive joystick control for use indoors as well as out may be necessary.

(v) *Environment*—it is important to consider whether the chair will be used indoors, outdoors, or both. Kerbs and steep hills may have to be negotiated and access in and out of the house may have to be adapted.

(vi) *Transport of the chair*—some chairs fold more easily than others to fit into a car, for going on outings or holidays.

(vii) *Storage*—the larger buggies may need a garage or a hut with a power outlet for recharging the batteries.

REFERENCES

Cochrane G M, Wilshere E R 1982 Equipment for the disabled: wheelchairs, 5th edn. Oxfordshire Health Authority, Oxford

Department of Health and Social Security 1982 Handbook of Wheelchairs and Bicycles and Tricycles, MHM 408

Harpin P 1981 With a little help, volume V1 Mobility. Muscular Dystrophy Group of Great Britain, London

18

Foot care
R. Gerber

A high proportion of the elderly population requires some form of help with foot care and many turn to the National Health Service (NHS) for advice and treatment. Chiropodists are recognised as specialists in problems of the feet, and although NHS chiropody is available, there are waiting lists in most areas and a form of rationing exists. Due to the wide range of foot health complaints suffered by the elderly patient group, mismatching problems to personnel is not uncommon. This means that appropriate help can be difficult to find, and since access to chiropody treatment is not always automatic, frustration often leads to criticism of the service.

The importance of chiropody to the continuing mobility of the growing elderly population is generally accepted, yet knowledge of the scope of the modern chiropodist within the NHS remains vague. It was stated recently that chiropody was the single service most lacking throughout the country and one of the utmost importance to the general health of the elderly.

WHO ARE CHIROPODISTS?

Chiropodists are specialists in problems of the feet. In the UK, chiropody is not a closed profession and so anyone can set up in practice as a 'chiropodist'. This means that the degree of skill on offer can vary widely. They can, however, be divided into two categories — state registered and non-registered.

Non-registered chiropodists

Non-registered chiropodists are a large group of unknown number and variable levels of training. They are represented by several associations, but accurate lists are difficult to come by. Mostly they are to be found in the private sector where, unlike registered chiropodists, they are not subject to a strict code of ethics regarding advertising etc. Some voluntary and commercial organisations do employ non-registered chiropodists but they are excluded from employment in the NHS.

State-registered chiropodists

Chiropodists have been state registered since 1964. Practising chiropodists who had received training before this time were admitted only on application and examination by the Board. Since 1964 state registration has been automatic, on application, for those who have completed a course at one of the schools recognised by the Chiropody Board. On completion of the course, employment is possible in private practice, NHS, industry or commercial organisations. Graduates may go on to take teaching qualifications, and since 1983 a degree course has been available.

State-registered chiropodists who work in the private sector are listed in an annual register which is available at public reference libraries.

FOOTCARE FOR THE ELDERLY AND WHO PROVIDES IT

Normal feet are expected to carry the full weight of the body through all of the functions expected of them without pain. Feet are furthest from the centre of the arterial blood supply, least well served with venous drainage and are supplied by the most peripheral nerves. Not unexpectedly, as time passes things can and do go wrong with feet, the forefoot being particularly vulnerable. It is in this area that most of the common adult foot problems occur.

AGEING FEET

As with the rest of the body, feet deteriorate with age to varying degrees.

Osteoarthrosis is an almost inevitable part of the ageing process, but does not always cause trouble apart from stiffness. This degenerative joint disorder causes deterioration of cartilage and formation of new bone at joint surfaces resulting in knobbly joints and restricted movement. Normally, no serious problems occur unless the affected joints are subjected to undue stress such as walking in excess of the norm or, more commonly, obesity.

With age, degenerative changes occur in the arterial system resulting in a diminishing supply of oxygenated blood to the tissues of the lower limb and foot. Drainage problems due to venous incompetence can also occur, for example varicose veins, and are a common cause of foot and ankle oedema.

There are also age-related changes to the skin resulting in a thinning of both the dermis and epidermis and a slowing of nail growth. There is a reduction of sweat and sebaceous secretion, causing dryness, and a diminution of the fat content of the underlying subcutaneous tissues which reduces natural padding. This subsequent loss of padding on the plantar aspect of the forefoot can be particularly troublesome. Many elderly people complain of feeling as if they are walking on pebbles, even when no local lesions are in evidence.

There are no specific lesions which occur exclusively in old feet but the presence of lesions on a foot displaying degenerative changes can lead to more serious complications such as infection and ulceration.

Many elderly people have skeletal deformities which cannot be cured by chiropody. Nonetheless, much can be done to improve their mobility by relieving local symptoms. In the long-term management of such cases, improvement of foot function can be achieved by the provision of appliances or by modifications to normal footwear.

The simplest form of footcare is the daily

washing and careful drying of the feet in order to maintain the skin in a healthy condition, plus the regular cutting of toenails. Several very good booklets on footcare for the elderly are available. For a wide variety of reasons many elderly people are unable to perform these tasks for themselves and in such cases help must be asked for from more able-bodied members of the family or close friends. Patients in hospitals and residential homes may require the help of a member of staff to perform these simple routine tasks.

Normal toe nails should be cut relatively straight across but following the shape of the end of the toe; care should be taken to keep scissors well away from the nail grooves. This is more easily done after bathing when the nails are soft, and should always be done in good light. The nails should not be cut so short as to expose the nail bed, as this can be very uncomfortable and lead to infection. All rough and sharp edges should be carefully filed. Dry skin is a feature of ageing feet, and the use of emollient creams, especially around the heel area, can be helpful in preventing fissures.

If no one is prepared to help or the need is beyond the scope of untrained personnel, help must be sought from a chiropodist either in the private sector or NHS.

Inability to cut their toe nails can be a source of discomfort, pain, misery and embarrassment to elderly people. Neglected feet are quite common among this age group and in some cases can severely restrict mobility.

Elderly people, or anyone involved in helping with their footcare, should regularly examine feet for signs and symptoms of more severe problems. In the presence of colour change, temperature change, increased dryness of skin, hard ridged brittle nails, hairless and shiny appearance of the skin, itching, swelling, pain, discharge from breaks in the skin or complaints of throbbing, professional help should be obtained. Where a patient has corns, callous, hypertrophic or deformed nails, she should be treated only by a chiropodist.

Chirodopy is of great importance to the general health of the elderly, and effective management of their foot problems makes a valuable contribution to the quality of their lives. The chiropodist's aim is to help maintain patient mobility for as long as possible.

HIGH RISK PATIENTS

Although chiropodists specialise in treatments of the foot, their knowledge extends beyond the foot itself, as many of its problems are related to particular systemic diseases. If, apart from normal degenerative changes a patient presents with specific effects from a particular systemic disease, the chiropodist would view that patient as falling into the 'high risk' group. There are a number of conditions which would qualify a patient as 'high risk' (Table 18.1).

Table 18.1 High risk group conditions

High risk group conditions	Associated Problems in the foot
Diabetes mellitus	Ischaemia due to atherosclerosis or diabetic microangiopathy leading to ulceration, infection, gangrene and amputation. Peripheral neuropathy due to sensory impairment leading to trauma, ulceration and infection. Motor involvement causing muscle weakness and deformity. Autonomic dysfunction causing dry skin leading to fissures and possible infection. Increased susceptibility to infection leading to cellulitis and possible gangrene
	Trauma is the main precipitating cause of infection in an ischaemic and denervated foot caused by, for example, ill-fitting footwear, improper cutting of nails, thermal burns, injury whilst walking barefoot etc. (*Fig. 18.1–18.4*)
Peripheral vascular disease	Ischaemia due to large vessel involvement of lower limbs causing intermittent claudication, rest pain, skin atrophy, hard, brittle nails, susceptibility to ulceration and infection leading to gangrene. Acute ischaemia due to thrombosis or embolism. Inflammatory arterial disease, for example Buerger's disease,

	polyarteritis nodosa, vasospastic disorders, for example Raynaud's disease, chilblains
Diseases of the veins	Caused by: phlebothrombosis, thrombophlebitis and varicose veins, causing oedema and therefore susceptibility to ulceration in infection
Oedema	Due to varicose veins, congestive cardiac failure, lymphoedema, liver disease, kidney problems etc., causing increased susceptibility to trauma, ulceration and infection
Diseases of the nervous system	Motor and sensory impairment causing trophic changes leading to ulceration
Rheumatoid arthritis	Causing gross deformities, peripheral neuropathy, nodules, ulceration, increased liability to infection due to vasculitis and possible systemic drug therapy
Steroid therapy	Poor response to inflammation and impaired healing
Anticoagulant therapy and some blood disorders	Prolonged coagulation time

Elderly patients will sometimes display the effects of combinations of more than one of these conditions.

Many high risk patients with no obvious clinical evidence of complications may only require routine conservative treatment and advice. These patients are extremely vulnerable and the importance of good hygiene and well-fitting footwear is always stressed, the aim here being to prevent trauma and the formation of any lesions. Local response in degenerated tissue to corns, callosities and trauma is very different to that of normal tissue and can quickly result in ulceration, infection, gangrene and eventual amputation. These patients must be monitored regularly as they may at any time present with acute symptoms.

Where serious complications are already present it is important that wherever possible these patients should be brought to clinics where specialist facilities are available in order to cut down further risk of infection. The benefits, physical and psychological, derived by semi-mobile patients from outings such as visits to the chiropody clinic are numerous. Where family or friends are unable to provide suitable transport arrangements, several voluntary groups can be called upon to help out. Where an ambulance is the only feasible form of transportation, visits can sometimes be combined with hospital outpatient appointments or visits to day hospitals.

As stated earlier, a domiciliary chiropody service is available but restricted to totally housebound patients. All patients in the 'high risk' category should only be treated by state-registered chiropodists.

FOOTWEAR

Examination of footwear and advice is a routine part of chiropody treatment. No long-term management plans can be made without thorough examination and assessment of the patient's footwear.

Forefoot deformities are common among the elderly population and many of these are the result of wearing badly fitting shoes during formative years. Comfortable, well-fitting shoes are vital to the continuing mobility of the elderly, and much can be done to improve the fit of mass-produced footwear. The commonest single cause of corns and callosities is ill-fitting shoes. Shoes should be long enough, wide enough and deep enough. Adjustable fastenings, such as laces or straps and buckles, are advisable so that the heel can be held in the heel seat, preventing excessive movement forwards into the toe box during walking. The widest part of the foot should coincide with the widest part of the shoe. Heels should not be too high; 3.8 cm ($1\frac{1}{2}$ in) is about the maximum height if overloading of the forefoot is to be avoided. The area of the heel base is also important, as the larger it is the more stable a base it will provide during walking. When buying shoes, patients are advised to choose a shop where a trained fitter is available in order to avoid costly mistakes.

Ideally each patient should have two pairs

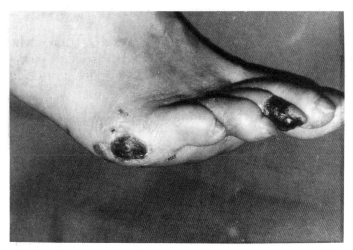

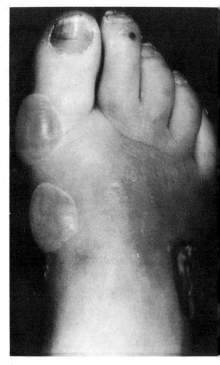

Fig. 18.1 Male insulin dependent diabetic displaying a degree of ischaemic ulceration on 5th metatarsalphalangeal joint and pregangrenous 3rd toe due to microangiopathy

Fig. 18.2 Female insulin dependent diabetic displaying infecting ulceration with cellutis. Thermal burns and small ischaemic area on 2nd toe

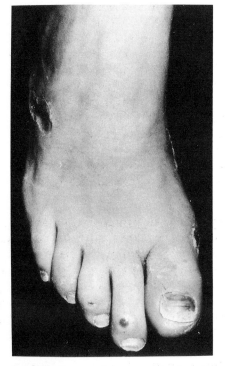

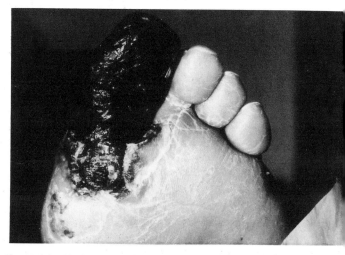

Fig. 18.3 Same patient one month later, cellulitis clear, ulcers healing, but area on 2nd toe increasing in size

Fig. 18.4 Male insulin dependent diabetic displaying severe ischaemic changes. This patient eventually had a mid-tarsal amputation

of leather shoes kept in good repair and a pair of slippers.

Some elderly people spend most of their time indoors wearing slippers or soft slip-on shoes. This type of footwear can be the cause of falls and should never be allowed to become sloppy or down at heel. It is important that they fit well, are not too loose and preferably have some form of fastening, for example, velcro etc. Where fastening is impossible, a style which comes high up on the front of the foot is advised. Well-fitting shoes can prevent the formation of lesions, even when deformities are present, by not interfering with foot function.

In the long-term management of some elderly patients it is desirable to protect bony prominances with silicone shields and to replace lack of natural padding by providing cushioned insoles. These treatments can only be effective with well-fitting shoes. Where gross deformity makes the wearing of mass-produced footwear difficult, modifications can be made, for example, balloon patches for gross hallux valgus with exostosis, or upper insertions to increase depth in the toe box to accommodate deformed or overlapping toes. There are many more shoe modifications too numerous to describe here.

Many old people complain of 'cold feet', and in an effort to solve the problem wear more than one pair of socks or stockings. One pair of well-fitting socks or stockings of suitable material without bulky seams or darns washed daily is a better solution. Thermal insoles are now available from chemists and shoe shops, are relatively inexpensive, take up little room in the shoes and are very effective insulators.

Elderly patients are always discouraged from wearing garters and where bed-socks are worn, are advised that they should always be loose fitting.

The chiropodist will be able to supply elderly patients with information about local stockists of extra-wide fitting shoes. He will also provide names and addresses of mail order firms specialising in footwear for particular problems, for example, felt bootees and machine-washable shoes.

Where surgical footwear is prescribed, more comfort can often be achieved by incorporating padded insoles or silicone shields provided by the chiropodist.

SUMMARY

As can be seen, elderly people's footcare needs cover a very wide spectrum.

1. There are those who only require help with basic foot hygiene and simple nail cutting, for whom skilled treatment by a chiropodist is unnecessary.
2. There is a large number who require fairly regular relief from local symptoms and advice in order that comfort be maintained and the occurrence of more serious foot problems avoided. Here appropriate care should be undertaken by a chiropodist either in the private sector or the NHS.
3. Due to increasing longevity there is a growing number of elderly people with underlying medical conditions whose mobility is heavily reliant on regular specialist treatment by a registered chiropodist in order that distressing and costly hospital admissions be minimised.
4. There are also elderly people whose conditions go beyond the scope of the registered chiropodist's practice, whose early referral for surgical intervention can sometimes be vital.

The demand for NHS chiropody has always exceeded supply. Despite the opening of two new schools of chiropody, the expansion of several others and the limited success of the introduction of footcare assistants the situation continues. This is to a great extent aggravated by the growing elderly population which it serves. There are, of course, a number of other factors which also influence the situation, but these are too complex to explore in this chapter.

It has been shown that a wide range of

personnel in both the public and private sector may offer footcare treatment of one form or another. Since chiropody is particularly scarce, the importance of appropriately deploying the limited resources available makes sense. At local level, responsibility for all Health Board Chiropody services rests with the area chiropodist. Requests for details of the service or any complaints should be addressed to him.

Where criticism of the service comes from a fellow professional the problem is often one of communication. For example, in a busy hospital how is the chiropodist contacted in order that his treatment of a particular patient enables the continuing management of that patient by other therapists? If all else fails details of the chiropodist's whereabouts at any given time (within reason) should be available from the administrators at the office of the area chiropodist. Having found him, clear arrangements should be made in order that a two way flow of information exists for the future. It is only through co-operation and understanding that any improvement will take place.

REFERENCES

Kemp J, Winkler J T 1983 Problems a foot: need and efficiency in footcare. Disabled Living Foundation
Neale D, Adams I 1985 Common foot disorders: diagnosis and management, 2nd edn. Churchill Livingstone, Edinburgh

19

Clothing

J. Maclean

Most people buy the type of clothes they like from the shops they choose without limitations except perhaps financial or geographical ones. Many older people have additional limitations imposed upon them by problems of ageing, illness and/or disability. The effects of these are very varied, ranging from difficulty with small fastenings to a total inability to dress; from minor mobility problems to being completely housebound or having difficuly with laundry and care of clothes. These and other clothing problems which frequently affect the elderly can often be alleviated by an occupational therapist.

An important role of the occupational therapist is to encourage people to lead as normal a life as possible within their limitations. In relation to clothing this encompasses a wide range of tasks starting with selecting and buying clothes, dressing and undressing independently, and laundering and caring for clothes in general. With ageing, these tasks may become more difficult. It is important that everything possible be done to minimise the problems and thus make life easier for the elderly people concerned.

Clothes fulfil several functions: they protect us and help keep us warm or cool depending on the climate; they also say something about the person wearing them — they are part of the identity of the individual.

Some people may not care much about what they look like, but everybody wishes to wear clothes in which they feel comfortable, both physically and psychologically.

As a general rule, when people grow older

their social circle diminishes. People retire from work, their freedom of choice to participate in interests outside the home may narrow, especially if they have mobility problems, and they may lose relatives and friends through bereavement. It is important, therefore, that factors such as clothes, which contribute to maintaining individuality, are given the utmost attention. This is of great importance in continuing care where people no longer have their own home to reflect their identity. All that remains to an individual is the limited number of personal items she can keep in an instition, along with the clothes she wears and the things she does.

Some institutions discourage residents from wearing their own clothes, but where possible residents should be allowed and encouraged to select, wear and care for their own clothes. It is distressing to treat a patient who does not want to wear 'hospital' clothing: the patient knows it is not her own and feels uncomfortable wearing it. In addition, it is often unsuitable and ill-fitting. It is no wonder that in such a situation patients tend to withdraw from participation into the isolation of institutionalisation.

The ideal is set out in DS85/75 (Minimum Standards in Geriatric Hospitals and Departments): 'All patients should have the necessary range of clothing, either personally owned or provided by the hospital on a personal basis'.

Attention to clothing is important, too, for elderly people living at home. Independence in dressing is not only morale-boosting; it may make the difference between returning to the community and being admitted to long-term care. It is also vital that elderly people feel they have clothes which are attractive enough to wear outside the home, otherwise they are less likely to go out and thus further limit outside interests and social contacts.

PROBLEM AREAS FOR THE ELDERLY IN RELATION TO CLOTHING

Limitation of range of movement

This may cause problems for many elderly people due to general loss of the integrity of joints, for example pathological changes caused by conditions such as rheumatoid disease or osteoarthrosis. The main clinical features of these disorders are joint stiffness, pain and loss of muscle power, and in advanced stages deformity of the joints involved. When hands and wrists are affected, the major functional problems are in gripping clothes to pull them on or off and in coping with small fastenings, e.g. small buttons, hooks and eyes, and zip tabs. If the elbows and shoulders are involved, reaching above the head and round the back is limited.

Solutions to these difficulties are to decrease the number but increase the size of fastenings; to choose garments with front fastenings rather than back ones; and to avoid garments which have a lot of stretch.

People with generalised upper limb stiffness may find it helpful, when putting garments over their head, to place their elbows on a table, hold the garment in their hands and bend the trunk to get their head into the garment. This reduces the amount of flexion and abduction required at the shoulder joint (see Fig. 19.1).

Limitation of range of movement can also affect the hips, knees, ankles and spine. Osteoarthrosis is a common condition in

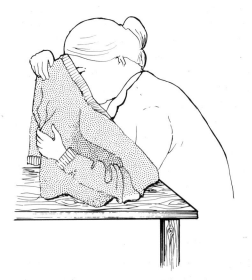

Fig. 19.1 Leaning elbows on a table helps an elderly person get garments over her head

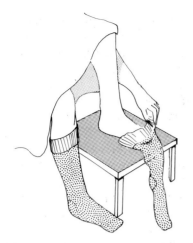

Fig. 19.2 Use of a small stool may help an elderly person reaching her foot

elderly people and these joints are its major targets. The main problem is bending down to reach the feet; this makes it difficult to put on socks, stockings, shoes, trousers and underpants. Placing the foot on a low stool and reaching down may help as this places less stress on the hips and spine (see Fig. 19.2). If this is not helpful, a stocking aid and/or long-handled shoe horn may be used. If the two can be combined, so much the better, as this reduces the number of aids required.

Generally, clothes which can be put on over the head, e.g. dresses, skirts and underslips, mean less bending than those which have to be pulled up over the feet. In all cases where joint stiffness is a problem, it is best to dress the stiffest side first, thus leaving the more mobile limbs to complete the task.

Joint stiffness may also affect the speed of walking. An elderly person walking to the toilet will take longer to get there; it is therefore important that she can deal efficiently with clothing on arrival in order to avoid accidental incontinence.

Cerebrovascular disease

This causes major and often multiple problems for elderly people in relation to clothing. Strokes usually result in hemiplegia and loss of balance, both of varying degrees of severity. If the dominant hemisphere is involved there may be problems with speech and comprehension; if the non-dominant hemisphere is involved, dressing apraxia and associated difficulties may be present. Muscle spasm, often worse on exertion, can add to these problems. If a neurodevelopmental approach to treatment is employed, the patient will have to learn a new system of dressing which involves maintaining the affected side in a reflex-inhibiting pattern. Many elderly patients find this confusing, especially if they also have the additional difficulty of receptive dysphasia. If a rehabilitative approach is used, the patient will have to learn to compensate for the inability to use one half of the body. Either way, the main rule is to dress the affected side first, and thus leave the more mobile limbs to complete the task.

The problems of one-handedness may be helped by having garments with front or side fastenings. Buttons or closed-end zips are the easiest to deal with. Open-ended zips, of the type seen on casual jackets, are almost impossible to manage using one hand. A larger than normal opening or reasonably stretchy fabric may help.

Tights, stockings and corsetry are the most difficult garments to deal with. There are no easy solutions. Bras may be elasticated or have front fastening, or they can be fastened at the front and then swivelled round to the back before putting the arms through the straps. The use of stocking or tights aids may add to rather than diminish the problem, as two hands are often needed to put the stocking on the aid. Corsetry may be adapted but this is often unsatisfactory. Many elderly ladies are used to wearing corsets, so as to have suspenders to hold up their stockings, in this case a light non-elastic suspender belt or liberty bodice may be a satisfactory alternative. If the lady can reach her feet it is possible to put on stockings, provided they have been carefully caught up between the thumb and fingers, placed over the toes, then gradually pulled up.

The frustration of dressing with the use of only one hand should not be underestimated. It is important that the occupational therapist teaching hemiplegic patients to dress should select garments which are likely to be relatively easy to put on. This will reduce the frustration and solve some of the possible problems before they emerge; at the same time it will boost the self-confidence and morale of the patient.

Balance may be a problem for a hemiplegic patient, especially in the early stages. It is important that the patient dresses sitting on the bed or a stable chair with arms, and that her feet reach the floor comfortably when she is seated. It is also important that clothes are placed within reach.

Dressing apraxia and associated problems cause a variety of difficulties. Clothes which the patient recognises as her own and are in a simple style, help a little. Coloured tags stitched to the garments to indicate the back, and presentation of clothes in the correct order, may all help with this problem; practice in dressing will give reinforcement. It must be noted, however, that some elderly people suffer from a very severe form of dressing apraxia and will never be able to dress independently. In this case it is important to involve carers as early as possible in order that they receive adequate advice and guidance before they have to cope unaided; this can make the patient's return home less traumatic.

Involuntary movements

Tremor is the commonest involuntary movement to affect elderly people. Its two major forms are resting and intention tremor. Resting tremor is seen most commonly in Parkinson's disease; it involves mainly the hands and forearms. It can sometimes be temporarily controlled when the patient is carrying out a task. However, after such control the tremor tends to return with increasing amplitude. It is vital that the clothes worn by the patient are easily put on and fastened, thus maximising the use of the limited time she can control her tremor.

Simple styles with fewer, larger fastenings which are within the field of vision and can be easily handled, are best. The other features of Parkinson's disease, such as stiffness and hypokinesia, are also helped by these solutions.

Intention tremor becomes apparent on specific movement, and this obviously affects dressing. The easiest solution is to wear clothes which have no fastenings, e.g. trousers and skirts with elastic waistbands, sweaters, casual shirts and blouses.

Any type of tremor is tiring; it is therefore important that the effort of dressing be reduced in order that the patient has enough energy to cope with other tasks.

Breathlessness

This is a very common feature of many chest and heart conditions, which tend to worsen with age. Severe breathlessness causes problems with dressing because the effort involved uses up the patient's limited oxygen supplies, and rest pauses may be required. Many breathless people feel more comfortable in loose non-restricting garments, which are also easier to put on.

Incontinence

Incontinence in the elderly is probably more common than is realised, mainly because many elderly people find it embarrassing to discuss. It may be caused by many different factors associated with bladder and bowel conditions, but it may also be secondary to factors such as confusion, dementia, limited mobility, or drugs. When a person is incontinent it poses social, psychological and practical problems. It is vital that patients who have other problems, e.g. joint stiffness, which slow their speed of access to a toilet, have clothing which is easy to cope with.

If the patient has a catheter, the catheter bag should be accommodated in or under the clothing. This is easy if reasonably wide trousers are worn, as a bag can be strapped to the leg. In the case of ladies wearing skirts the use of a leg bag may be impractical, as it would have to be strapped to the thigh. A large hidden pocket inside the front of a skirt to accommodate a bag, providing that the bag is emptied at regular intervals, need not be cumbersome. This problem deserves careful consideration by occupational therapists and other staff, as most people are appalled at the thought of carrying around a catheter bag full of urine, either on the front of a walking frame or on the side of a wheelchair.

People who use incontinence pads also have clothing-related problems. Most firms who manufacture incontinence pads also produce pants to accommodate them. To be comfortable they must fulfil certain criteria: they must be the correct size to minimise the amount of possible chafing; fastenings must be easy for the patient or carer to deal with; and they must give good protection with maximum circulation of air to the skin. Other clothes worn over the pads and pants must be loose enough so that they do not show their contours and can be easily taken off and replaced.

Incontinence poses the additional problems of extra laundry: washing garments as soon as possible after soiling helps minimise smells and stains (see also p. 200).

Sensory loss

Loss of sensation in the hands gives rise to difficulty with fastenings which cannot be seen, e.g. back zips or collar buttons. The use of a mirror or clothes with front fastenings help here. Loss of sensation in the feet is common in vascular conditions in elderly people. It is important that socks, stockings and footwear do not chafe or constrict the limbs, as this can cause problems of skin breakdown, and the resultant healing process is often protracted. Tight elastic, e.g. in sock tops, should be avoided to reduce the risk of oedema in the limbs. Loss of sensation in other areas may also give rise to problems of pressure. Clothes with bulky seams, hard zips and buttons should be avoided. Elderly people with any type of loss of sensation

should be taught to inspect the areas involved and advised to avoid wearing clothing and footwear which produces redness or abrasion of the skin.

Visual handicap

This is found to varying degrees in many elderly people. Patients with this problem may have difficulty in identifying the back and front of a garment and in establishing if it is right side out. Clues such as seam edges and labels help to establish the correct way to put a garment on. Elderly people with visual impairment may also need some help in buying a garment if they are unable to distinguish colours and see styles. Once they have purchased it, however, they may be able to identify the garment by touch.

Confusion

Confusion in elderly patients may be short or long-term, mild or severe. Using familiar clothes and dressing in a non-distracting environment may help. The occupational therapist should also establish what the patient calls a garment (e.g. sweater, jumper or pullover, trousers or slacks) and use that term when dealing with the patient. Careful consideration should be given as to whether or not dressing aids should be introduced to a confused patient, as they may add to rather than reduce difficulties.

General mobility

General mobility may be diminished as people get older; this, along with some of the problem areas previously discussed, may pose difficulties for elderly people getting to and from shops to buy clothes. It may be that the person is unable to drive and has to rely on public transport, which is often difficult to cope with because of the distance from home, waiting time and high steps for access. This is a vast problem for people who are unsteady on their feet and for those who use walking aids. On arriving at a shopping area the shops may be a considerable distance from bus stops; there may also be stairs to negotiate within the shops. All of this is tiring and requires a great deal of effort.

The use of taxis, whilst convenient, is expensive and adds a considerable amount to the cost of clothes. For elderly people with this type of problem there are two main solutions. Firstly, someone else can buy clothes on their behalf. However, many people find it difficult to buy for someone else. The range of shops available may be limited because some shops will not refund money for unsuitable goods. Sale items, especially, often fall into this category. It is always advisable to ask, before purchasing clothes for someone else, if the shop will refund money or exchange unsuitable goods.

The second alternative is the use of mail order catalogues. This enables elderly people to select clothes of their choice in their own homes. A criticism sometimes levelled at mail order shopping is that it is relatively more expensive; this has to be weighed up against possible bus or taxi fares and the effort involved in getting to and from shops. Another advantage of mail order shopping is that garments can be tried on at home. Many elderly people have difficulty in coping with small or communal changing facilities, which often have no seats. Payments for clothes can be spread over a period of time if necessary, and several catalogues can be used, thus increasing the choice. Some mail order firms now cater specifically for older people and for those with a fuller figure.

Suitability

Clothes must be suitable for the individual wearing them and her life-style. It is important that elderly people do not look or feel out of place because of the clothes they wear; their clothes should be acceptable for the age group and general fashion trends for the elderly. This allows a good deal of leeway for personal choice; it may be that one elderly lady will find a jogging suit both acceptable and suitable for her needs whilst another may

not be happy unless dressed in a more formal way.

Comfort

There are several factors which contribute to the comfort of a garment; these include the fabric; style, size, appearance and its acceptability to the wearer. The number and type of garments will also contribute to comfort. Dressing as well as wearing should be considered in relation to comfort. Warmth is important, especially as many elderly people move more slowly and subsequently the body's own heat-generating capacity decreases. Elderly people are also at risk from hypothermia.

Fabrics which trap and retain air, e.g. wool, piled, knitted and woven fabrics, are all warm. Quilted fabrics are also ideal, as their construction effectively combines two or more layers of usually light-weight material. Many people equate weight or bulk of fabrics with warmth, but two thinner garments are more effective in maintaining heat than one thick one. However, two garments also take twice as much effort to put on. Many elderly people solve that problem by putting on and taking off two garments at a time, e.g. two jumpers. Lined garments also increase warmth.

Heavy and bulky garments are not only limited in their warmth, but also restrict movement in general and lead to problems in dressing for elderly people with stiff and painful joints.

Absorption

Absorption of fabrics should be considered, especially for those elderly people who have to make an additional effort in getting about; they may perspire more heavily than normal and if perspiration is not absorbed this causes discomfort and odour. Natural fibres are very absorbent; nylon and similar man-made fibres are not.

The dilemma which faces people in this situation is that clothes require to be washed more often to keep them fresh, and some natural fibres are more diffiult to wash, e.g. hand-wash woollens. A balance has to be found between the comfort of an absorbent natural fibre which may be more difficult to wash and the relative discomfort of a man-made which is easy to wash. Many fabric mixtures currently available answer this problem very adequately as do machine-washable woollen garments.

Elasticity

Elasticity of fabrics can both help and hinder dressing and increase or decrease comfort.

Very firm elastic garments, e.g. elastic stockings, are difficult to deal with, especially for elderly people with weak grip or painful joints. Some types of corsetry also fall into this category. Corsetry fastenings can be adapted using webbing, D-rings and Velcro (Figs. 19.3, 19.4).

Less constricting elasticity of fabric is an advantage as it allows stretch of garments when dressing or moving about; they also return to their 'proper' state after stretch. It is vital that any thread used in the construction, repair and reinforcement of these garments is also stretchy in order to avoid tearing of the garment. Knitted fabrics, wool jersey and crimplene all have more stretch than woven fabrics. Elderly people who use a wheelchair or walking aids and those who have difficulty getting out of a chair will all find stretch fabrics more comfortable. They are also a better and more attractive solution than merely buying clothing a few sizes larger than is necessary.

Texture

Texture of clothes and fabrics may be a problem for some people who dislike the feel of certain materials and for those who have extra-sensitive areas, e.g. following herpes zoster. Some people dislike the feel of, for example, brushed nylon which is used in the manufacture of warm garments such as night-dresses. In cases where people suffer from extra sensitivity, fabrics must be selected with

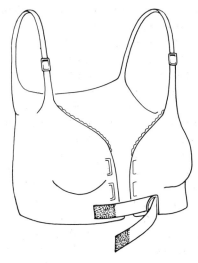

Fig. 19.3 Straps with Velcro and D ring

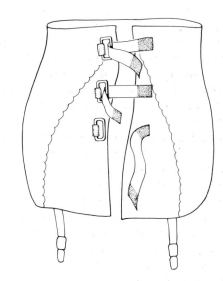

Fig. 19.4 Adaptation to bra and corsets to ease dressing

care in order to provide maximum comfort for the wearer.

Durability

Wear and tear on fabrics can be increased by the use of crutches, prostheses, calipers and wheelchairs, and by other factors such as frequent washing. It is vital that clothes are selected for maximum wear and value for money.

Compact woven fabrics are stronger than knitted ones. Cheaper garments often have poor seam allowance and construction and are usually a false economy. Garments which have a mixture of natural and synthetic fibres have the advantage of comfort and durability combined. Lining in a garment also increases its life. Garments which are likely to be subjected to additional strain, e.g. when dressing, may be reinforced by extra stitching when the garment is new. Areas such as armhole seams, buttons, buttonholes, zips and pocket corners are all worthy of this attention. Thread suitable for the type of fabric must be used.

Laundry

Laundry of clothing can be a difficulty for many elderly people, especially when increased washing is necessary because of incontinence, dribbling or food spillage.

Machine washing is ideal, but many elderly people cannot afford to install a washing machine. Hand washing is difficult and time consuming. It is very important that elderly people are encouraged to read care labels on garments at the time of purchase. Many of today's fabrics are relatively easy to care for. They should be washed before they are too grubby; pre-wash soaking may reduce the effort of hand washing, and short spins or drip drying minimise the amount of ironing required.

Limitation in mobility and diminished stamina also give rise to difficulties in getting to dry cleaning and launderette facilities.

Safety

Safety of garments and fabrics is vital for elderly people. Those with loss of sensation should avoid garments with hard seams in order to prevent abrasions.

Flame resistance is important in night-gowns, dressing gowns and other long, loose garments, especially if there is danger from an open fire.

Loose garments, ties and belts should be

chosen with care so that they cannot get caught when walking, transferring etc.

Slippery fabrics may be a problem for those elderly people who sit a lot of the time and are unable to push up in a chair. In this situation either the clothes or the seat cover must be non-slip.

Dressing difficulties

These can be minimised substantially by careful selection of clothes.

Generally, factors which facilitate dressing for someone coping independently will also aid a carer. Fewer fastenings within easy reach, stretch and lined garments, wrap-over skirts, and garments with wider armholes, sleeves and legs all help to minimise the effort required in dressing (see Fig. 19.4).

Elderly people with deteriorating health will not always be in a financial position to buy new suitable clothing; however the above guidelines may apply equally to selection from their current wardrobe.

ADAPTATION OF CLOTHING

The most useful clothing adaptations are often the simplest ones. Adaptations fall into five major categories:

1. Replacing one type of fastening with another
2. Removing unnecessary fastening
3. Increasing the size of an opening or fastening
4. Altering the position of an opening or fastening
5. Addition of features to assist in dressing.

1. The commonest replacement fastening is velcro, which can be substituted for buttons, zips, and hooks and eyes. Velcro is available in a wide colour range and colour matching is important in order that the adaptation is unobtrusive. When using velcro, small pieces are easier to align than long strips, which can be awkward and frustrating to deal with. It is best to stitch the hooked side so that it is

under the looped side in fastening. This decreases the chance of the hooks catching on garments and becoming clogged up with fibres. Buttonholes must be stitched up and buttons sewn on top of them so that it looks like a normal fastening.

Buttons may also be replaced by press studs. In order to be strong the press studs must be fairly large, which makes them more obvious. In areas where there is no strain, smaller press studs may replace buttons in the same way as velcro.

2. Some or all buttons can be left permanently fastened in a cardigan and it can be put on over the head. It is neater if the open edge of the cardigan is stitched to the button border; this prevents buttonholes looking 'pulled'. This type of adaptation can only be achieved with stretch fabrics.

The use of elastic thread to sew cuff buttons on shirts helps people who have loss of muscle power in the upper limbs. Elastic thread has the disadvantage that repeated stretch tends to make it fray.

3. Increasing the size of an opening may be necessary if excessive strain is placed on a garment when dressing. A zip may be replaced by a longer one; this is easy if the zip is in a seam, as the opening can be enlarged by unpicking some of the seam. If the zip is in a faced opening; care must be taken to make a new facing with matching fabric; otherwise it looks obvious. The same adaptation can be carried out on the shoulder seam of a dress or a raglan seam of a sweater.

Increasing the size of the fastening can be achieved by using larger buttons, which often fit through existing buttonholes. Care must be taken not to make these too tight; buttonholes can, in some cases; be enlarged but this should only be tackled by an experienced dressmaker.

Zip tags can have loops or rings attached to them in order to make them easier to grasp.

4. Alteration of the position of an opening or fastening may be achieved by making a side opening, e.g. in a dress to replace a back opening; this is easily achieved if the seam allowance is good. Front openings may be difficult to make because of lack of front seams or because of collars or facings on a garment.

Additional openings may be required in some garments, e.g. provision of a zip in the inside leg seam of trousers in order to gain access to a catheter bag or prosthesis; this is usually best stitched neatly by hand, at least on one side, as it is difficult to sew by machine.

Provision of an additional opening in corsetry is useful in some cases and may be achieved by opening the garment, neatening the raw edges and sewing on tapes and D-rings or inserting a zip.

The problem of fastening bras can be overcome by adapting the bra to open at the front; again the use of tapes, velcro and a small D-ring often help here (see Fig. 19.3).

5. The most common additions to a garment are tapes attached to the inside of it in order that the wearer can get the garment over her feet and pull it up. It is important that the tapes are made of a soft fabric and that they can be hidden from view after use.

There are many garment adaptations which may be carried out. The main questions which should be asked about any proposed adaptation are: will the adaptation help the individual in dressing and undressing and will it be unobtrusive? If the answer to either is no then it is not worth doing.

The same questions must be asked about dressing aids. These should only be used if they are easy to operate, uncumbersome and resistant to wear and tear.

The most commonly used dressing aids are stocking aids, long-handled shoe horns, dressing sticks and button hooks. Some of them are quite difficult to use and should be selected with care by the occupational therapist. If an aid is to be used as a temporary measure, e.g. a stocking aid following a hip replacement operation, it is important that it is discontinued as soon as the patient is able to achieve the task without its use: this encoures active increase in range of movement.

When clothing for elderly people is considered, many factors have to be taken into account about the clothes and the problems, wishes and expectations of the people wearing them. There can be no hard and fast rules or definite answers and each case must be considered on its own merits. Some general points do apply, however: clothing must be attractive, suitable and comfortable as well as easy to put on and take off, and easy to care for.

Attractive clothing and independence in dressing cannot halt the progress of illness or advancing years; it can, however, boost the morale and self-confidence of elderly people.

Occupational therapists would do their elderly patients and clients a disservice if they did not acknowledge the importance of clothing. It is vital that we make every effort to solve any clothing problems our elderly patients may have to their satisfaction.

FURTHER READING

Dean F 1982 Clothing needs of the elderly person. Disabled Living Foundation, London
Elphick S 1970 Incontinence — some problems, suggestions and conclusions. Disabled Living Foundation, London
Gammell A M, Joyce F 1966 Problems of clothing for the sick and disabled. Disabled Living Foundation, London
Harpin P 1982 With a little help, Vol II. Muscular Dystrophy Group of Great Britain
Hoffman A M 1979 Clothing for the handicapped, the aged and other people with special needs. Charles C Thomas, Illinois
Jay P 1985 Help yourselves, 4th edn. Ian Henry Publications, Hornchurch
Macartney P 1973 Clothes sense for handicapped adults of all ages. Disabled Living Foundation, London
Ruston R 1982 Dressing for disabled people. Disabled Living Foundation, London

20

Recognising problems of sexuality

L. Harris

For all of us working and training in the health care professions today, the need to look at the 'whole person' rather than just the problem areas is emphasised time and time again. We know we must look beyond the obvious, to try to gain some insight into that person's life. If any one patient group has suffered before this ethic came along, it is the elderly. We are now aware that the needs of the elderly patient are greater and more varied than those of most other patients we work with. If the needs of our elderly patients or clients are to be successfully met, we must build up a past/present/future picture, essentially to determine their personality and life-style prior to their illness. An accurate history is essential for any treatment to be effective.

SEXUALITY AND THE ELDERLY

One area that many health care professionals consciously or unconsciously overlook when working with elderly people is sexuality. Even in these days of sexual permissiveness, there are few people who think of sexuality as a life-long need.

We do know that there are obvious physical changes which will inhibit sexual responses; yet there is no known age limit to an active sex life. There are, of course, major factors which will affect an elderly person's sexuality, these being:

1. Age
2. Physical health
3. Marital status (this seems to be especially important for women)
4. Social situation, i.e. living in own home, residential care or hospital.

Research by Pfeiffer and Davis (1972) has also indicated that a high level of sexual activity in youth could correlate with continued sexual interest and activity in later life.

Psychological changes occurring in the elderly

To understand problems related to sexuality in the elderly, we must first look at the psychological changes which occur. These vary greatly between individuals. Any combination of the following will affect most people as they grow older.

1. Retirement with subsequent loss of income and status
2. Ill health (physical or mental)
3. Social isolation due to:
   a. geographically scattered family
   b. loss of partner
   c. ill health
4. Grief and bereavement.

The ability to cope with change and loss, and to adapt appropriately to them, seems to be the key to growing old happily. The elderly have to face many changes in their lives — physical, cognitive and social. How they cope with such changes will depend largely upon their personalities, past life experience and social support. Those who work with the elderly will see that there are many different strategies for coping with change or loss. For some elderly people, to continue to lead active and constructive lives will be the best way. Others will be unable to accept change and may become dependent or manipulative towards those around them. It is often families rather than professionals who will bear the brunt of maladaptive behaviour.

We can see how, for some people, the years after 65 can be filled with stress, ill health, and loneliness. This is reinforced by a 1975 Edinburgh study which showed that 50% of admissions to psychiatric hospitals were aged 65 years or over.

Sexual attitudes

To understand the patterns of presentation of problems related to sexuality, we must first of all consider the moral attitudes of this generation. In general terms they are a generation who rarely discussed sex, had no access to information or education, had slight knowledge of contraception and little awareness of sexually transmitted disease.

Sexual intercourse outside marriage was seen as sinful, and with no legal abortion, illegitimate children were often brought up by married members of the family, by grandmothers, or were adopted. There are many known cases of the mother of an illegitimate child being admitted to a psychiatric hospital. Therefore with this ethic of not speaking, thinking or reading about sex, how do the older generation cope with today's permissive society? Many elderly people are embarrassed and shocked by the media; others see it as part of the general decline in society's morality. A few more liberated elderly people welcome today's permissiveness as freedom which they were denied.

Perhaps by understanding the morals instilled into the elderly from youth, by considering the repression and guilt which accompanied them, we can begin to understand why many elderly people have problems related to sexuality. These problems can present in many different ways.

SEXUALITY RELATED TO PHYSICAL AND PHYSIOLOGICAL CHANGES

The physiological changes in the elderly which relate to sexual activity are easily defined. Like most other changes occurring in the elderly there is a reduction, or in some cases loss, of ability. The accompanying emotional changes are more difficult to define as the elderly are not keen to discuss their sexual feelings openly and honestly. Most research, therefore, shows wide fluctuations.

Physiological changes

1. *Male*
   a. increased difficulty obtaining and maintaining an erection
   b. decreased power of ejaculation
   c. reduced volume of ejaculate
   d. longer refractory period.

2. *Female*
   a. thinning of vaginal skin
   b. loss of elasticity of vaginal wall
   c. increase in time for lubrication to occur
   d. shorter orgasmic phase
   e. vaginismus may occur.

The few studies which have been carried out concerning emotional changes show marked difference in desire between men and women. Most women claim to lose the desire for sex at an earlier age than men. However, physiologically women have fewer difficulties and can continue to respond sexually until late in life. The fact that most women depend on their male partner to initiate sex may explain this discrepancy.

There is no doubt that many couples, as they grow older, simply close the door on the sexual part of their relationship. The menopause or other physiological changes, e.g. prostate problems, may provide a stepping stone out of a sexual relationship for those who have had long-term unsuccessful sexual experiences.

For those who choose to continue to have an active sex life, they should be seen as normal, healthy people. We must also remember that the non-coitus part of sex becomes increasingly important as physiological changes occur. Touching, stroking and holding may become as fulfilling as sexual intercourse and orgasm.

Causes of sexual problems

1. Physical or physiological changes
2. Unsuitable circumstances, e.g. residential care or hospital
3. Anxiety, especially after illness
4. Poor communication and understanding within the relationship
5. Depression resulting in loss of libido
6. Imbalance of sexual needs between partners
7. Change in body image e.g. after mastectomy or amputation, resulting in low self-esteem
8. Reduced sensory input e.g. vision, touch
9. Loss of partner.

All of these problems will be reinforced if there is poor communication between the partners or with the professionals with whom they have contact.

Anxiety is a major cause of sexual difficulties. This is especially common after illness, e.g. post-coronary or cerebral vascular accident. There may not just be the person's own anxieties but also those of his or her partner to deal with. Partners often fear the exertion associated with sex will exacerbate the patient's symptoms or cause a relapse. Therefore there may be guilt associated with resuming active sex. Appropriate guidance and counselling taking the couple's individual needs into account should alleviate much anxiety.

Unsuitable circumstances are another important factor in sexual difficulties. A couple living in their own home may have become less inhibited once their children have left home. However, when one or both partners are in an institution — hospital, nursing home or residential care — they will probably feel restricted and inhibited even in the non-coitus aspect of sex. Little consideration is made within institutional care for the sexual needs of the clients. Few institutions have adequate accommodation for married couples, or even individual bedrooms where a couple could feel secure in touching and holding. Most elderly people do not demonstrate their feelings openly in public and many couples would benefit from personal space where they could feel secure and be demonstrative.

Where there is an imbalance of sexual needs within the couple little can be done without honest communication between partners. Often wives will tolerate such a situation, seeing it as their duty.

Coping with physical disability

After any major illness or operation there may be anxiety or doubt about resuming a sexual relationship. The following are guidelines to show how a patient may be affected. A worried patient or client should always be encouraged to discuss the problem with his or her doctor.

1. Prostatectomy. Side-effects may be impotence or retrograde ejaculation. The patient should be reassured that he can still experience and enjoy orgasm.

2. Hysterectomy. Patients may experience vaginal dryness which can be treated with hormone replacements or local creams. A hysterectomy should not effect sexual enjoyment, although most patients believe it will. Counselling and reassurance should give the patient enough confidence to resume a sexual relationship.

3. Hip replacement. Anxiety may be the greatest problem after a hip replacement operation. Patients may need some guidance on positioning and 'permission' from doctor.

4. Hemiplegia. Again anxiety may be a major problem. The rise in blood pressure which occurs during intercourse could be dangerous for the patient. Medical advice is essential. It may be possible for the patient to take hypertensive medication prior to intercourse. Advice on positioning and taking a less active role will be useful. Counselling will relieve the partner's anxiety that sex may cause a relapse.

5. Acute cardiac problems. As with a hemiplegic patient, the acute rise in blood pressure may be dangerous. A very rough guide is that if six weeks after a myocardial infarction the patient can climb a flight of stairs, and walk without distress around the block, then intercourse should be possible. The patient will be advised to take a less active part, and to seek medical approval. Anxiety is often present but again medical 'permission' may be enough to counteract it.

6. Hypertension. The patient should be advised to avoid exertion and be aware of the rise in blood pressure during intercourse. Hypertensives can be taken prior to intercourse, but the patient should be advised to take a less active role and to rest afterwards.

7. Asthma. Intercourse may precipitate an attack, but it may be possible to take antispasmodics before or during intercourse. There is often prolonged breathlessness immediately after sexual intercourse. Counselling will alleviate both patient's and partner's anxieties.

8. Acute respiratory disorders. With respiratory disorders there may be accompanying cardiac problems. Advice as for (5) Acute cardiac problems and (7) Asthma.

9. Clients under dialysis. Advice as (6) Hypertension.

10. Diabetes. Diabetics may experience local irritation. During intercourse there may be painful irritation due to inflamed foreskin or vaginitis. Use of a lubricating jelly or treatment with oestrogen may help vaginal dryness. Vaginitis which is the involuntary spasm of the muscles surrounding the entrance to the vagina, can be treated by vaginal muscle training.

11. Rheumatoid arthritis/osteoarthritis. Advice on positioning is useful. The patient may need advice on how to take a less active role. It is often possible for the patient to take analgesics before intercourse.

12. Amputee. Advice on positioning and techniques are useful. Patient must be aware of rise in blood pressure. Altered body image may cause anxiety, poor self-esteem. How the patient has adapted to amputation will affect his or her sexual relationship.

Often practical advice and appropriate counselling will be enough to relieve anxiety. Medical approval or 'permission' is important. However, many patients feel that they are not 'normal' to still have an active interest in sex and may feel too inhibited to seek advice.

Therefore we must be sensitive to their needs and the cues which they may give us.

SEXUALITY RELATED TO PSYCHIATRIC ILLNESS

It is common in both organic and functional illness for a patient to have a strong sexual component to his or her presentation. In illnesses which result in organic impairment there are similar patterns of presentation.

Organic illness

Senile dementia (arteriosclerotic/cerebrovascular):

Toxic confusional state

Often the problems which stem from organic impairment will be tolerated or 'covered up' by spouse or family. Therefore the difficulties may only come to light through ill health of one partner. Common difficulties are:

1. Disinhibition
2. Patient becomes too demanding on partner creating an imbalance of sexual needs
3. Content of speech can become sexually explicit or suggestive
4. Inappropriate initiation of a sexual relationship
5. Inappropriate masturbation or exposing sexual organs.

Partners who are experiencing any of the above problems may feel embarrassed or guilty confiding in family or professionals. In institutional settings such behaviour is likely to lead to rejection by fellow residents and possibly by untrained or inexperienced staff.

Pre-senile dementia:

Alzheimer's disease
Jakob-Creutzfeldt's disease
Pick's disease
Toxic confusional state
Korsakov's psychosis.

When organic problems occur in a person under 65 years of age, they can be more serious as the accompanying physical deterioration is absent. Therefore, the person's true level of impairment may not be obvious to family, friends or indeed to those in the health care professions. Often the younger patient with organic problems will retain good social responses, dress appropriately and adopt very clever mechanisms for covering up their problem areas. Therefore a sexual problem may be difficult to sort out from all the other concurrent difficulties.

The patterns of presentation of sexual problems in under-65s with organic impairment are very similar to those described above for the over-65s. There will be a similar increase of stress on the partner and tension within the family. Again, disinhibited behaviour is the most common symptom. Speech and behaviour can be erotic, and there will be increased sexual demands on the partner. However, because these difficulties in this younger age group are more readily accepted by professionals, spouses or families may be more inclined to seek help, for example, from the GP.

Functional illness

A patient who is suffering from a functional illness is more likely to have acute signs and symptoms and be admitted to a psychiatric unit. Sexual problems may be seen as the presenting problem on admission, or as part of a more complicated history.

Depressive illness: (reactive/endogenous). There may be a strong sexual component to a depressive history, usually linked to feelings of worthlessness and guilt. These may present clinically as:

1. Feelings of guilt about a sexual relationship in the distant past, perhaps extra-marital
2. Feelings of unworthiness, e.g. not being a 'good' husband or wife as they have refused to have sexual intercourse (past or present)
3. Feelings of guilt about practising 'different' forms of sexual intercourse, e.g. anal intercourse

4. Guilt stemming from an illegitimate child or extra-marital affair
5. In females, guilt over initiating a sexual relationship
6. Fixed ideas or hypochondriacal delusions, e.g. pregnancy or cancer as a result of sexual activities.

Manic-depressive psychosis. The sexual component can be similar to that described in the depressive history. In the manic phase, however, there is a more obvious sexual component. Patients will often present with disinhibited, flirtatious behaviour. Their speech content is erotic and there may be accompanying irritability of mood. As with patients with organic problems there may be increased demands on the partner, or initiation of sexual relationships.

Paranoid/paraphrenic states. Paraphrenia is a term which has been used to describe an illness characterised by delusions in a setting of well-preserved intellect and personality, in which there are often auditory hallucinations. These fixed ideas or delusions in the elderly commonly involve money and family relationships; however, sexual delusions have been seen as part of this clinical picture.

Sexual delusions which present most commonly are:

1. Pregnancy
2. Fixed idea that the patient has been sexually 'interfered with'
3. Hypochondriacal delusions, e.g. cancer of the bowel caused by anal intercourse in the past.

Schizophrenia is rarely experienced by elderly people. It is generally felt that normal sexual expression in schizophrenics is inhibited by the effects of long-term phenothiazine treatment and by abnormal patterns of social interaction.

Treatment

In looking at the relationship of sexual problems to psychiatric illness, we can see how the sexual component is part of a more complicated clinical picture. Active treatment, chemotherapy and ECT, will hopefully produce a lessening of symptoms. Residual symptoms will require more specific treatment.

THE ROLE OF THE OT IN HELPING THE ELDERLY WITH SEXUAL PROBLEMS

Any occupational therapist who has close patient contact could find herself dealing with a patient's sexual problem. A patient will often ask an occupational therapist something which he or she is too embarrassed or frightened to ask a doctor. This is not surprising as the basis of our relationship with the patient is the solution of practical problems. We must carefully consider the best way to deal with a problem which has probably taken much courage to reveal. First of all, we must come to terms with our own views of sexuality and the elderly. Society sees it as a joke — the 'dirty old man' or women who are 'mutton dressed as lamb'. If as therapists we can overcome this view and see their sexuality as an important need, then we are half-way to understanding our patients' problems.

How can an occupational therapist help?

1. Simple counselling (patient alone and/or with spouse)

Sensitive counselling about sexual problems appears to be the most effective method of helping the elderly. The greatest difficulty can be to encourage open and honest discussion on what a couple's sexual needs are. They may never, as a couple, have discussed what they find most pleasurable or satisfying.

Education may be appropriate, as the couple may feel what they are doing is wrong. Reassurance that they are 'normal' or the giving of 'permission' may be enough. The effects of anxiety should be explained, as sexual responses will often be inhibited after any major illness.

If a couple are prepared to adapt to their physical limitations and are able to communicate their needs and feelings to each other, then they can continue to enjoy mutual pleasure and satisfaction.

2. Advice on aids/positioning

The use of aids seems to be a less effective method of treatment. However, advice on positioning may be especially important for patients with recent physical disability.

Aids which may be useful are penile splints to help maintain an erection and reduce anxiety in male patients. Women may find the use of a vibrator for clitoral stimulation effective. However, few older patients respond to the use of aids.

Practical advice on positioning and techniques seems to be more effective. Simple advice, e.g. pillows under stiff or painful joints, or women taking a dominant position can take much anxiety out of the relationship. Encouragement to take time over stimulation, even if intercourse is not possible, may mean both partners can achieve orgasm without penetration. Emphasising the importance of touching and closeness may be enough to meet the couple's needs, and will reduce 'performance' anxiety.

3. Refer to specialist

As therapists we must always be aware that our elderly patients may have problems related to sexuality. Some patients may find it difficult to be open about their fears and drop heavily guarded 'hints'. If the occupational therapist feels embarrassed or unable to deal adequately with the problem, then she must refer it to someone who can deal with it. If she does not, then she will realise her patients' worst fears, and they may never find the courage to air the problem again.

CONCLUSION

In this chapter we have looked at how problems of sexuality can directly or indirectly affect elderly patients with physical or psychiatric problems. It is clear that there is a need for increased awareness of these problems by all health care professionals.

As occupational therapists we can offer advice and support on a practical basis. More importantly we must be aware that these problems may exist, but are suppressed through embarrassment or fear that the partner would be angry or embarrassed. An active sex life need not stop at 65 years of age, nor after a physical or mental illness. Therefore we must consider how illness can affect a person's sexuality, be sensitive in our approach to sexual problems, and most of all, see our patients as normal, healthy individuals.

We must be aware of our own feelings towards sexuality and any negative feelings we may have regarding sexuality as a lifelong need.

If our true concern is the quality of life of our patients or clients, then we must regard their sexuality as a pleasurable and fulfilling part of their lives.

USEFUL ADDRESS

SPOD (Sexual Problems of the Disabled)
The Diorama
14 Petro Place
LONDON NW1 4DT

REFERENCES

Bancroft J 1983 Human sexuality and its problems. Churchill Livingstone, Edinburgh

Bancroft J 1983 The treatment of sexual problems. In: Kendell R, Zealley A (eds) Companion to psychiatric studies. Churchill Livingstone, Edinburgh

Duddle C M 1982 Sex and the elderly. Geriatric Medicine January

Duddle C M 1982 Sexual problems of the elderly — some practical solutions. Geriatric Medicine, February

Fransella F 1982 Psychology for occupational therapists. The British Psychological Society and the Macmillan Press Ltd, London

Kaplan H S 1974 The new sex therapy. Brunner/Mazel, New York

Kendell R E, Zealley A K 1983 Companion to psychiatric studies, 3rd edn. Churchill Livingstone, Edinburgh

Pfeiffer E, Davis 1972 Sexual behaviour. In: Howells J G (ed) Modern perspectives in the psychiatry of old age. Churchill Livingstone, Edinburgh

White C B 1982 Sexual interest, attitudes, knowledge and sexual history in relation to sexual behaviour in the institutionalised aged. Archives of Sexual Behaviour II: 11–21

Winn R L, Newton N 1982 Sexuality in aging — a study of 106 cultures. Archives of Sexual Behaviour II: 283–98

21

Death, dying and bereavement

A. Fraser
K. Kennedy
K. Rumney

Dying is normal — a natural thing to do. . . everyone does it

Since the late Victorian era, when good drains, clean water, good food and hygiene were insisted upon, death has become increasingly the province of older members of society. Developments in medical science, public health and the control of infections enable us to live much longer. Consequently the major causes of death, apart from war and natural disasters, have become the degenerative and neoplastic diseases.

From Figure 21.1 it can be seen that more than half the deaths are caused by diseases of heart and brain, such as myocardial infarctions, strokes and cardiac failure. Approximately a quarter of all deaths are due to cancer which encompasses a large number of maligant diseases such as leukaemia and cancers of the major organs. 15% of dying people have respiratory diseases such as emphysema and bronchitis. Neurological conditions, infections and accidents make up the remaining 7%. Sudden death, as experienced in many of the circulatory disorders, does not present the medical profession with options. However, slow, lingering terminal illness challenges all professionals in the medical and paramedical field.

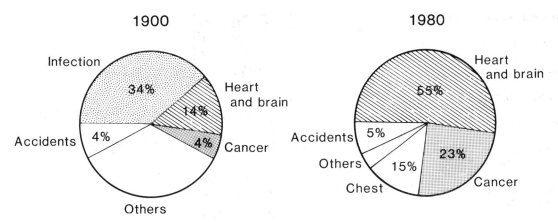

Fig. 21.1 Causes of death (UK)

Where do people die?

Since the turn of the century there has been a dramatic change in the places where people eventually die. When dying was an everyday occurrence the vast majority of people were looked after by their families before dying at home.

Figure 21.1 clearly shows that in the last few decades the numbers of deaths in hospital have more than doubled, mainly owing to family dispersal, carers being in full-time employment and the increased number of elderly people living alone.

The medical profession has somehow succeeded in convincing the general public that it is better to die in a hospital setting. This attitude is mixed up with the increased expectation that modern science ought to have some sort of answer to all or most of mankind's problems.

It is generally accepted that busy medical and surgical wards, while giving good medical and nursing care, are not the ideal places for patients nearing the ends of their lives. This is vividly described by the following dying patient:

> I huddle warm inside my corner bed,
> Watching the other patients sipping tea.
> I wonder why I'm so long getting well,
> And why it is no-one will talk to me.
>
> The nurses are so kind. They brush my hair
> On days I feel too ill to read or sew
> I smile and chat, try not to show my fear.
> They cannot tell me what I want to know

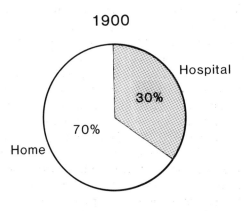

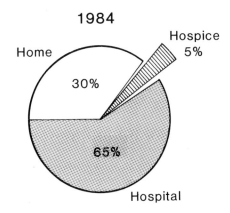

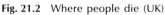

Fig. 21.2 Where people die (UK)

The visitors come in. I see their eyes
Become embarrassed as they pass my bed.
What lovely flowers they say, then hurry on
In case their faces show what can't be said.

The Chaplain passes on his weekly round
With friendly smile and calm untroubled brow
He speaks with deep sincerity of life.
I'd like to speak of death, but don't know how.

The surgeon comes, with student retinue
Mutters to Sister, deaf to my silent plea.
I want to tell this dread I feel inside
But they are all too kind to talk to me.

Twycross, 1975

DEVELOPMENT OF HOSPICE MOVEMENT

The hospice movement has grown out of the increasing need to provide palliative care to terminally ill patients of all ages. Hospices — 'places of rest for travellers' — have been in existence since the beginning of time, but the modern generation of hospices recognises the important needs, physical, emotional, social and spiritual, of the terminally ill. To date (1985) there are 96 terminal care units in the UK. Several more are in the planning stages. Many have beds for in-patients, a home care service which is an advisory service for patients and carers, and a day care unit. There is also a recognised commitment to education of medical staff, paramedicals, pastoral staff, volunteers and the general public.

Most hospices, though specialising in the care of patients with far-advanced cancer, also admit those with other conditions. Many patients, relieved of their pain and distress, can return home if there is continuing support and encouragement for themselves and their carers. Present figures show that at the hospice approximately one-third of all patients are discharged after treatment.

TERMINAL CARE FOR THE ELDERLY

Sensitive treatment of terminally ill patients is essential. They fear the unknown more than the known and every effort must be made to dispel unfounded fears. Patients rarely dread death but rather the manner of their dying.

All our efforts should be geared to the patients' need of 'dying to live' when time is short. The final weeks of life can be often a most rewarding and fulfilling period. Everyone needs reassurance that in the majority of cases, elderly patients approach death 'in control' and clear-minded.

Elderly patients, unlike younger people, tend to suffer from several disorders associated with the general wear-and-tear of life. In the terminal stage their needs are acute in nature. Good terminal care is concerned therefore with solving problems of suffering caused by disease, such as pain, constipation, diarrhoea, anorexia, dyspnoea, nausea, vomiting, pruritis, anxiety and depression.

Besides the symptoms mentioned there are many borne in silence and are thought to be too trivial to mention. When caring for the dying, nothing is trivial and attention to even the smallest problem can make a marked improvement to the patient's quality of life. The importance of pain cannot be exaggerated. Failure to control pain undermines any good work being done for the patient. Successful pain control with the skilled use of drugs enables most patients to remain pain-free, and improved methods of continuous medication, such as a battery-operated portable syringe-driver which infuses medication subcutaneously over many hours, can help patients to remain at home and mobile with only a daily nursing visit. Research into new substances that can soak up a drug and release it in a controlled dose over many hours continues apace.

Besides using drugs, nerve blocks, transcutaneous nerve stimulator and other procedures for the control of pain, the following factors are identified as capable of raising the pain threshold:

Physical	Emotional	Spiritual
Symptom relief	Empathy	Understanding
Sleep	Understanding	Companionship
Rest	Diversion	Prayer

Improved appearance	Mood elevation	Autohypnosis
Environment		Meditation
	Antidepressants	
	Anxiolytics	

Effective occupational therapy encompasses many of these factors. Recreating a sense of personal worth raises the pain threshold and the person's ability to cope with suffering.

Inevitably, in terminal care there are stresses on patient, carer and loved ones. Fay Fransella (1982) identifies the sources of distress in Table 21.1

Table 21.1 Common sources of distress

Fatally ill patient	Those who love patient
Awareness of impending death	Awareness of impending bereavement
Anticipation of loss	Anticipation of loss
Physical sequelae of disease process, e.g. tumours, lesions, nausea, incontinence, breathlessness, unpleasant smells	Empathic concern, aversion, etc
Frustration and helplessness as disease progresses	Frustration and helplessness as disease progresses
Uncertainty about the future welfare of the family	Uncertainty about the future welfare of the family
Anticipation of pain	
Empathic concern	Caring for patient, nightsitting, tiredness etc.
Changes in roles with family, friends, etc.	Changes in roles with family, friends, etc.
Changes in abilities as illness progresses	Empathic concern
Changes in appearance as illness progresses	Empathic concern, aversion, etc.
Uncertainties about dying	Empathic concern
Dying	Empathic concern
	Discovery of death, directly or indirectly
	Practicalities, funeral, etc.
	Grief
	Role changes
	Reconstruction of life

DILEMMA OF TELLING

As Dame Cicely Saunders remarks:

> The truth gradually dawns on many, even most, of the dying even when they do not ask and are not told. They accept it quietly and often gratefully but some may not wish to discuss it and we must respect their reticence.

If patients do ask, however, we have a duty to make an appropriate answer and not hide behind the excuse that 'that patient couldn't take it', because of our own anxieties or feelings of helplessness. Dr Derek Doyle (1984) states that the central issues are not in fact 'what to tell' but 'when to tell', 'whom to tell', 'how to tell' and 'who should tell'.

Very often it is the patient's general practitioner or hospital consultant who decides what to tell the patient, and in certain cases instead of the patient, the nearest relative is informed. They in turn will often withhold the information from the patient in the well-intentioned attempt to save the patient anguish. The truth, although very painful to patient, carers and medical staff, can allow free discussion of important information, mutual support and meaningful exchanges. There are many instances when keeping up a facade adds to the considerable strain on all concerned.

Since some medical treatments can in themselves cause considerable distress, many people might choose to spend the last few months of their lives in the greatest possible comfort, even if, in so doing, they live for a few weeks less. The quality of life is as important to many people as the extension of it.

A doctor is inclined to tell as little as he sees fit, both about the nature of any illness contracted and about the likely pros and cons of differing approaches towards a cure.

Even where the patients suffer from poor memory and slight confusion, every unhurried effort should be taken to discuss fully in layman's terms the information the patients need to know. Armed with this knowledge they may act as though they have not been told. This is their decision — often made through shyness, embarrassment, or being protective to others — and does not necessarily indicate ignorance of the true situation. Unless they are fully informed, however, they cannot conclude unfinished business or make unhurried, rational decisions about their own future.

Ultimately the patient's wish for care in the terminal stage must be carefully considered; but other factors such as carer support, suitability of access and nursing problems, must be taken into account.

For those who wish to be cared for at home, community help such as home helps, and/or provision of aids may be needed. Attendance at a luncheon club, day centre or hospice day care unit may be of benefit. Close teamwork by those involved in care of the patient is vital, and good communication and a flexible approach is important at all levels.

ADJUSTMENT TO APPROACHING DEATH

When all active measures cannot effect a cure, the patient will experience various emotions as impending death is faced. Many stages have been recognised in a wide range of publications, but the mnemonic DIABDA which Sylvia Poss (1981) identifies from Kübler–Ross's 1969 work, jogs the memory and contains the main points of the adjustment process. It must be stressed that people do not necessarily travel from stage to stage; and many never reach the final acceptance of death. However, it is helpful for health care professionals to recognise the adjustments which are being made by patients at this difficult time. The emotional stages described are also experienced in many other life crises, e.g. natural disasters, sudden disability such as CVA or bomb outrages, divorce and bereavement.

Denial

The sudden shock of bad news creates a sense of disbelief. 'This can't happen to me.' 'It just isn't possible that I am so ill.' 'I'm fine, never felt better.' 'I'm going on holiday next year.'

Isolation

This time of bleakness is characterised by a terrible feeling of being alone which persists even when surrounded by loved ones. 'I've never felt so lonely although I have kind visitors.' 'I feel like a cork tossing on the ocean.' 'I try to hide what I'm feeling, so that I don't upset my family.'

Anger

The person experiences feeling of anger, frustration and a rage of resentment. This is when the wish to retaliate is at its strongest. 'Why am I being punished?' 'Nothing's fair in this world.' 'Why can't you do something for me — nobody else cares.'

Bargaining

A stage of negotiation with reality that often gives people phenomenal willpower, enabling them to prolong life and achieve a certain objective. 'If only I can be spared to see my son from Australia.' 'If I could go to heaven it would be worth all this.' 'If I could see my daughter through university, I'd not mind so much.'

Depression

A time of great sadness, worry about near relatives, an overwhelming misery and a sense of weakness and fatigue. 'Why am I still alive?' 'There's nothing left to live for.' 'I'm so useless now.' 'Life isn't worth living.'

Acceptance

Now there is a sense of taking the future as it comes and of calm after the storm. 'Please take this bracelet as a memory of me.' 'Thank you for all you've done for me.' 'My wife is being so brave. I think it has helped her to

know where the insurance documents are.'
'I'm not leaving you much but I am leaving
you my love, as your heritage. May it give you
courage.'

OCCUPATIONAL THERAPY

Common aims in terminal care

1. To improve and maintain quality of life
2. To maximise the patient's abilities.

Each person will have different ideas about
what makes life worth living — the ability to
see her own street or garden, to care for a
pet, to struggle to the pub for a drink with
pals, or the chance to live dangerously. These
ideas may change from day to day as the
patient's physical condition and mood vary,
but her basic needs for life will not. The
occupational therapist works with the patient
and carers to discover what makes life worth
living at these different levels and adjusts the
treatment accordingly.

Most needs can be met by information,
advice and attention to detail.

a. Basic physical needs (e.g. warmth,
physical comfort, food). At this stage in a
person's life aids may be given purely for
comfort and conserving energy rather than
maximising independence and mobility, e.g.
duvet lighter than blankets, an ejector chair,
advice on suitable clothing, small attractive
meals for someone with a waning appetite, or
provision of a liquidiser where food is difficult
to swallow.

b. Safety and security. This area covers the
range of personal, psychological and financial
needs highlighted by ill-health. Aids may be
provided; e.g. rails, toilet frames, alarm
systems, entryphone facilities. Easy access to
doctor, grocer, lawyer and social worker may
be needed.

c. A sense of belonging and affection. At
this time of adjustment to many changes,
people can withdraw and become isolated
from those around them. Well-meaning carers
may even encourage this by denying access to
friends and neighbours, and shielding the

person from 'anything that would worry
them'. It is essential that the person maintains
social contacts for as long as possible. Sharing
in important decisions and even just giving
advice can maintain a sense of worth, usefulness and belonging. There is a fine line
between tender loving care with an objective
approach and smothering over-protection.

Often overlooked amongst the activities of
daily living is the importance of touch as a
basic form of communication; the support of
another's arm, a gentle hug or holding hands
can give a feeling of care and reassurance.
Sexual activity and physical closeness is often
shunned at this time for fear of 'catching the
disease' or being too stressful for either the
patient or partner. Any acceptable intimacy,
however, can give comfort to both where
words may be difficult.

Carers also need support and advice and
may not know how to ask for it. Simple questions from the occupational therapist such as
'Who else can help you?' or 'Have you asked
them?' may help to draw them out, for as
Averil Stedeford (1984) points out, 'under
acute stress, people do not always think
clearly and tend to muddle on in isolation'.

d. Respect and self-respect. Acute awareness of failing abilities can accentuate feelings
of inadequacy and worthlessness. It is
important to recognise the need to maintain
or re-build self-esteem.

e. Self-actualisation. Occupational Therapy
can provide opportunities for new experiences, creativity and humour which can so
easily be overlooked or lost as the person's
abilities and energies decline (Maslow, 1968).

THE GENERAL ROLE OF THE
OCCUPATIONAL THERAPIST IN TERMINAL
CARE

Aims

a. To ensure that basic physical needs are
provided
b. To develop social contacts and enable
patients to give as well as receive

c. To advice and facilitate maximum independence in activities of daily living
d. To establish a close rapport with patients and actively involve them in decision-making to achieve their own goals
e. To demonstrate to patients their own capabilities
f. To maintain, improve or rebuild self-esteem by introducing tasks that are of value and worth to others
g. To improve local function: e.g. reduce oedema, improve joint range, maintain good posture
h. To assess patients' ability to return home or continue living at home
i. To alleviate over-introspection, boredom and anxiety which compounds suffering
j. To broaden interests and experiences while horizons are narrowing
k. To provide and facilitate emotional, psychological and spiritual support to patients and those who care for them by reducing tension at home and by visiting after bereavement
l. To be aware of local community support and refer patient, if necessary, to the appropriate agency
m. To continually assess the patient's physical and mental abilities.

These aims are met by assessment, treatment planning and activities.

1. Assessment

a. Assesssment of physical abilities

During prolonged illness there may be frequent form-filling and detail-giving to different medical personnel. To spare the patient further questioning in the terminal phase it is important to build up a picture of the patient from several sources. Access to the patient's files, attendance at team meetings, contact with the primary care team and initial talks with the patient will enable the occupational therapist to gather sufficient information, sparing the patient further intrusion. The patient's non-verbal cues can be as revealing as the spoken word. In an informal way through activities of daily living the occupational therapist can observe and assess physical loss, sensory loss (vision, hearing, sensation), co-ordination and work tolerance.

b. Assessment of mental abilities

Memory, concentration, motivation, perception and adaptability can be effectively assessed by specific recreational activities. Previous occupation, present interests, and the patients' attitude and understanding of their illness are all important factors.

c. Continuing assessment

The nature of terminal illness is often characterised by relapses and remissions which are unpredictable. A flexible approach will enable the occupational therapist to take into account the patient's fluctuating health, modifying activities accordingly.

2. Treatment planning

a. Planning use of aids and equipment

Correct and careful positioning of patients is of the utmost importance to make maximum use of their available energy and to eliminate unnecessary fatigue. Here patients must decide on their own priorities and may willingly accept help in one area while denying it in another; e.g. wheelchair, newspaper stand, adapted cutlery, to achieve the task in hand. However, before introducing an aid or piece of equipment the advantages must be carefully considered. In terminal illness it may not be appropriate to introduce equipment to which the patient has to adjust. It may be better in the circumstances to consider a different activity altogether — one more suited to the patient's abilities. Aids and equipment can be:
(i) facilitative — e.g. typewriter, cantilever table, trolleys, communicators for the hard of hearing, clamps, vices
(ii) supportive — e.g. correct seating, foot-

stools, gel cushions, lap cushions to prevent pressure on sensitive parts of the body.

b. Special considerations for planning activities

Listed below are some of the more common problems which an occupational therapist will need to take into consideration when planning treatment.

(i) Sore or dry mouth. This is common in terminally ill patients and is due to a number of factors. Frequent drinks are indicated for patient comfort and for easing speech. Iced drinks are especially soothing.

(ii) Diarrhoea and constipation. These conditions will certainly cause anxiety in all patients (resulting in poor concentration) and especially those who have to cope with stoma care. If a patient is observed to be in discomfort (they may not mention it), air-rings, a change of seating or an activity with more standing is indicated.

(iii) Wig and hair loss. Extra care needs to be taken during dressing and some recreational activities.

(iv) Skin sensitivity. The skin may be fragile, oversensitive and irritated. Plastic gloves should be used when working with food and certain substances such as adhesives.

(v) Nausea and vomiting. Both can be triggered off by use of perfumes and other strong smelling substances. Careful activity planning and extra ventilation may be needed when cooking, candle-making or varnishing.

(vi) Position of syringe-driver. This is important to note during patient handling.

(vii) Sleepiness and fatigue. Encourage the patients to pace themselves during activity. Many will wish to work through their fatigue and others wish to rest.

(viii) Clumsiness of hands. This may be caused by inactivity over a long period, nerve involvement, medication and other conditions such as rheumatoid arthritis. Avoid intricate activities in these circumstances.

(ix) Lack of power. Lightweight activities are indicated unless the patient wishes to complete a specific task and is willing to accept the brute force from another person. (viii and xi are often seen by the patient as impending paralysis leading to total dependence. This is not necessarily so; therefore reassurance is essential.)

(x) Dizziness. Correct support of the patient when sitting and posture positioning on movement will help to lessen this unpleasant symptom.

(xi) Dyspnoea. A well-ventilated room with a table fan can be of benefit. Sanding of wooden items may be contra-indicated in some cases. Use of strong-smelling substances should be avoided.

(xii) Excessive sweating. Activities where grip is important may be affected, e.g. canework.

3. Activities

Suggestions

A wide range of activities can be undertaken at home, hospital and in a day unit:

a. Individual activities—making jewellery, flower arranging, typing, solving crosswords, completing jigsaw puzzles, preparing software for a computer, growing plants, polishing the silver, looking at illustrated books, tidying drawers, making bird-boxes, using a camera or binoculars.

b. A complete task which is part of a larger project — preparing vegetables for a meal, making cushion covers, clerical tasks, winding wool, putting ties on gift tags, repairing children's toys, compiling questions for a quiz.

c. Group activities where there are interchangeable tasks — making a doll's house and furniture, helping with a collage (see Case history III), planning and building a model railway, making guys for a bonfire, playing percussion instruments.

Outings to places of interest are much appreciated by patients who may be housebound or have limited mobility. Birthdays and anniversaries should be celebrated in the appropriate manner.

1. ROLE OF THE OCCUPATIONAL THERAPIST IN THE COMMUNITY

The occupational therapist sees the patient and carer in their own social setting and is therefore first and foremost a visitor to the home and second an occupational therapist delivering a service. Occupational therapists should be aware that they may be one of many professional people providing care to the patient, even though they may not meet them.

Terminal Care

a. Short term. If the patient is referred in the later stages of an illness, there may be as few as one or two visits possible in which to assess, supply aids and advise on specific problems. As time may only permit a superficial relationship with patient and carer, the occupational therapist must have readily available information of local resources, and liaise with members of the primary health care team and others.

b. Long term. If the patient is already known to the occupational therapist, as in the case of someone with a progressive illness, a close relationship may have been established and the occupational therapist may be the most appropriate person to work with the patient and carer through their adjustments to face coming death.

Bereavement

a. Carers. The closeness of the relationship between the occupational therapist and carer will determine whether the bereaved person is visited after the patient's death. Making a point of personally collecting any aids on loan can allow an opportunity for a final visit if the occupational therapist wishes to say goodbye or is concerned about the carer.

b. General. Elderly people referred to the occupational therapist may have been recently bereaved. It is important that occupational therapists are able to recognise needs in this area, and where appropriate refer them to CRUSE, a local bereavement counselling service, or a social club to relieve loneliness.

Case history I

Mrs H., a 75-year-old widow, was referred to occupational therapy by her general practitioner with a request for 'toilet aids'. Her diagnosis was given as 'liver failure secondary to cirrhosis (patient does not know her diagnosis)'.

She had recently been discharged from hospital to the care of her daughter who wished to look after her for as long as possible. The daughter knew the diagnosis but did not want her mother to know.

On the first visit the occupational therapist was met at the door by the daughter who looked stressed and exhausted, and who whispered 'we don't want her to know what's wrong with her — we don't want to upset her'. The daughter, standing in the hall, then went on to explain the difficulties her mother was having, getting up from the toilet and in and out of the bath. After some persuasion, the occupational therapist was finally introduced to Mrs H. who was lying on her bed looking frail and emaciated, with a deep yellow colour to her skin. On further discussion it appeared that most of her difficulties arose from weakness and nausea on effort.

The occupational therapist decided to supply an adjustable toilet frame, bathseat and board, high-backed chair with a spring seat, bed blocks to raise the height of the bed and an adjustable canti-lever table. Time was an important factor and the aids were chosen to conserve energy and to assist the daughter in handling her frail mother with the least effort.

The aids were delivered, adjusted and installed by the occupational therapist the following day. Because of Mrs H.'s fatigue, the occupational therapist gave careful instructions to the daughter on the correct use of the aids, and so as not to tire the client further, it was decided to leave Mrs H. resting until she needed to use each item.

The next day, the occupational therapist visited to assess progress. The aids had been used successfully with beneficial results for both mother and daughter with the exception of the bathseat. The effort involved in getting from board to seat was so great, they had both decided it was enough for Mrs H. to remain sitting on the board and to be washed thoroughly by her daughter.

Over a cup of tea the daughter confessed that although her mother was so tired, she was also bored at times and this the daughter found very upsetting as she was not able to spend much time sitting with her mother. The occupational therapist suggested activities for Mrs H. that would be helpful to her daughter and give Mrs H. a feeling of usefulness. Noticing an overflowing box of photos on a bookshelf the occupational therapist suggested that Mrs H. could sort out the family photograph album—an activity which would be light-weight, and would provide an excellent opportunity to reminisce as well as doing something useful. Mrs H. agreed to this 'to please her daughter'.

The occupational therapist visited a week later to find that Mrs H. was now confined to bed. Her daughter described how her mother had spent short periods of time sorting through the photos and both had enjoyed sharing memories, thus bringing them closer together. Whereas initially, she had not wanted her mother to know she was dying, the daughter began to realise by comments made, that Mrs H. probably knew, but did not want to upset her daughter. The daughter then commented on how alike they were. She promised to contact the occupational therapist if any further aids or advice were needed. Mrs H. died two days later. The aids were returned to the occupational therapist and the case was closed.

2. ROLE OF THE OCCUPATIONAL THERAPIST IN RESIDENTIAL CARE

Roles may differ widely in residential and nursing homes with the terminally ill, but all aim to improve the quality of life. The occupational therapist may be involved in:

a. Therapeutic activities—individual or group

b. Activities of daily living—individual residents may be assessed for difficulties with bathing, toileting, dressing, eating etc.

c. General safety and suitability of home for elderly residents—providing aids and adaptations or in an advisory category only

d. Education and skill-sharing with staff covering such aspects as bathing and dressing with the disabled, lifting techniques, reality orientation, and understanding death and bereavement.

3. ROLE OF THE OCCUPATIONAL THERAPIST IN HOSPITAL

Hospital occupational therapists may work in many settings with elderly people in the terminal stages of an illness. As one occupational therapist stated 'It is rare for an elderly person to be diagnosed as terminal — they all are. It's more a question of when'. The occupational therapist works as a member of a multidisciplinary team to assess and plan a treatment programme for the patient.

Acute assessment and longer stay units

a. The occupational therapist is involved in rehabilitation, in working with the patients to improve their ability to function as independently as possible so that they can be discharged home.

b. Patients may have many admissions over a long period of time, enabling the occupational therapist to build up a strong rapport with them and their relatives. The occupational therapist may have an important role in supporting and advising the relatives throughout the patients' illness.

c. The occupational therapist may be involved in home visits when preparing the patient for discharge and may need to liaise with the community occupational therapist and other local services.

Continuous care units

Where the patient is in need of continuous care and it is apparent she will not be discharged home, the occupational therapist will be involved in improving and maintaining the quality of life, either working with groups or individually with patients.

Case history II

Mr B. was an alert, heavily built widower aged 78 years. A retired miner, he was suffering from advanced Parkinson's disease, osteoarthritis, a right-sided hemiparesis with spasticity and dysarthria, urinary incontinence and congestive cardiac failure. Mr B. lived with his 50-year-old unmarried daughter, Miss B., in a first floor flat. She was in full-time employment.

At the flat a home help attended Mr B. twice daily, 5 days a week, providing him with breakfast, lunch and hot drinks.

The community occupational therapist had been involved with the family over many years as Mr B.'s condition deteriorated. As Mr B.'s hospital admissions increased, close partnership between community and hospital occupational therapists became vital.

Initially, Mr B. was admitted to hospital for urinary incontinence, decreasing mobility and reassessment of drug therapy. At this early stage the hospital also provided for holiday relief admissions.

When living at home Mr B. attended the day hospital twice weekly for physiotherapy, occupational therapy, relief from social isolation, and a weekly bath. He enjoyed dominoes and other social activities there.

Mr B.'s management difficulties increased as he deteriorated further. The strain on his daughter was immense but she was resistant to the concept of 'shared care' which the hospital offered her. This would have allowed for Mr B. to be at home for four weeks and in hospital for two.

During a short hospital stay the occupational therapist provided adapted trousers and long johns which could be put on as one garment. It was decided to dispense with the wearing of pyjama trousers as incontinence and considerable sweating made their removal distressing. Miss B. was shown ways to move and dress her father more easily while Mr B. was encouraged to assist her as much as possible.

An appropriate communications board was set up with the support of the speech therapist, when staff found it difficult to understand Mr B's speech. A light-weight specially-made cushion prevented pressure sores between his knees as his spasticity increased and he became more immobile.

After a hoist was recommended by the hospital occupational therapist, Miss B., with the support of a male relative, spent time with the therapist practising and gaining confidence in hoist management and then coping with her father in the hospital under supervision. From the start Mr B. had complete faith in the hoist, being familiar with the principles involved from his working days, and actually directed his daughter. They worked together as a team with years of experience behind them.

At hospital Mr B. was encouraged to feed himself with the help of adapted cutlery, plate guard and non-slip mat. There was little drooling at this stage and although eating was messy, the activity was nevertheless encouraged.

Miss B. was an exceptional lady, totally devoted to her father, who needed to be convinced that the hospital could supply the high standard of care she expected. Gaining her confidence and trust whilst dispelling her guilt took time and care. She visited him daily after work, travelling a considerable distance by public transport, and worked for his return home. Gradually, she established a close rapport with the occupational therapist and was able to speak openly about Mr B.'s increasingly impatient and aggressive behaviour towards her.

At home, nursing aids and a laundry service were provided and a district nurse attended daily. Miss B. happily undertook the major share of caring for him, but the months of rising at 6 am to wash and dress him before going to work were taking their toll. She spoke of her social isolation which the years of selfless caring had resulted in. She shared her guilt at 'failing' with the therapist when she finally accepted shared care and then his final permanent admission to hospital. This was due to his complete immobility arising from irreducible spasticity in the lower limbs with the development of contractures and bedsores.

Tentatively at first, she responded to the therapist's encouragement to believe in her achievements and to regard her father's hospitalisation as one in which they shared his care with her. Amid her guilt, she spoke of the hoist with pleasure because it had enabled her to care for her father at home for the last 2 months. She talked of the spare time and energy that posed problems for her now. The therapist encouraged her to think more positively about her future social life and the time ahead. A considerable number of aids were removed from the home at her request.

Mr B. died after a chest infection 2 weeks later. His death was not unexpected and Miss B., though deeply grieving, found comfort in the fact that she had cared for him for so long. Throughout, the therapist was aware that those who care for their relatives most actively have a higher degree of guilt, but in time they can achieve immense comfort from their efforts which eventually facilitate the healing process.

4. THE ROLE OF THE OCCUPATIONAL THERAPIST IN A HOSPICE DAY CARE UNIT

In recent years with the world-wide development of the hospice movement there has been a growing acceptance of the important contribution which occupational therapists can bring to this area of care. They work on the wards, and with patients attending the day care unit. The occupational therapist is likely to be a co-ordinator, assessor, planner of treatment programmes and an educator to professionals and volunteers.

Co-operation between all professional staff and volunteers — e.g. hospice chaplain, physiotherapist, chiropodist, hairdresser, beautician — provides consistent support for patients and staff alike. In these small terminal care units there may be slight changes in traditional roles. All staff have to be flexible in the hospice setting, where there is no place for interdisciplinary rivalry.

In most hospices volunteers are a valuable resource and can provide the day care unit with extra help. They are likely to be trained and supported by the occupational therapist, and work with patients under supervision.

The occupational therapist provides opportunities where active participation is involved. Flexibility of programming allows for sudden fluctuation of the patient's condition, and can enable participation in a selected activity, often within a short time of dying. Patients are encouraged to report any small change in their condition. All small worries, pains and complaints are taken seriously and acted upon swiftly by medical staff in order to lessen the patient's general anxiety.

The aims of treatment will include tender loving care and in some cases a positive decision to discourage physical activity. Quick accessibility to materials and equipment is important when time is short. Reliable methods of obtaining specific items must be established.

Case history III

Dorothy, 70 years old and living on her own, was referred to the day unit after being discharged home from the hospice ward. She was suffering from advanced cancer with metastatic spread to liver and kidneys from an unknown primary. Dorothy was a business woman still running her own small company from home. During an initial visit to the ward prior to discharge the occupational therapist was able to establish contact with the patient and talk generally about her interests. On her attendance at the day unit an idea for a collage depicting all aspects of life was discussed by all patients. When completed, this would be used in a teaching resource centre. Dorothy quickly organised the ideas and took over the project. She sent all over Britain for articles to hang on 'The Tree of Life' and many visitors came to view it. Not only did she fix money onto the branches but also added coloured blobs signifying the blood, sweat and tears of making a living. Dorothy proved to be an incessant talker and was somewhat trying to other patients. The collage, fixed to a free standing screen, was positioned in the main area of the day unit. Without isolating Dorothy from other patients, this arrangement provided her with her own corner and her chatter was considerably reduced. At first she stood to work but later worked from a chair, pacing her efforts throughout the activity.

Dorothy also started to learn calligraphy with guidance from an artist, and entertained other patients with recitations, and surprised herself by enjoying a game of bingo.

Up to the time of her final admission she was attending the day unit for 3 days a week. As an in-patient she carried on attending when well enough and then in the final week of her life she handed the completed collage over to a volunteer to paint in the background.

Headstone on a London grave:

> God give me work
> until my life shall end
> And life
> till my work is done

IMMINENT DEATH

To enable the reader to support the patient and others involved in her care, it is helpful to understand the changes that occur as life draws to a close.

When death is imminent the signs are almost the same whatever the underlying cause, i.e. whether it is chest disease or cancer, heart disease or kidney failure.

Patients become weak and weary. They may not necessarily sleep much more but they often speak of overwhelming tiredness and exhaustion. The smallest movement becomes an effort, with the result that no amount of gentle encouragement will persuade them to eat or drink.

Colour rapidly fades from the face, hands become blotchy, cold and clammy, and sometimes there is slight mental confusion. Like any of us in a deep sleep the patient may mutter incoherently, jerk as if in a dream, and waken with a start, disorientated and sometimes a little frightened.

Usually the final days and hours of life are filled with a well-deserved sleep. The watching relatives know only too well that this serene sleep will end in the loss of their loved one and sometimes tend to blame drugs for what is happening. Jerking of limbs, coughing and sighing may be interpreted as 'fighting for breath'.

In the final day or so the breathing changes as the patient slips into a coma. It becomes shallow with occasional deeper sighs and then enters the final phase with even longer spells when there is no breathing at all. At this time when the patient appears to be in coma, unable to feel pain and apparently unable to respond to anything happening in the room, she will probably recognise the voice of a loved one or squeeze the hand held in hers. It is important that nothing should be said by the bedside which could in any way upset the patient, and that at all times someone should endeavour to sit by the bedside firmly holding the patient's hand.

Up to half a minute may lapse before a small breath comes, followed by a few deeper ones, only to be succeeded by another time of absolute silence until the breathing does not resume and death has come.

Many people fear they will not recognise this moment, but this is seldom the case. All colour drains from the lips, the eyes immediately lose their lustre and moisture, breathing stops, the pulse in the neck is no longer seen and a deep peace descends.

The booklet 'What to do after a death — practical advice for times of bereavement' is available at Citizens' Advice Bureaux and other government offices throughout the country. This booklet, one for England and Wales and another specifically for Scotland is a mine of practical information needed at this time.

BEREAVEMENT

'Grief is like a surgical wound — painful and ugly at first, gradually fading but still easily damaged and hurt, never disappearing and always a reminder of a time of profound shock, change and fear. Time does not heal — it only makes the scar less visible to onlookers' (Doyle 1983). Bereavement is a time of adjusting to the loss of a loved one — knots that were formed by shared experiences have to be gradually untied during the grieving process. There are sudden changes in social status, economic security, health and the whole pattern of life, when a partner or close friend dies. Elderly people have to face the loss of not only contemporaries but also of younger relatives, occasionally, even great grandchildren. All medical professionals must be aware of the factors affecting bereavement, the times of danger (see stages of grief), and possible ways of alleviating some of the suffering: they should be constantly on their guard lest they follow the trend in modern society of ignoring a person's silent grief on the false assumption that he or she seems to be coping because they are not seeking help.

Factors affecting grief outcome

1. Time to prepare for death

Sudden, unexpected death produces the most profound emotional shock and grief reaction. This reaction will lessen if the carer has spent some time looking after the patient as some of the grieving will have taken place prior to death.

2. Bereaved person's sense of usefulness in caring for the deceased

The more 'useful' the carer can be made to

feel the less will be the grief. The modern tendency to admit gravely ill people to hospital will deprive the carer of the opportunity to demonstrate their love and devotion to the patient.

3. Bereaved person's perception of personal support received

Several studies have shown that the bereaved person's perception of the support given to them is more important than the amount of support actually given.

4. Bereaved person's personality and health

Most people cope with grief in the same way that they have coped with other episodes of loss, whether of job, status or popularity. Predictably, those with dependent personalities who have leaned heavily on their lost one will intuitively seek someone else on whom to depend. The person with an inflexible, obsessional personality will find adapting to a new way of life especially difficult. It is essential to appreciate that many bereaved people will need to ventilate anger against medical staff, against God or against the patient for dying inconsiderately. It is equally important that the medical team do not defend, retaliate or attempt to rationalise, but instead that they permit an outpouring of anger, guilt and/or relief.

Features of grief

During the first months after loss, the bereaved person may experience a number of physical symptoms suffered by their dying loved one and inevitably suspect that they are to suffer a similar fate. A thorough medical examination in an understanding manner will do much to lessen anxieties. Most bereaved persons in the first few months suffer a disturbed sleep pattern with vivid dreams and bouts of profound misery. More than half will have auditory and visual hallucinations of the dead persons behaving exactly as they did in life. An explanation of these phenomena in advance, reinforcing that this is a normal aspect of bereavement saves much sadness and silent fear.

Stages of grief

Many people have described the course of grief (Kübler–Ross 1969), Parkes et al 1972; Doyle recognises five periods following loss, but bereaved people do not necessarily follow or progress through these periods, rather they can be used as a guide to understand behaviour at this time.

1. Time of relief

This follows immediately after death and usually lasts for a few days. It is characterised by happiness for the deceased ('thank goodness he will have no more suffering') together with personal relief ('I couldn't have coped much more'). There is also a sense of unreality and numbness ('I just can't take it in').

2. Time of shared realisation

This follows the funeral and usually lasts only as long as near relatives remain with the bereaved person. For a week or so they create a sense of support and acceptance and shared pain. They help with the practical problems, and sometimes try to force decisions at this time, e.g. to move house, dispose of treasured items etc., but these should be resisted.

3. Time of bleakness

There is a profound sense of loneliness, aloneness, of insecurity and self-pity with much criticism of self and of professional helpers. Friends may tell the bereaved person how well they look and this good outward appearance belies very often the anguish inside. Worries about health, finances and problems of living accumulate.

4. Time of reminiscence

This may start at three months and continue for a year or more. Reliving of the events before death and reminiscing are an attempt to recapture the happy emotions of the past. Visual and auditory hallucinations may be experienced. Most breakdowns occur around seven months after bereavement. This may be significant if an occupational therapist is visiting the bereaved person on another matter.

5. Time of resolution

The bereaved person begins to make a deliberate effort to make a fresh start as new interests, hobbies and friendships are cultivated. Anniversaries and other memorable dates are still extremely painful but this state is characterised by the expression 'life must go on'.

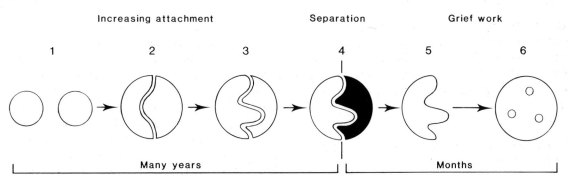

Fig. 21.3 Lifetime relationship affected by bereavement

Morbid grief reaction

Occasionally, profound grieving can lead to physical and psychological problems. The physical manifestations, such as breathlessness, weight loss or palpitations, become more severe. The psychological problems may include transient hypochondriasis, phobias, alcoholism, mania, deep depression and continued grieving. In all these states professional advice should be sought.

Figure 21.3 (Stedeford 1984) shows clearly the development of a relationship and the grief work to be done when this close involvement with another is brought to an end. The bereaved person must eventually gain a new identity and life-style. It should be noted that in most cases the griever emerges from bereavement as a 'bigger' person: broadened, rounded and matured by the experience.

Conclusion

Bereavement is an experience of change and adjustment, involving considerable suffering, but having within it the potential for continued growth.

APPENDIX I

SURVEY OF OCCUPATIONAL THERAPISTS' PERSONAL EXPERIENCES

In helping to research the background information for this chapter, a random group of occupational therapists working in the community, hospital settings and hospice care, agreed to take part in a series of informal interviews.

The discussions centred around their feelings, thoughts and amount of personal involvement allowable in working with people who are dying. Several common themes emerged, some particular to each field and some which seem common to all occupational therapists engaged in this kind of work.

Common themes

1. One of the most difficult situations for all occupational therapists interviewed was when the family did not want the patient to know their diagnosis. Occupational therapists felt that this collusion put a distance between them and their patient, and interfered with their ability to assess and realistically plan a treatment programme.

2. Most occupational therapists expressed a feeling of helplessness when they were unable to 'do any more for the patient — i.e. give aids or do anything that could be measured in practical terms. Community occupational therapists tended to discontinue visiting at this point, but hospital occupational therapists were more able to hand over to other members of the care team and at least chat to the patient, experiencing more of a feeling of continuity.

3. Patients did not often discuss thoughts or feelings about dying with the occupational therapist, but more commonly asked for information about their illness. This, however, depended on whether they regarded the occupational therapist as a 'medical person' — more common for occupational therapists in hospitals, who wear uniforms. If the patient knew her diagnosis, occupational therapists were able to share information, but if not the patient was steered towards the doctor.

4. Occupational therapists who had experienced personal loss themselves were able to share their experiences with patients and relatives, whereas occupational therapists who had little or no experience of this kind tended to be worried about 'saying the wrong thing' or feeling they had 'no right' to talk to patients about their feelings regarding loss or grief.

5. All the occupational therapists spoken to were affected in some way by at least some of their patients dying. Some described taking their feelings home with them, some had good support in the hospital or office so could leave their feelings at work, and one occupational therapist denied being affected at all while clearly showing signs of grief even while speaking.

Community occupational therapists

1. They seldom work as a member of the primary care team, i.e. GP, district nurse, health visitor, and often work in a secondary role. Particularly with these kinds of referrals, occupational therapists could easily feel they were working in isolation with little support from other members of the health care team.

2. The pressure of high case loads tended to prevent occupational therapists from becoming more deeply involved with their clients than assessing for and providing aids. One brave occupational therapist wondered whether in fact she used the excuse of the limited time to avoid getting more involved with 'difficult' clients.

3. Most community occupational therapists said they felt unskilled in initiating a discussion with the client or family about the client's imminent death, but all said they would talk about it if the client or family initiated the discussion.

4. Most occupational therapists expresssd concern about the gap in the services for the bereaved carers who not only lost their loved one but also all the contacts and support they received while the client was alive. Many used

the excuse of picking up the aids as a way of justifying another visit, but were not able to continue visiting after that.

Hospital occupational therapists

Hospital occupational therapists as a rule come in contact with dying patients more often than do community occupational therapists. At first they tend to find this upsetting, especially as in many cases they have spent some time working closely with the patient and sharing their hopes and fears for the future. Gradually, however, they develop their own personal and unique ways of dealing with these losses. One occupational therapist stated 'I always experience a sense of loss when a patient dies. I find myself looking for the patient on the ward and I'm a little shocked to see someone else so fast in their bed. But you always have to move on to other living people who need you, so you can't allow yourself to get too involved — someone else will do the grieving for the person who is gone'. Another occupational therapist described how her uncle with a terminal illness came into the hospital where she worked. She visited him frequently over a period of weeks whenever time allowed, popping into the ward during the day, usually in uniform, and until he died was concerned for him and his comfort. It was not until she attended his funeral amongst friends and relatives that she finally experienced the pain of her own loss, and was suddenly overwhelmed with grief.

A third occupational therapist said in conversation that she did not usually discuss death or dying with elderly patients whereas she did frequently with the younger ones. She tended to believe that elderly people 'knew all about it already' and therefore did not need to discuss their thoughts and fears. Even as she said this she began to wonder if this was an assumption based on her own difficulties.

Hospice occupational therapists

Although hospice occupational therapists work specifically with dying people they are no less affected by the deaths of their patients. As one occupational therapist stated 'It is impossible to prepare yourself for the death of a patient no matter how ill the person is, or how quietly they slip away. If I have established some rapport with them, the finality of their passing affects me. It is as if they are on a journey and everyone else is left behind at the station'.

Conclusion

It has previously been stated that as occupational therapists we are treating the whole person. It is impossible not to bring ourselves into this kind of work and we will be affected despite the ways we learn to protect ourselves. It is therefore essential that we develop supportive relationships with other occupational therapists and members of the care teams in which we work. We must find a healthy balance between becoming too involved with each patient to be able to let go without great pain, and developing a professional barrier that does not allow our humanness through. Being touched by our patients is their gift to us. Being able to accept this legacy and then move on is our most valuable skill, and can only improve the quality of our lives and theirs.

APPENDIX II

USEFUL SUPPORTERS AND CARE AGENCIES

General practitioners, health visitors, district nurses and social workers should always be asked for help first. Social work departments can assist with claiming benefits, occupational therapy support and practical advice. In alphabetical order:

Benevolent societies

Patients who served in the Forces and who need some financial assistance could approach SSAFA, the Earl Haig Fund and RAF Benevolent Fund.

British Red Cross Society

Look in the telephone directory — it can often help by loaning useful equipment, such as commodes, air-rings, urinals, walking aids, back-rests and wheelchairs etc.

Care — Cancer aftercare and rehabilitation society

Secretary: G.W.Poole
Lodge Cottage
Church Lane
Timbsbury
Bath
Telephone: 0761 70731

A self-help group of ex-cancer patients and their friends who help cancer patients to return to a normal life. Branches have been formed in Hastings, Huddersfield, London, Worthing and Edinburgh.

Colostomy Welfare Group

38–39 Eccleston Square
London SW1V 1PB
Telephone: 01 828 5175

Aims to help the mental, physical and spiritual adjustment of those who have had or are about to have a colostomy. All officers of the association have colostomies and can give advice from personal experience. Home and hospital visiting is an important aspect of their work. This group has branches in various parts of the country.

CRUSE — The national organisation for the widowed and their children

Cruse House
126 Sheen Road
Richmond
Surrey TW9 1UR
Telephone: 01940 4818 (9047)

Edinburgh Branch:
3 Rutland Square
Edinburgh EH1 1AS
Telephone: 031 229 6275

Offers a counselling service to help with the emotional difficulties of bereavement. A network of local branches exists throughout the country.

Friends and neighbours

Caring for a dying loved one is a testing time. It need not be a test of endurance and stamina. Housework and errands can normally be done by a friend or good neighbour, leaving energy for the task of nursing and sitting with the one who is dying.

Do not hesitate to restrict visiting. The dying rarely have the strength to entertain guests. It is the true friend who will sit in silence by the bedside of a dying person who is too weary to speak, but never too ill to enjoy the warmth of human companionship.

Hospice Information Service

St Christopher's Hospice
51/59 Lawrie Park Road
Sydenham
London SE26 6DZ

Supplies details of all hospices, home care services, symptom relief teams and pain clinics in the UK.

Ileostomy Association of Great Britain and Ireland

Central Office
1st Floor
23 Winchester Road
Basingstoke RG21 1UE
Telephone: 0256 21288

A mutual aid association for those with a permanent ileostomy. Their main object is to help people with an ileostomy resume a full life as soon as possible. They will visit patients in their home or in hospital. There are over 50 divisions throughout the country.

Leukaemia Research Fund

43 Great Ormond Street
London WC1N 3JJ
Telephone: 01 405 0101

Exists to encourage, promote and assist research into leukaemia and similar blood disorders. Supports research in over 40 centres in Britain. There are 160 local branches throughout the country. Does publish some information leaflets for patients with lymphomas and leukaemia.

The Leukaemia Society

186 Torbay Road
Rayners Lane
Harrow
Middlesex HA2 9QL
Telephone: 01 868 4107

The society was formed by parents, some of whom had leukaemic children, with the object of helping others in the same position. Membership is now open to adult sufferers and their families. Help is available in different parts of Britain.

Malcolm Sargent Cancer Fund for Children

Administrative Office
6 Sydney Street
London SW3 6PP
Telephone: 01 352 6884

Exists to give financial aid and support to children suffering from cancer, and their families, either in their own homes or in hospital. An application for a grant is made by the GP, social worker or district nurse and money is available for a wide range of needs. In addition to individual grants the fund maintains its own social workers in Belfast, Birmingham, Edinburgh, Liverpool, London, Manchester and Newcastle. May be of help to grandparents coping with children's illness.

Marie Curie Fund

Head Office
124 Sloane Street
London SW1Y 9BP
Telephone: 01 730 9157

21 Rutland Street
Edinburgh EH1 2AE

The foundation is mainly concerned with providing skilled nursing care to cancer patients. This is available through 11 residential nursing homes and a nationwide home nursing service, particularly at night to enable the carer to get a night's sleep.

The Mastectomy Association

25 Brighton Road
South Croydon
Surrey CR2 6EA
Telephone: 01 654 8643

This association is a group of women who have had a mastectomy and who are willing to talk with, and reassure other women who have recently had a breast removed. The association is nationwide but is centrally organised.

National Association of Laryngectomy Clubs

39 Eccleston Square
London SW1V 1PB
Telephone: 01 834 2857

The basic aim of the laryngectomy club is to give patients the opportunity to meet and practise speaking in a sympathetic environment. It also gives support for those about to undergo an operation or those who are recovering from surgery.

National Society for Cancer Relief

Michael Sobell House
30 Dorset Square
London NW1 6QL
Telephone: 01 402 8125

The main object is to give practical help to cancer sufferers in need. Much of this assistance takes a financial form. Special grants are given to help pay heavy debts, fuel bills, nursing and convalescent home fees, day and night nursing, fares for treatment and relatives for visiting. Application is made via the hospital social work service, social services departments and community nursing service. They also support a number of Macmillan continuing care units and their home care services.

Neighbours — see Friends

Pain clinics

Ask your General Practitioner.

Private nurses

These agencies are listed in Yellow Pages. It is important not to engage a private nurse until you have had discussions with your GP and community nurses.

Samaritans

They can be telephoned outwith a time of personal crises. It sometimes helps to talk to an anonymous voice at the other end of the phone. Number is in Telephone Directory or Yellow Pages.

Spiritual helpers

Many patients have felt little need of spiritual comfort when life was good to them. Suddenly all has changed and often people begin to think of religion — what lies ahead and what life is all about. The patient is strongly advised to take the opportunity of sharing her suffering and shaky faith with her own or local clergyman.

Stoma Advisory Service

Abbott Laboratories Ltd
Queenborough
Kent
Telephone: 07956 3371

Although run by a manufacturer this group will provide independent advice and publishes useful booklets.

Tenovus Cancer Information Centre

College Building
University Place
Splott
Cardiff CF1 1SA
Telephone: 0222 483500

This centre was set up to inform the public about cancer. It is associated with Tenovus, a group supporting cancer research.

The Compassionate Friends

25 Kingsdown Parade
Bristol B56 5UE

This is an organisation of bereaved parents who through their own experience offer help to other bereaved parents.

The Urinary Conduit Association

c/o L. Kennifick
Christie Hospital and Holt Radium Institute
Wilmslow Road
Withington
Manchester 20

Provides information for patients who have had a urinary diversion.

Voluntary sitters

There may be a scheme in your area.

Wessex Cancer Trust

Royal South Hants Hospital
Graham Road
Southampton S09 4PE
Telephone: 0703 34288 — ext 447/448

An independent charity established to raise money for cancer care and research in the Wessex region. It operates as an 'umbrella' organisation for the region, promoting research, care of cancer sufferers as well as public education.

REFERENCES

Doyle D 1983 Coping with a dying relative. MacDonald, Edinburgh

Doyle D 1984 Terminal care and bereavement. In: Barber J H (ed) General practice medicine. Churchill Livingstone, Edinburgh

Fransella F 1982 Psychology for occupational therapists. Macmillan, London

Kubler-Ross E 1969 On death and dying. Tavistock, London

Maslow A 1968 Toward a psychology of being. Van Nostrand Reinhold, New York

Parkes C M 1972 Bereavement, Tavistock London

Poss S 1981 Towards death with dignity. George Allen and Unwin, London

Saunders C M (ed) 1978 The management of terminal illness. Edward Arnold, London

Stedeford A 1984 Facing death, patients, families and professionals. William Heinemann Medical Books, London

Twycross R G 1975 The dying patient. CMF Publications, London

William C 1983 All about cancer. John Wiley, Chichester, Sussex

FURTHER READING

De Beauvoir S 1964 A very easy death. Librarie Gallimard, Paris; 1969 Penguin Books, London

Bower F L, Brown M S 1980 Nursing and the concept of loss. John Wiley, London

Flanigan K 1982 The art of the possible — occupational therapy in terminal care. British Journal of Occupational Therapy 45(8): 274–6

Holland A 1984 Occupational therapy and day care for the teminally ill 47(11): 345–8

Pincus L 1976 Death and the family. Faber & Faber, London

Sarton M 1981 A reckoning. Norton, London

22

Different types of housing and homes

I. Duncan

INTRODUCTION

Suitable housing is an important factor in the health of any individual. The young, the strong and the healthy may not spend much time reflecting on the importance of housing to health, but for various groups in society poor housing can have far-reaching consequences. The effect of poor housing on children is well documented. For older people, as well, housing is a significant factor in the maintenance of health and independence.

By the very nature of things older people tend to live in older housing. Some are living up three or four flights of stairs in the same flat into which they moved when they were first married. The children have grown up and left home long ago, and many older people are occupying houses which are far too big for their needs, and which lack modern amenities (out of 616 884 households in Scotland with at least one pensioner living in them 20 470 have no bath at all (Age Concern 1984). Old houses are hard to heat and require increasingly expensive repairs.

PROBLEMS CAUSED BY UNSUITABLE HOUSING

Whilst many old people remain independent and active for many years after retirement, there is inevitably a decrease in the pace of life. Arthritis, heart disease, obesity and other health problems may lead to impaired mobility. This results in people becoming housebound because they no longer have the energy to climb up the hill to the nearest shops, or up and down the steep stairs of the block of flats. They are then deprived of any regular exercise and also of the company and stimulation they need. Without these important elements the old person may start on the downward spiral of loneliness, apathy and ill health which will often end with an admission to hospital.

Hospital staff will be familiar with the kind of patient who is admitted because in the GP's words she has 'gone off her feet'. After a few days she will make good progress with physiotherapy, regular meals and an improved drug regime. When she is told she is ready for discharge she will become anxious. She does not want to go back to the third floor flat where she will see no-one except her twice weekly home help. She will be unable to light her coal fire and her house will be damp and cold. She will never get out to the shops and above all she will miss the company. She will once again be a prisoner in her house.

Often in a case like this, there is no suitable alternative. A quick solution is rarely possible, but in the long term, prevention of such a situation arising is better than crisis management once the damage is done.

THE IMPORTANCE OF ENVIRONMENT AND DESIGN IN HOUSING OLDER PEOPLE

In recent years much more attention has been paid, by those designing houses, to the needs of elderly people. Moreover, it is recognised that the location of the housing is almost as important as the actual design. Level ground, easy access to shops (including post office, bank, and chemist) and a good bus route are important in helping older people to retain their independence and maintain as normal a pattern of living as possible. A site just off a main road is ideal, giving access to the main facilities, whilst retaining the degree of privacy and peacefulness which older people enjoy. Where access to a main shopping area is across a busy road, the proximity of a pedestrian crossing is also important.

Most older people find a two or three room house or flat is sufficient for their needs, but the dearth of two room houses in ordinary housing stock has meant that many retired people have remained in four or five room houses. Where new houses are being built, older people are competing with young marrieds or single parents for smaller housing, and there is no doubt that more smaller houses need to be provided by local authorities.

Some local authorities are now making special efforts to provide more 'single person housing', and since 31% of elderly people live on their own (Age Concern 1984) they will benefit from the increase in specially built housing for single people. Some authorities also encourage older people living in large houses to transfer to smaller ones, thus freeing underused larger houses for families.

These kinds of initiatives help retired people to think about their housing needs before increasing age and disability make moving house difficult. Planning ahead can help to prevent many of the problems caused by unsuitable housing. Consideration can be given at leisure to the kind of house which will be suitable when age and disability begin to restrict mobility. This is the stage when local authority tenants should be indicating their need of a smaller house, and when those in rented or privately-owned housing should be putting their names down on the local authority housing list to increase their choice of future housing. One reason for this is that many housing associations specialise in housing for elderly and single people, and local authorities make 50% of the nominations for housing association property.

KIND OF HOUSING NEEDED BY OLDER PEOPLE

Some of the questions to be asked when older people are moving house are:
— Is it in a suitable location?
— Is it the right size?
— Will it be easy to maintain?
— Has it many steps or stairs and are they easy to negotiate?
— Does it have a bedroom and bathroom at ground level?
— If an upstairs flat — does it have a lift?
— Is the garden small enough to be managed easily?

Other points to be taken into consideration are proximity to relatives, or to the area where the old person previously lived. Older people may find making new friends more difficult than younger people and may not want to move too far from their circle of friends. On the other hand, if an older person chooses to move nearer to a son or daughter, then this is best done when she is still active enough to enable her to make new friends in her own age group, which may prevent her becoming too dependent on younger relatives.

THE GROWTH OF SPECIALISED HOUSING

In the last twenty years there has been a great upsurge in the provision of purpose-built housing for older people in Britain. In England this began in the 1960s, and important landmarks were the issue of Ministry of Housing and Local Government Circulars which laid down standards and designs for housing for the elderly (MHLG Circular 36/67 HMSC 1967) and 'Housing standards and Costs: Accommodation specially designed for old people' (Circular 82/69 HMSO 1969). In Scotland the growth came later following the Housing Act of 1974 and the Scottish Development Department Circular 120/75 which laid down standards for sheltered housing. This was superceded by the Scottish Housing Handbook No. 5, Housing for the Elderly (Scottish Development Department 1980).

Previously, some voluntary societies had provided 'almshouses' and some local authorities had designated some houses as 'pensioners' housing', but the real growth has been in the 1970s and 80s.

The purpose of specialist housing was to build houses appropriate to the needs of elderly people. Many of these needs have already been mentioned. In addition, a number of design features were included which would make the life of an older person easier such as (Scottish Developed Department 1980):
— Handrails on both sides of common stairs
— Bathroom doors opening outward and fitted with locks operable from outside
— Non-slip finish on bathroom floors
— Fitted hand holds beside bath and WC
— Electrical sockets at least 500 mm above floor level
— Central heating in all rooms.

The two main categories of housing incorporating these design features are (1) Amenity housing and (2) Sheltered housing.

Amenity housing

The main need of many retired people is for a small house, suitably designed and located, and easy to manage. Amenity housing fulfils this need. In addition, as the houses are usually grouped together, older people can visit their neighbours easily and become part of the community, whilst remaining independent in their own house. Many developments of amenity housing are built in a cottage-type design and are very popular. They differ from sheltered housing in that they do not provide communal facilities and there is no resident warden. When some of the tenants become frailer there may be the possibility of linking them into a nearby sheltered housing development or to a radio or telephone alarm system.

Alarm systems

The provision of alarm systems in people's own homes and in specialist housing is a growth industry and the technology is constantly improving. Earlier systems provided flashing lights outside the old person's house to raise the alarm, or alerted someone at a central point to the fact that an old person was in difficulty. More sophisticated systems now provide two-way speech communication.

One of the most important factors is the way in which help is provided in response to a call for help. Modern technology is of no use without a good back-up system to respond to the old person's needs. Some systems are linked up with sheltered housing schemes or old people's homes; others with a team of mobile wardens provided by the local authority; and yet others through the telephone to relatives or neighbours.

Sheltered housing

Design and size

Sheltered housing has all the design features described above. In addition it has some or all of the following facilities:

— A common room — which provides a focal point for social events and which has its own kitchenette attached so that teas and coffees and even full meals can be served there.
— A laundry — with automatic washing machines, dryers, a large size sink, and an ironing board. Most laundry rooms are also provided with chairs as the sheltered housing tenants often use this as a place to chat whilst waiting for their washing to be ready.
— One or more guest rooms — for the friends and relatives of tenants to stay overnight. One of these rooms may double as the room for the relief warden whilst on overnight duty.
— A bathroom with a bath suitable for assisted bathing — for those who need the services of a district nurse.
— An alarm system — which connects each flat to the warden's house. Pull cords to activate the alarm are usually provided in the living room, bedroom, bathroom and kitchen, and the warden can communicate

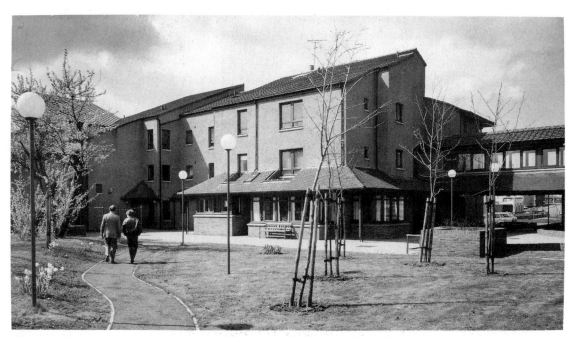

Fig. 22.1 Sheltered housing in Motherwell — features include covered walkways connecting buildings, level access, and raised flower bed

with the tenant through the two-way speech system. Pressure mats linked to the alarm system are often provided in each flat and these are placed near the entrance to the bathroom and record movement in the flat. This enables the warden to check whether tenants are up and about without disturbing their privacy.

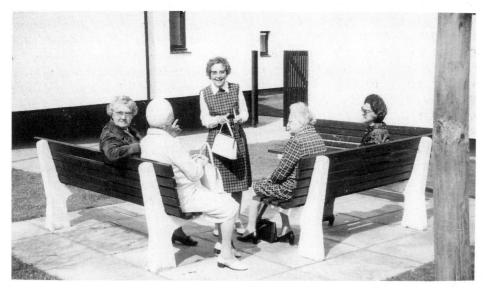

Fig. 22.2 Tenants of sheltered housing congregate in the sunshine for a chat

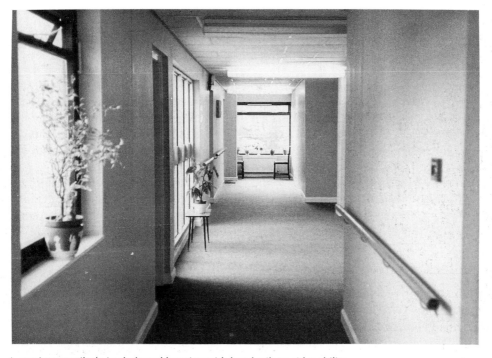

Fig. 22.3 A spacious vestibule in sheltered housing with hand rails to aid mobility

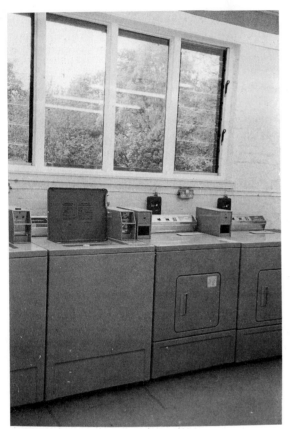

Fig. 22.4 A well-equipped laundry is an asset to sheltered housing tenants

Sheltered housing developments vary in size and may be part of a larger development which contains amenity and/or mainstream housing. Very large developments are becoming rarer, since experience has shown that these are more difficult to manage. Developments of fewer than twenty houses are expensive to run. Probably the best size for sheltered housing is between thirty and forty units.

The role of the warden

The warden plays a crucial role in sheltered housing. A good warden is the key to successful management of a development. She (or in a few cases, he) lives in a family-sized house, attached to the sheltered housing and linked to every house by the alarm system. A portable hand-set enables her to be in contact with the alarm even when she is away from her house and visiting a tenant. Her role has often been described as that of a good neighbour. As well as being on call, she keeps an unobtrusive eye on the welfare of the tenants and liaises with health, community and social services, and also tenants' relatives. She is responsible for the maintenance and upkeep of the development, alerting the housing authority to any problems which may arise. She will also help the tenants to organise social activities. The use of the common room, and the formation of a tenants' committee, is often dependent on the encouragement given to the tenants by the warden. Wardens normally have two days off a week and a relief warden is needed to cover in her absence. Some authorities use mobile wardens to respond to calls whilst a warden is off duty, and dispense with the need for a relief warden who actually sleeps in the development.

Problems experienced in sheltered housing

Many old people who move into sheltered housing receive a new lease of life, but a few do not settle because they have not fully understood the nature of sheltered housing. Those who would resent the surveillance of the warden (however unobtrusive) and do not wish to partake in the community life of the development would be better off in amenity housing.

Allocation of sheltered housing needs to be based on the fullest possible information about prospective tenants so that a reasonable balance of age and ability is kept within the sheltered housing. A development of fit and active 65 to 70 year olds will become an over-loaded development of over-eighties in fifteen years time, and therefore initial allocations should have a wide spread of age, health and ability to maintain a good balance. If the tenants are too fit the services of the warden become an unnecessary expense. If too many of the tenants are frail, then the warden is overburdened and subjected to intolerable stress. Whilst a number of frailer people can be accommodated in new developments, later on when there is a vacancy it is common practice to select someone who though needing support is not necessarily the frailest person on the list. To fill all vacancies with frail people is to add to the burdens of the warden in a steadily ageing development. It cannot be too strongly emphasised that the warden of sheltered housing is not employed to provide care for the tenants, but to call on others (relatives, home helps, community nursing services) to provide the necessary care. In an emergency the warden may provide temporary care but she should not be expected to do this except in an emergency.

Probably the most difficult problem to deal with in sheltered housing is that of coping with the mentally infirm. 10% of old people over the age of 65 suffer from some degree of mental infirmity (Gray & Isaacs 1979), and even if only a few tenants suffer from this disability on admission, others will show signs of dementia as they grow older. This can pose a problem for both wardens and other tenants. Many wardens will have had to deal with the night wanderer who rings other people's door bells in the early hours of the morning, with tenants who burn their saucepans and set off the fire alarm, and with those whose mental deterioration leads to a neglect of their personal hygiene which becomes a source of complaints from tenants. Though many wardens can cope with one or two such tenants for a short time, if they have good support from medical and domiciliary services, in the long run the old person and her relatives may have to be persuaded that more care is needed than these services can provide. The co-operation of the psychogeriatricians and the social services is of the greatest importance in this area. It is worth noting that a special sheltered housing development for the elderly mentally infirm was opened in Bromley, Kent in 1984. Experience gained there will no doubt lead to more of this kind of specialist housing.

Very sheltered housing

Very sheltered or extra-care sheltered housing is similar in design to sheltered housing with one or two additions. It may have larger communal areas, since the tenants will spend more time within the development. Similarly, a hobbies room may be included in the building to encourage activities which more able elderly people would be pursuing by going out to clubs or adult education classes. A dining room may also be provided, since the provision of at least one meal a day is one of the distinguishing marks of very sheltered housing.

In this kind of housing up to a third of the tenants may be quite frail and may need not only meals, but also a degree of personal care. This may be provided in various ways including an adequate supply of specially designated home helps or care assistants, and a special arrangement with the community nursing service which may provide a district nurse who spends some time each day in the very sheltered housing. A greater degree of warden service is also required. This may be achieved by having two resident wardens and extra relief wardens so that there are always two members of staff on call. Alternatively, wardens may be non-resident and work on a shift system, although this will subtly change the nature of the development since the wardens are no longer housed in the development and are therefore not quite so much part of the community.

Abbeyfield houses

Another option for elderly people is the group living provided by the Abbeyfield Society, which caters for people who are lonely and want somewhere to live which provides friendship, comfort and security. Abbeyfield houses are normally large family-sized houses where each resident has her own bed-sitting room, and communal meals are provided by a resident housekeeper. Volunteers provide meals on the housekeeper's day off. This level of staffing cannot provide for residents when they become frailer and more disabled. Some 'extra care' houses are now being provided with extra staffing so that people can move on from the ordinary Abbeyfield houses when they need a greater degree of personal care.

Care housing

A further housing provision for frail elderly people has been developed in Scotland, extending the Abbeyfield type of house. Care housing has many of the same characteristics as sheltered housing but is different in five significant ways:

— Each tenant occupies not a complete flat but a bed-sitting room with, if possible, a private shower and toilet
— The ratio of staff to tenants is higher than in sheltered housing
— The cost of all meals is included in the overall charge for housing
— It can consist of a number of ordinary council flats or houses which have been adapted for the purpose.

Because of its small size and higher staffing ratio it can provide accommodation for people who are past the stage of being able to manage in sheltered housing, but who do not need the intensive 24-hour care provided in an old people's home.

Care housing aims to provide housing for frail elderly people on a domestic scale, and because it is small it can be more flexible and vary with the needs of the people who live there. It is also a local resource, only taking applicants from the surrounding area and encouraging tenants to keep up their links with the community.

A development of care housing caters for between six and ten tenants who will have their own rooms which they furnish themselves and where they can maintain their own privacy. They make their own breakfast and snacks in their rooms but join together for

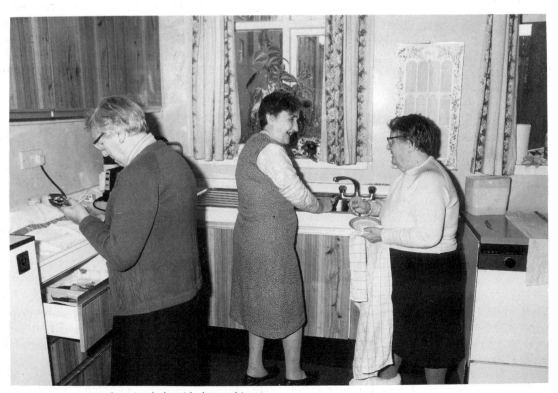

Fig. 22.5 Tenants in care housing help with the washing up

two main meals a day. There is also a communal sitting room. As in sheltered housing there is a warden and a relief warden, and home helps and the community nurses are involved. The warden has a closer relationship with the tenants since she cooks the main meals and may eat with them. Part of her job is to encourage the tenants to take as much part as possible in the running of the house by joining in household tasks and taking responsibility for decisions about the communal life together. A regular tenants' meeting at least once a month helps to encourage participation. A close link with the area social work department helps to identify problems experienced by the older people at an early stage and prevents crises which might involve the need for someone to move on to an old people's home. Many of the tenants can, as in sheltered housing, stay in care housing to the end of their lives.

OTHER ACCOMMODATION FOR OLDER PEOPLE

All the accommodation described above is essentially a housing provision and is provided by local authorities and housing associations or is privately owned. Other forms of accommodation are available and these may be divided into three categories: lodgings and family care, residential care homes and nursing homes.

Lodgings and family care

Many older people live in lodgings, and this may vary from room and board in a private household to accommodation in a small hotel or guest house. The quality of the accommodation and food varies enormously, as does the cost to the individual. The largest concentration of such accommodation is found in big cities and seaside towns. Most older people living in this kind of accommodation have arranged it themselves, but there is now an increasing involvement of local authority social work departments in recruiting special landladies for dependent elderly people to ensure that the quality of the accommodation is suitable for the needs of the old person. Such 'family placement schemes' cover a range of long- and short-term accommodation from ordinary lodgings right up to family care, where an older and frailer person may live with a family who look after her needs, and receive a special payment from social work departments for this provision of care.

Residential care homes

This traditional provision for older people has changed over the last twenty years. With the development of sheltered housing and the increase in the elderly population, old people's homes are catering for older and frailer people than in the past. Many of those going now into homes are over 80, and a significant proportion will be mentally infirm and need a degree of nursing care.

Modern purpose-built old people's homes are being designed as groups of smaller units. Five such units catering for eight to ten people may be grouped together and use communal catering facilities and staff. There are still, however, many of the older large Victorian homes built far from shops and transport and there the residents have to share rooms.

Residential care homes are run by voluntary organisations, private companies and local authorities. Applications to the former are made direct to the home or the company concerned and addresses can often be found in the Yellow Pages under Retirement homes. Local authority homes are administered by social work departments and usually operate a selection procedure based on priority need. In England these homes are often known as Part III (from Part III of the National Assistance Act 1948, and in Scotland Part IV (from Part IV of the Social Work (Scotland) Act 1968). Now that legislation is being changed, these terms will no longer be accurate and, at any rate, it is much better to refer to them as residential homes for the elderly.

All private and voluntary residential homes are required to be registered by the local social work authority (under the Residential Home Act (1984) in England and Social Work (Scotland) Act 1968 in Scotland). Registration deals with space standards, staffing and the nature of care provided, and there is an inspection of each registered home at least once a year. Information and advice on registered homes in any locality may be had from the headquarters of the social services department for that area.

Nursing homes

Most nursing homes are privately run and provide both residential and nursing care. Some specialise in various kinds of medical conditions whilst others cater for long-term geriatric patients. Some provide a high degree of nursing care whilst others are not very different from residential care homes except that they have qualified nursing staff. Nursing homes require twice yearly inspection which is regulated by Health Boards. The relevant legislation is the Residential Homes Act 1984 for England, and the Nursing Homes Registration (Scotland) Act 1938 and Nursing Registration (Scotland) Amendment Act 1981. Information about nursing homes may be had from the local health board.

PAYING FOR ACCOMMODATION AND AVAILABLE BENEFITS

All people on low incomes are entitled to housing benefit which is administered by the local housing authority. Older people may get help with both rent and rates from this source. Where an elderly person is on supplementary benefit she should apply first of all to her local social security office, even though the payments for housing will be made by the housing benefits section. At present people on supplementary benefit have their rent and rates paid in full.

In sheltered housing, as well as rent and rates, a service charge is paid to the housing authority. This covers warden service, communal facilities, upkeep of grounds etc.

The whole service charge is taken into account for the calculation of housing benefit except for any charge made for heating and lighting. Whilst the cost of sheltered housing may seem high to older people, the majority of elderly people qualify for some help from housing benefit.

For people in lodgings, family placement and care housing who qualify for supplementary benefit, the total cost of board and lodgings will be paid up to a set limit for each area. In addition to the local limit, an extra sum known as the extension is paid for every elderly person. The old person will receive in addition a personal allowance from DHSS for her personal needs.

For people in residential homes who qualify for supplementary benefit the same provisions apply except that the limit for charges is set nationally. The nursing home rate is also set nationally and is determined by adding together the rate for residential homes and the rate for the attendance allowance.

In the past, people on low incomes have not considered applying for private residential home or nursing home care because they did not have the money to pay. The change in the board and lodgings regulations at DHSS have made it possible for people on supplementary benefit to have the same range of choices as those on higher incomes, since all charges (unless they are abnormally high) can be paid by DHSS allowance.

MAINTAINING INDEPENDENCE

The range of housing options described above makes it possible for older people to choose the kind of accommodation most suitable to their needs. Unfortunately this does not always happen. It may be that the choice in the area where they live is limited by lack of suitable resources. Or they may be persuaded by anxious relatives or those who provide medical or social work care, to accept a place in a home when they do not really wish to do so.

Those advising elderly people about accommodation need to bear in mind the following points:

1. Housing is a basic human right and a 'home of one's own' is important to everyone, regardless of age or disability. It follows, therefore, that choice of suitable accommodation for elderly people must take into account the necessity for sufficient personal private space whether it be in a housing development or in a home.

2. Older people need time to make decisions and it is important that decisions to give up a house and move to other accommodation should not be rushed. In particular, irrevocable decisions to move should not be made at the time of a bereavement, when the old person is undergoing an emotional trauma which impairs his or her ability to make decisions.

3. For an old person, living alone entails an element of risk. This may be a risk which the old person is prepared to take even when others are not. Care should be exercised in persuading an old person to move to an environment where the total responsibility is taken by others. The ability to take risks and retain some responsibility for decisions relating to day-to-day living is important to us all. When we deprive old people of these rights we often deprive them of the will to live.

Ideally, all old people should have the final say in choosing suitable accommodation for themselves. They should also be encouraged to remain independent as long as they can. For almost everyone, support in one's own home is the ideal situation, for then the person can retain responsibility for at least some of the decisions of everyday living. Suitable housing is an important factor in retaining that independence.

REFERENCES AND BIBLIOGRAPHY

Age Concern 1984 Old people in Scotland; Some basic facts. Edinburgh

Butler A, Oldman C, Wright R 1979 Sheltered housing for the elderly: a critical review. University of Leeds, Department of Social Policy and Administration Research Monograph, Leeds

Butler A et al (ed) 1983 Sheltered housing for the elderly; policy, practice and the consumer. George Allen and Unwin, London

Department of the Environment 1979 Better Homes: the next priorities. HMSO, London

Gray B, Isaacs B 1979 Care of the elderly mentally infirm. Tavistock Publications, London

Greve J, Butler A, Oldman C 1981 Sheltered housing for the elderly: report on study. University of Leeds, Department of Social Policy and Administration, Leeds

Heumann L, Boldy D 1982 Housing for the elderly: planning and policy formulation in Western Europe and North America. Croom Helm, Kent

Home Life: A code of Practice for Residential Care 1984 Report of a Working Party sponsored by Department of Health and Social Security Centre for Policy and Ageing, London

Scottish Development Department 1980 Scottish Housing Handbook No. 5: Housing for the Elderly. HMSO, London

Willcocks A J (ed) 1982 The care and housing of the elderly in the community. Institute of Social Welfare, Stafford

23

The statutory agencies: the role of the community health care team

C. Mason

It has been noted elsewhere in this book that the current trend in the care of elderly people is away from the hospital into the community. In the Scottish Health Authority's document 'Priorities for the Eighties' (HMSO 1980) a recurring theme is 'the need to care for more patients in the community'. Interestingly, this conclusion is reached from two opposing standpoints.

Firstly, for economic reasons it appeals to the Health Service. To improve hospital efficiency in the use of resources, there is a drive to increase the annual throughput of patients. This is largely achieved by reducing the length of stay in hospital, with early discharge back to the community. Treating people at home rather than admitting them to hospital also makes significant savings for the acute health services and is encouraged where possible. This is very pertinent with regard to elderly people. Mention has been made in earlier chapters of studies done on the effects of hospitalisation on the elderly. The likelihood of long-term care becoming the only solution for someone originally admitted with an acute medical problem is high. In other words not only is it cheaper to treat elderly people at home but the chances of their managing to continue living in the community are much higher, thus costly long-term care is avoided.

Secondly, probably the more important standpoint for occupational therapists and other health professionals is the well-being of their clients. To that end, elderly people should be helped to stay in their own environment for as long as possible amongst their family, friends and familiar surroundings.

The belief that individuals should be encouraged and helped to maintain their identity and independence in their chosen setting, is the core philosophy of the community health care team.

The maintenance of elderly people in the community is rapidly, and perhaps not surprisingly, developing into an industry in itself. A large number of people from statutory and voluntary agencies offer a wide range of expertise, advice and practical help. This chapter deals with the team of people employed by the statutory agencies. The voluntary agencies are covered in the next chapter.

Before discussing the roles of individual members of the health care team it is appropriate to look at the context in which they work and the need for and value of teamwork in this setting. Taking the context in its broadest sense this covers the elderly person, her environment and the community in general.

Firstly, let us consider the elderly person who, in the context of this book, is the main concern of the community team. It is the needs of this individual that dictate the selection of the team. For some people a team of two, perhaps a district nurse and home help, may be all that is needed, whereas a person with a complexity of health and social problems may require help from as many as eight different professionals and services.

As with the general population many elderly people are pleasant, open to suggestion, accepting of advice and help, perhaps even distressingly passive. However, some may be cantankerous, abusive and aggressive, taking every opportunity to play one member of the team off against another. They may be from differing social groups or different ethnic origins and live in vastly different home settings with varied family help and social support.

Irrespective of their physical and social circumstances, they will still have expectations about their future life. For some this may be simply to live quietly, managing for themselves. For others it may be something as dramatic as running in a marathon. They will experience hope, excitement, disappointment, loneliness. Age is no barrier to feelings and desires, though younger people often fail to acknowledge this.

Working with elderly people in the community can be many things. It can be challenging, enjoyable, frustrating, fulfilling — the list may seem unending. Above all it is varied. The clients are living in their own surroundings and can consequently maintain their individuality. If the needs of the individual dictate the selection of the health care team involved with them, then they must also dictate the aims of each worker in the team. It follows, therefore, that the work will be varied by the range of personalities and situations encountered.

There are many benefits in working with elderly clients in the community as opposed to the hospital setting. Assessment of a person's abilities is more realistic in her own familiar surroundings. In hospital there is always an element of guesswork about whether a daily living activity will be managed better when the patient is at home — whether signs of confusion, in fact, result from strange surroundings rather than the patient's mental state. At home these factors are not relevant and a clearer picture of a person's abilities can be gained.

In the home there are usually lots of pointers to indicate how the elderly person is coping, for example, the state of the house: is it untidy, dirty? Is the person dressed if you call at midday? Is the dress appropriate? Seeing client's belongings around them will give clues about their life, their family, their hobbies and interests.

In the community the worker meets the client on a more equal footing. The authoritarian hospital model is reversed. The client is on her own home ground and in a position of control. The professional worker is, in effect, a guest in the house and must build a good relationship with the client in order to gain her co-operation in whatever treatment or action is decided upon.

At this point it may be useful to take note of a change in terminology from patient to client. The latter tends to be used more frequently in the community. It better fits the philosophy of choice and independence, since its definition in this context is an 'employer of any professional man' (Oxford Concise Dictionary). This suggests an active role rather than the patient model which, by definition, is a 'person under medical treatment', a more passive role with strong clinical overtones.

Relatively few elderly people are maintained at home solely by the efforts of the statutory agencies. The majority are reliant on family, friends, or good neighbours for care and support. Frequently those offering the help and support are elderly themselves. The daughter of an eighty-eight year old lady may well be nearing seventy herself, and in other circumstances would be considered elderly. Yet she has a full-time commitment caring for her mother. It is essential that visiting professionals acknowledge the importance of the carer and her needs. While concentrating on establishing a good working relationship with the client, it is all too easy to see the carer only as the person who lets you into the house, makes you a cup of tea while you are there and shows you out again. Yet her need to talk, perhaps about her frustrations at being tied to the elderly person or her fears about her ability or strength to carry on, is often as important to the overall success of the situation as the needs of the elderly person. Supporting the carers is an essential part of the role of the health care team.

There are of course disadvantages to working in the community. The environment is more difficult to dictate. People choose their own life-style and professionals have to accept a high level of risk if that is the client's choice. In an institutional setting, safety has to be a major consideration. If an elderly lady has always had occasional rugs lying on her floors, often no amount of persuasion will make her remove them. The professional worker can only point out the potential hazard and continually encourage removal of the rugs. At the end of the day, however, the choice lies with the old lady.

The help and support offered by family and friends is more difficult to manipulate than in a hospital setting where the actions of the staff can be dictated by the treatment team or the doctor. Through anxiety, lack of understanding, or even guilt, family or friends can be overprotective, not allowing the elderly person to try things but rather encouraging her to sit and vegetate until she really is unable to perform even basic daily living activities. It may be difficult to get a reasonable assessment of a person's abilities because she is not allowed to try. It may also be difficult because the relative or friend insists on answering all the questions and monopolising the conversation!

Professional workers must develop their interpersonal skills and their objectivity to cope with the conflicting situations they encounter. They must learn not to be judgemental, imposing their own standards, but to help people to attain and maintain their chosen life-style so far as is reasonable and possible.

Two main statutory agencies have legislative responsibilities for providing services to elderly people in the community, namely, the National Health Service and the local authority through their social work (or social services) department. Unfortunately, their divisions of responsibility while perhaps clear and logical on paper are, in practice, often less than helpful in actually meeting the needs of an individual client who cannot be labelled as a 'health problem' or a 'social problem'. Elderly people in particular cannot be categorised in this way. Their health problems are invariably inter-related with their social circumstances.

The financial stringency under which these agencies now find themselves operating has a further detrimental effect on the services provided. The need to husband shrinking resources leads to a rigid demarcation of responsibility. The client is the person who suffers, frequently falling between two stools. The variations in hierarchical structure, funding and overall aims, bring about fragmentation which must be overcome by better co-operation and joint planning. Happily this has been recognised at government levels. Papers recently produced by the Scottish Office give recommendations and guidelines for joint planning and support financing between health and social services as well as voluntary organisations. In these proposals the elderly are a key client group for joint planning.

The manifold variety of professions working in the community confuses the picture further. The development over the years of professional standards and training in various areas of care, has led to a multiplicity of professions. These are confusing to elderly people. Indeed, they are frequently confusing to the professionals themselves since there are often areas of overlap between their different roles.

Earlier in this chapter it was said that as many as eight different professionals and services may be involved with one elderly person whose health and social needs are complex. To the client some of these will be unmistakable. The chiropodist or home help, for example, will be known and remembered because on the whole their roles are clear and understood. Similarly, the district nurse, a traditionally familiar figure wearing a recognisable uniform, will be remembered. There is likely, however, to be confusion between health visitors, occupational therapists and social workers, whose tasks are less well defined and understood and who wear no distinguishing uniform to label them.

Elderly people cannot be blamed for being bewildered about who is doing what and who to tell about which problem. Each professional has an obvious responsibility to explain to the client what help she can offer. But more than this, she has a responsibility to co-operate with the other professional involved to eliminate inappropriate overlap, reduce the number of people involved and maximise the potential of the service offered to the client. Teamwork is essential if the best use is to be made of the resources and skills available.

The members of the health care team are from different professions and organisational backgrounds. To avoid confusion of approach to the problems of an elderly client it is important that they work together. They need to have a consensus over the aims of treatment so that all are working towards the same goals.

To take an extreme, though not unknown, example: a community occupational therapist, aiming to help maintain her client's independence in her own home, may be planning an expensive alteration to the house, while at the same time the client's general practitioner is in the process of arranging for a long-term hospital bed to be made available. It may well be that the occupational therapist and the general practitioner each have information, not available to the other, which has caused them to pursue divergent courses of action. With communication this contradiction of treatment aims would be avoided.

A basic component of teamwork, therefore, must be communication. There is a need to share information and ideas, not only about the client, but also about each other's roles. It is only from understanding and acceptance of another professional's role and competence that a basis of trust can develop. Interprofessional trust is essential if areas of overlap are to be eliminated.

THE MEMBERS OF THE COMMUNITY HEALTH CARE TEAM

The following section contains information on the roles of the various members of the community health care team. No hierarchical choice is implied by the order of the professions. However, since this book is essentially about occupational therapy and the care of the elderly the section on occupational therapy has been placed first and is rather fuller than other sections.

Since chiropody has a chapter to itself it has not been included in this section, though the chiropodist is, of course, a relevant member of the community team.

1. The community occupational therapist
2. The community physiotherapist
3. The district nursing service
4. The general practitioner
5. The health visitor
6. The home care service
7. The social worker
8. The speech therapist.

The community occupational therapist

In common with other members of the community team the main aim of the occupational therapist when working with elderly people is to work towards and maintain as high a level of independence as possible given the physical, emotional and social circumstances of the individual client.

Community occupational therapists are, on the whole, employed by local authorities and work from the local offices of social work (social services) departments. In some areas they are employed by health boards and may be seconded to social services or work from a health base. The job title also varies in different parts of the country. In Scotland, community occupational therapist is the accepted title whereas in other parts of the country they may be rehabilitation officers, or social workers for the disabled. Irrespective of title, though, and unless they are employed in a specialist post, it is usual to find that 60% or more of a community occupational therapist's caseload is composed of people over the age of 65.

Community occupational therapists usually accept referrals from any source including the clients themselves or their relatives. The majority of referrals do, however, come through the primary health care team of general practitioner, health visitor or district nurse. For referrals with inadequate, or non-existent, medical information, occupational therapists will, where possible, contact the client's general practitioner for more information.

Because of local variation in both the demand for occupational therapy services and the number of occupational therapists employed, the service offered and speed with which a visit is made will vary.

Maximum information about the client's condition and needs is essential to ensure that the most needy are visited most quickly.

Coming to terms with increasing frailty or with acquired disabilities resulting from such conditions as rheumatoid arthritis or stroke is a major task for elderly people as much as it is for younger folk. New limitations and frustrations are distressing to an age group where the ability to accept change is perhaps lessened. The occupational therapist can play a major role in helping her client to understand her disability, to accept the limitations that cannot be changed, to develop and maximise the abilities that remain and to minimise the handicapping affects of the disability. Sensitivity on the part of the occupational therapist is very important in helping an elderly person accept help with dignity.

The occupational therapist will first visit to assess the client. It may take several visits before she has a full picture of her client's needs. Elderly people, in particular, need time to learn to trust the occupational therapist, to admit they have difficulties and to accept help.

The initial assessment will be done with particular reference to the presenting problem. It is often the case, however, that the presenting problem is only one of a range of difficulties, ironically often a relatively minor one, perhaps because the person making the referral was only aware of the one area of difficulty or was unaware of the full range of help that might be available. The occupational therapist must be alert to this and look to identifying any needs other than the presenting problem.

Earlier in the chapter it was stated that

assessment of an elderly person in her own home is realistic. An alert occupational therapist can glean a lot of information purely by observation before ever asking the client any questions.

— Where is the house? Is it near shops, the doctor's surgery, the community centre, the chiropody clinic? Is it an area of mostly elderly people or an area with a mixed population where younger neighbours may offer help?

— What style of house is it, a mansion or a flat? What is the access like, are there flights of steps, long paths? If there is a garden what state is it in?

— If the elderly person answers the door herself, how long does it take her? What does her walking sound like — a slow shuffle, a limp? Can she open the door without difficulty or does she struggle with the lock and handle? Can she hear what you say when you introduce yourself? Does she understand?

— How mobile is she as she moves back into the house? Does she use a walking aid and does she use it safely? Does she sit down with ease or does she drop back into a chair piled high with cushions? Is she breathless from the exertion?

During an assessment it is often necessary to ask the elderly person to demonstrate how she manages to do essential daily living activities. This can be very tiring for her, but the number of activities it is necessary to have demonstrated can be minimised by transferring knowledge about one area to another. If the elderly person has difficulty getting up off her chair it is likely she will have similar problems with the WC or her bed. If she has problems bending to put her shoes on how does she manage bending for other purposes such as switching on plugs or picking up articles she has dropped?

It may well be that the client does not admit to difficulties through fear of admitting perhaps to herself that she is not able to manage. It may be though that she has forgotten for the moment that she has difficulty. From her observations the occupational therapist can suggest other areas which may be difficult.

Providing advice about easier or safer ways of doing things or, where necessary, gadgets to help, can increase an elderly person's independence in daily living activities. This in turn can prove a major boost to her morale and self-esteem. Too often elderly people are expected to accept that they will become less and less able to do things, and consequently more dependent, as they grow older. The occupational therapist, through her advice and practical help, can encourage them to realise that this is not necessarily the case.

The solution to the client's difficulties may require more major provision such as bathroom alterations, provision of a ramp and/or rails at the door or a stairlift to reach an upstairs bedroom and bathroom. This may involve liaison with salesmen, tradesmen and architects. The occupational therapist has the responsibility for ensuring that her client's needs are being catered for in the best way within the resources available. In order to do this she must be able to understand architectural plans, tradesmen's tenders and the planning process in general. Having a property adapted can be distressing for the client. The occupational therapist must support her through the whole process and keep her well informed at all stages up to and including completion of the work and the safe usage of the adaptation.

The occupational therapist will not only concentrate on the practical aspects of her client's life: her social and emotional needs are equally important.

There is questionable value in managing to dress oneself and make breakfast if for the rest of the day there is nothing to do but sit in solitude. Independence can be unattractive if it means the withdrawal of the cheery company of the home help because one can now manage better for oneself. Outlets for perhaps pursuing hobbies and interests need to be investigated. There may be clubs or classes that the elderly person could attend or it may be appropriate for someone to visit them regularly in their own home as a friend.

Many of the voluntary organisations provide valuable help in this way. The occupational therapist must be aware of the resources, both statutory and voluntary, that are available in her area in order to help her client to meet her own needs.

Liaison with and referral to other professionals and agencies is an important part of the occupational therapist's task. It may be that the client has continence problems which the district nurse could advise on or help with. Perhaps the occupational therapist feels that the client would benefit from attending a day hospital for some intensive treatment, in which case she would contact the general practitioner. Fostering good communication and developing mutual trust and understanding with other professionals working in the same locality is essential to the role of the occupational therapist as part of the wider community health care team.

The community physiotherapist

Physiotherapists have a major role to play in the maintenance of the physical functioning and mobility of elderly people.

As the trend towards care in the community grows, and thus the need to help elderly people maintain a good functional level in their own home, the community physiotherapy service is increasingly in demand. The practicality of transporting elderly people to hospital out-patient departments, often long distances from their home, has for a long time been questionable. Apart from the expense and organisational difficulties of the transport, the stress of the journey for an elderly person all too often outweighs the benefit of the treatment.

Community physiotherapists, employed by the National Health Service, may work in physiotherapy clinics or health centres or provide a domiciliary service actually visiting and treating patients in their own home. Increasingly, new health centre buildings include premises for a physiotherapist who can provide advice and treatment to the health centre patients.

In making a referral the doctor may ask for treatment for a specific purpose, but the physiotherapist has professional autonomy to decide what actual treatment to give, how frequently it should be given and when it should be terminated. It is worthy of note that physiotherapists can provide a valuable diagnostic service for musculo-skeletal problems which doctors may make use of.

Physiotherapists working in the community with elderly people will be particularly involved with their mobility. This will include the achieving and maintaining of a good range of movement and muscle power, good balance and a co-ordinated reciprocal walking pattern. This is particularly relevant following the onset of a new illness such as a stroke or Parkinson's disease. Carers can be involved profitably in treatment sessions so that they can continue the encouragement between sessions. The physiotherapist will assess for and arrange the provision of walking aids, should they be required to increase the safety of the patient's mobility.

Physiotherapists play a valuable part in prevention. Teaching people who are at risk of falling how to get up off the floor is a practical way of helping an elderly person to avoid a potentially critical situation. Teaching lifting techniques to carers prevents back problems and muscle strains; it will help them cope safely and cause less physical stress to the elderly person.

The district nursing-service

The district nursing service provides a nursing and care service to elderly people in the community. It is staffed by district nursing sisters, enrolled nurses and nursing auxiliaries.

The district nursing sister is a registered general nurse who has undergone a further period of training before working in the community. She is responsible for deciding what nursing care a patient needs, for seeing that this is provided and for evaluating the treatment and changing it or terminating it, whichever she considers is appropriate.

The district sister may have enrolled nurses

and nursing auxiliaries working with her. She will be responsible for delegating work to them and supervising that work. The enrolled nurse, who will also have done a period of further training to work in the community, will undertake the full range of nursing tasks. The nursing auxiliary can undertake only basic nursing care such as would be expected of a relative. In many areas the nursing auxiliary helps elderly people to get up in the morning, to go to bed at night or perhaps to have a bath.

The work base of the district nursing service varies from place to place. Probably the most common is the general practice, where district nurses will attend to the patients registered with the practice irrespective of where they live. However, where this is not practical, for example in rural areas or in urban areas where there are only one or two doctors in a practice, the nurses may work from a clinic, usually a children's clinic, and will cover a geographical area. Whichever base they work from they will be employed by the National Health Service, not the individual practices.

Nurses attached to general practices probably have better access, in most cases, to client records and to both formal and informal discussions with doctors and other team members such as health visitors. Nurses who work geographically do have contact with general practitioners but it is not necessarily so easy and is likely to be more formal and less frequent.

Changing trends in medical care have a direct effect on the district nursing service. The development of caring for terminally ill people at home requires the full co-operation of the nurses. In most areas, the district nursing service provides a night nursing service and, in many, a night sitting service also in order to ease the burden on caring relatives and to ensure the maximum comfort to the patients.

Increasingly general practices are employing practice nurses or have treatment room nurses attached to the practice. These nurses, though not part of the district nursing service and not usually district trained, have taken over part of the work originally done by district nurses—patients can now go to the surgery to have dressings done, stitches removed and injections given. The district nurse, as a result, can concentrate on the housebound patients, of which a large number are, of course, elderly. The general support and basic nursing care of frail elderly people in the community is increasingly a major part of her work. This will include the important area of continence, both from the health aspect of prevention and, where necessary, from the practical aspect of the management of incontinence.

The general practitioner

The general practitioner is responsible for the medical care of the patients registered with his practice. The trend towards community care gives general practitioners wider responsibility for the full care of their patients. Indeed, many people may now be treated at home who would previously have been admitted to hospital. If the family supports are willing and able to cope, people who have had, for example, a mild stroke may be nursed at home, using the full resources of the community health care team.

General practitioners usually have direct access to certain hospital diagnostic facilities such as peripheral X-ray and laboratory tests. In many areas they also have open access to physiotherapy services, either in the community or, where this is not available, in hospital departments. This allows the general practitioner to maintain control and co-ordination of their patient's treatment and allows a continuity of medical care in the community which is particularly valuable to elderly people.

The approach to the care of elderly people will vary from practice to practice and will often depend on the age structure and possibly the social structure of the practice caseload and the different pressures that they may create. Most general practitioners will endeavour to maintain some level of preventive surveillance of their elderly patients rather than just responding to patient identification of illness. This may involve occasional visits to the elderly, at risk person by the doctors themselves, or the health visitor's help may be enlisted to run screening programmes to identify those at risk.

There is no statutory requirement on general practitioners to visit their elderly patients, but on the whole they view this as a valuable preventive measure to be undertaken as and when surgery work allows.

The health visitor

The health visitor has a unique role among community health care professionals. Because her major role is in the prevention of ill health and the promotion of healthy living, a large part of her work is done with people who have no apparent health problems. This is unlike the other team members whose involvement with clients is primarily in response to some existing health or social problem.

Health visitors are qualified nurses who have undergone a further period of training. They may be attached to general practices or they may work from clinics or health centres where they provide a service to the patients of more than one doctor's practice.

Work with elderly people is only part of the health visitor's job. In many areas it is difficult for health visitors to give this work the time it merits. There is a legislative requirement that health visitors must visit all newborn babies. In their prevention role they have the responsibility for the early detection of ill health and consequently the surveillance of those members of the population at high risk. In areas of high social deprivation, work with children and their families so often has to take precedence over work with elderly people.

In some areas, in an effort to overcome this difficulty specialist health visitors have been appointed to work solely with the elderly. In other areas health visitors, using age/sex registers where they exist, are endeavouring to run screening programmes of various kinds to identify those elderly people likely to be at risk.

Liaison with and referral to other professionals is an important aspect of the health visitor's work. She must recognise the needs of the individual and arrange for help to be provided by the relevant services whether they be health board or local authority services.

Though the health visitor is a trained nurse, she does not become actively involved in the nursing care of an elderly person — that is the job of district nurse — but she will understand the person's problems and can offer support during times of stress. In this area her work may be as much with the carer(s) as with the elderly person.

The home care service

One of the most invaluable services for elderly people living in their own home is that offered by the home care service of the social work (social services) department.

The major thrust of the home care service is through the home helps, the majority of whom work with elderly people. Other services provided may vary from authority to authority but will usually include organisation of meals-on-wheels, liaison with lunch clubs, community laundry schemes, perhaps also warden schemes, nightsitters and family aide schemes.

The service offered by home helps has changed considerably in recent years and is continuing to do so. The traditional view of a home help as a charlady is no longer accurate. For many vulnerable elderly people living alone the home help is their most regular visitor. The practical tasks the individual home help undertakes will depend on the needs of her client. For the more independent people the home help may only be asked to do the heavier tasks of washing, shopping and some household cleaning while the client continues to manage her own cooking. But for others who are less able the home help will do cooking as well as cleaning, shopping and laundry. It may well be that the home help cooks not only the meal on the day she is with the client but also leaves food prepared for meals in between her visits.

But there is more that the home help offers than purely practical help. She brings news of the outside world to clients who are housebound. She can keep her client up to date with local information and interested with general chat. Being a regular visitor the home help is more able to keep an eye on her client's health, making sure medication is being taken and the client is eating properly. She can alert the other services if she feels her client's condition warrants it.

A home help is well placed to encourage her client to be as independent as is possible and practical. In this, home helps often work closely with occupational therapists. The home help can encourage her client to continue planning meals, managing her own money and doing her own cooking. Some elderly people may be able to go out but lack the confidence to do so. The home help can accompany them on short outings, perhaps to the shops, to help them realise what they are able to do. Having her bath while the home help is in the house may increase an elderly person's confidence and, in turn, her independence because she knows someone is within calling distance should she have difficulties.

The increasing number of elderly people who are mentally infirm but are maintained in the community places new demands on home helps who must develop new ways of working to support and help these people to live safely and happily at home.

Home helps undergo periods of training, the length and timing of which will vary from authority to authority. Basic subjects usually covered include budgeting, nutrition, basic first aid, mobility, home safety and security. Increasingly though, training is including such subjects as working with confused elderly people, attitudes to elderly people and reality orientation.

The hours and times that home helps visit will vary depending on the needs of the client and the home help resources available in her area. The most common timings are probably 2 or 3 hours on 2 or 3 days a week. The maximum of 7 days a week home help can be provided in some areas for people who are particularly in need. Home help hours can also be adjusted to include helping the client get up in the morning and preparing breakfast and/or the evening meal. The hours offered will be based on an assessment done by a home care organiser who is also responsible for supervising the home help. The assessment takes into account the person's needs, both physical and emotional, and the help that is already available.

Legislation allows for the local authority to levy a charge for the home care service. Most authorities do charge but the level varies: in some areas there is a flat rate; in other areas the amount paid is based on a financial assessment. Most authorities have discretional powers for dealing with people who feel they cannot afford or do not wish to pay the charges requested, but the charging system may mean that some people who would benefit from a home help receive no service.

The social worker

The role of the social worker with elderly people can take a variety of forms depending on the individual client's needs. This is a growing area of work for social workers. Work with children and families has for a long time received the major attention of social workers, much of this work being a requirement of the plethora of legislation relating to children.

However, the growing number of elderly people and the problems relating to increasing age, frailty and isolation have encouraged the development of better services for this client group.

Social workers are usually based in the Area offices of social work (social services) departments. Their work may be generic, in which case they will work with clients of all ages with a wide range of problems, or they may work specifically with elderly people. There are also social workers who work with special categories of clients, for example the blind or those with hearing problems, which will include elderly people.

Elderly clients seek help, or are referred, for

a variety of reasons, but most relate to difficulty in coping in their existing situation. The social worker may assess that the help required is purely practical, such as referral for meals-on-wheels or home help or intervention with the Department of Health and Social Security to ensure that the appropriate benefits are being received. Once these practical difficulties are dealt with, the client may then continue to manage her life for herself.

But for some elderly people their situation may be such that more drastic solutions, a move to sheltered housing or residential care for example, would seem to be the only way of easing their difficulties. The social worker must make an assessment of her client's situation, taking into account her physical and mental state, her living conditions and the supports available to her. These are likely to relate directly to the reason for the difficulties being experienced and must be taken into consideration when looking at possible solutions.

The social worker's task is not easy. She must endeavour to encourage elderly people to make their own decisions about their future rather than take the decisions for them. This can be particularly difficult when the course of action the client wishes to follow is not the one that would seem to be the best for her. It is often necessary to support clients in unsafe or unsatisfactory situations because that is their choice. It is very difficult, and rightly so, to gain compulsory admission to care for an elderly person. The social worker must liaise with other health care professionals and make referrals to other services to ensure as far as possible that her client can live as safe and satisfying a life as possible wherever she chooses to be.

If admission to residential care is the eventual outcome then the social worker has an important contribution to make. Research has shown that an elderly person's move to a residential home is more likely to be successful if they have been well prepared beforehand. Clients may feel they are giving up their identity and personal history when they give up the home in which they have lived for many years and maybe raised a family. The fear of relinquishing independence and the ability to make decisions can make admission to residential care feel like the end of the road. The social worker must help the elderly person work through these feelings to enable her to view the move to residential care as a positive, helpful step. There will be practicalities to arrange — giving up the house, disposing of the furniture, finding homes for pets. Much of this work will have to be done by the social worker if the elderly person has no family willing or able to help.

The speech therapist

Speech therapists working in the community offer a service to all ages of clients. The elderly people with whom they work usually have communication problems resulting from illnesses such as cerebrovascular accidents, Parkinson's disease or other neurological conditions.

Speech therapy in the community is often provided in health centres, but for elderly people whose mobility is restricted the speech therapist will make a home visit.

The ability to communicate with others is an essential need for most people. Whether it is for practical purposes, such as giving instructions or asking for help, or for the enjoyment of social interaction, the ability to communicate is a basic human need. The work of the speech therapist is in turn essential to those for whom communication has become difficult.

An assessment of the client's communication difficulties should be made. It is necessary to make a differential diagnosis firstly, to ensure that the communication difficulty is not a result of dementia or confusion, and secondly in order to choose the appropriate treatment to offer.

For some, that treatment will involve direct work on speech, but for others, where this is impractical, the therapist will look at developing other means of communication, for example, with faint speech amplifiers, communication aids or the use of gestures.

Speech therapists have a valuable role to play in working with other community professionals on individual cases. They can help them to understand the reasons for the speech difficulty and suggest ways of overcoming the problem, for example by the use of more gestures. Family counselling too is important. Carers need help in coping with the problems and frustrations arising from difficulties with communication.

REFERENCE

HMSO 1980 Scottish Health Authorities Priorities of the Eighties (Shape Report). HMSO, London

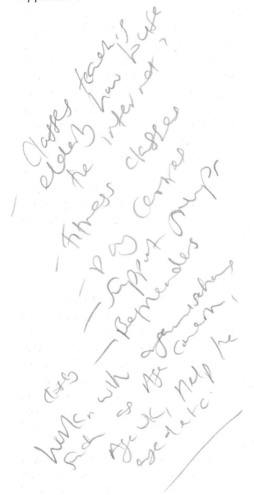

24
Voluntary organisations concerned with elderly people
G. Crosby

Voluntary organisations work in a variety of different ways to meet the needs of people over 65 years of age. They provide a service which ranges from social groups for the newly retired to 24-hour support for individuals and their families who are at risk in the community. In describing someone as elderly in this chapter we shall be considering those people over 65 years who, owing to failing health, are unable to carry out the normal everyday tasks they previously managed. For this reason they could be described as being at risk in the community. It is important to recognise that this group of people is a small percentage of the elderly population and voluntary groups offer help to many other people. Each organisation tackles an area of concern in different ways depending on its focus, for example, those organisations set up to help people with specific chronic conditions such as Parkinson's disease, Alzheimers disease and arthritis. Their membership and areas of activity are aimed to help all people suffering from the condition regardless of age. National organisations for the over-65 age group like Age Concern, Help the Aged and the Centre for Policy on Ageing are involved in campaigning for the rights of all elderly people.

Statutory provision

It is important to identify when, how and where statutory provision through the local authority should be provided. These responsibilities for the care of elderly people are in many aspects discretionary and open to varying interpretation throughout the United Kingdom. There are no hard and fast rules about the level of provision for such services as home helps, day centres and occupational therapists. It is important that the voluntary organisations enhance existing services, adding to the resources in an area rather than plugging gaps in the local authorities' provision caused by financial restraint.

The debate as to who should provide different services will no doubt continue for years to come. The controversy over the philosophy of self-help and community involvement, and the belief that help should be a right and available through statutory bodies, is politically emotive and has to be considered with great care. The present trend is to give voluntary groups every encouragement. It is of the utmost importance that liaison between statutory agencies and voluntary bodies takes place so the needs of elderly people are identified and met by well co-ordinated resources.

It is difficult to make generalisations about the role of the voluntary organisations, but in broad terms help available to elderly people can be divided into the following groups:

1. Administration of services by voluntary agencies on behalf of the local authority
2. Financial assistance
3. Support to individuals and their families
4. Day centres
5. Education of the public and government
6. Funding and volunteers — the problems

Administration of services by volunteers on behalf of the local authority

Legislation for provision of some services gives a local authority the opportunity of funding a service provision, but the actual day-to-day running of this is handed over to a voluntary organisation. An easily identifiable example of this is the meals-on-wheels service. The voluntary group involved in organising this provision varies in different parts of the country, the two most common being Age Concern and the WRVS. Under Section 10 of the Social Work Scotland Act 1968, a local authority may make available premises, equipment, vehicles etc. to carry out the functions delegated to a voluntary group. There are many benefits in using a group of volunteers for this task. It could be viewed as a driving and delivery job, but by using volunteers who genuinely wish to offer help to the community the job meets other needs. Volunteers delivering meals may be a housebound person's only contact with the outside world on any particular day. In befriending an elderly person the observant volunteer may be able to report back to the professional staff any deterioration in general health and behaviour, facilitating early involvement of the GP to avoid serious health problems.

Financial assistance

In providing any service it is necessary to define guidelines and criteria, ensuring those most in need receive the necessary help. There are always people whom the occupational therapist, district nurse or social worker feel require help, although they may not meet the exact criteria for statutory provision. The level of cut-off for services may vary from area to area depending on budgets, priorities and interpretation of legislation.

Some voluntary groups have welfare funds which help bridge gaps for those who just fail to qualify for statutory help. An example of this is the free installation of telephones for disabled and elderly people. Broadly speaking, to qualify for this provision the applicant must live alone, be totally housebound and be medically at risk. There are occasions when someone does not qualify for help under this provision but it is felt a telephone is necessary to summon help, such as an elderly person with a chronic chest condition. She may not be totally housebound but an acute attack of breathing difficulties requires the immediate attention of the doctor. In such circumstances organisations like the Chest, Stroke and Heart Association may grant all or part payment of telephone installation. Few organisations can take responsibility for regular payments. The financial outlay required would be too great for organisations whose funding depends on contributions and discretionary grants rather than guaranteed budgets.

Cancer Relief can help in this area by providing financial assistance to enhance a family's income so that additional costs incurred due to illness can be met. This could cover such items as heating costs and special diet needs, where the family do not qualify for supplementary benefit but nevertheless are experiencing hardship.

Support to individuals and their families

Support can be offered in a variety of ways: one-to-one counselling, group meetings, visiting services and additional care schemes.

Support groups tend to be small local concerns who specialise in a specific condition, helping both the carer and the individual at risk. Support offered will be determined by individual needs, general level of statutory services, geographical factors and ethnic variations.

In coping on a day-to-day basis with the effects of a condition such as rheumatoid arthritis many people gain comfort from belonging to a group where hopes and fears can be shared. They are strengthened by meeting people experiencing similar difficulties. Coupled with this understanding is the opportunity, through the organisation, to keep informed of current research into their condition, new developments in drug therapy, diets and general information through magazines and newsletters. Members of these groups benefit from being able to work, even in a small way, to raise money for research, offering help and hope for the future.

For those who care for their elderly relatives in failing health, the opportunity to meet others in a similar situation should never be underestimated. To share experiences with someone else who understands them can relieve stress and anxiety and help a carer continue with the pressures placed on her. The advice and skills of a counsellor offer an objective view of a situation which will help the carer come to terms with conditions that cannot be changed and may well deteriorate. On the other hand, the opportunity to share with someone who has been through the same experience, some of the guilt and inadequacies which go hand in hand with the restrictions and distress of watching a loved one gradually become weaker, whose personality may have altered and who is slowly deteriorating before death, is of inestimable value.

Local factors will dictate the best ways to offer support. Group meetings may be appropriate in urban areas where public transport is readily available. In a rural setting, however, it may not be possible to get people, on a regular basis, from remote farms to a central meeting place.

Telephone support offers several advantages. It is an immediate source of help, beneficial in all areas; overcoming the problems of distance, it is available to those who cannot leave their relative unattended, and relevant to the housebound individual who could not use transport even if it was available. This counsellor can be contacted at any time of the day or night in times of stress and despair. Knowing that help is available is reassuring in its own right, and experience shows that such a service is only used in emergencies or in times of dire distress.

Visiting and sitter services offer company to frail elderly people and their carers. By calling regularly they bring the outside world to the housebound, and provide practical help by allowing the carer to take a break to go shopping, meet friends and maintain some form of limited social life. This is essential, particularly for single carers, as it is so easy for them to fall into the trap of being so immersed in day-to-day care that subsequently they are left alone with no friends or interests and no idea of where to turn for help. There are some voluntary groups whose role is specifically designed to 'care' for a carer such as the Crossroads Care Attendant Scheme. This group is run locally throughout the country. Funded by grants it offers payment to the sitters but no charge is levied to the family receiving help.

Day centres

Day centres offer support to a wide variety of elderly people. Some travel independently to a centre to meet friends and have a hot meal and a chat, but these centres may also offer help to those who are 'at risk'. With this group of frail elderly people attendance may be a prophylactic measure to try and avoid the problems of hypothermia or malnutrition. The type of people, numbers and interests will determine the role of any group. General activities may include dancing, craft work, games, theatre visits and bus trips. The caring role of day centres can provide services such as bathing, hairdressing, chiropody, dentistry and physiotherapy. All these are most necessary for those people unable to use these facilities in their normal setting.

By providing such a variety of activities and services a day centre offers not only the opportunity to enhance the physical well-being of elderly people, but also the psychological benefits of belonging to a group and maintaining or making new friends. This aspect may be the only incentive an elderly person has to to get out of bed and make an effort to get dressed to go out.

Education of the public and government

Some voluntary organisations work locally, supporting elderly people in their own community. This is, however, only a part of their role. Several agencies such as Age Concern and Help the Aged, work at a national level, trying to instigate changes in policy which improve the quality of life for people over 65 years of age. They push for more acceptable retirement pensions, a real-

istic death grant, lower transport costs and better statutory services. The larger organisations often employ professional staff who link with local people, helping to set up and identify the needs of the area and taking the community's needs to national level.

The role of the staff is very varied and can encompass, as with Age Concern, a small administrative staff, training officers and development officers.

Training officers run courses, seminars and conferences to educate other professionals and volunteers working with elderly people and through this, aim to improve services and the quality of work carried out by others.

Development officers give advice to existing groups, help in setting up new groups, assist in recruiting volunteers, and encourage the local area to make use of existing statutory services. Through their publications, Age Concern and the other organisations in the voluntary sector offer information on a wide variety of topics that are of help to groups and individuals. Current lists of publications can be obtained from Age Concern.*

It is important that voluntary organisations act in a co-ordinated way with the statutory services and that they also work together. An example of this is Age Concern, Help the Aged and the Centre for Policy on Ageing. Each of these organisations has a different focus to their role, Age Concern in instigating services locally, the Centre for Policy on Ageing in providing research and information for the policy makers, and Help the Aged in fund raising here and abroad. By working together they assist one another in projects, and campaign together on certain issues nationally and internationally to achieve the aim of improving the quality of life for the elderly.

Funding and volunteers — the problems

In considering the role of voluntary groups it is important to consider the volunteers themselves. Voluntary work is a labour-intensive

* See Appendix I

job which requires individuals committed to the identified tasks. Being a volunteer is not something one can enter into on a whim. To provide a reliable support service requires commitment from each individual.

In discussing the type of people involved in voluntary work today, a changing pattern emerges. Long gone are the days when it was a middle-class housewife's pastime. The volunteers today may be retired healthy individuals with the energy and will to still feel useful to the community, the unemployed, those in sedentary office-based jobs, and members of the primary health care teams volunteering outwith their working hours. More men are volunteering but it is still a predominantly female occupation.

Some day centres invite local secondary school pupils to visit and help on a regular basis in pre-work experience, and some are involved in a small way in pre-work training schemes. Scout and Guide activities are often linked to voluntary groups and offer valuable help to various organisations.

The issue of funding can be a source of continual strain to voluntary groups, and the unpredictability can deter them from becoming involved in expensive long-term projects stretching over 10 years. Under Section 10 of the Social Work Scotland Act 1968 a Local Authority may offer a grant or loan to a Voluntary Agency, whose aim is to promote social welfare. Awards do, however, tend to be made annually and the amount given will depend on the local authority's own budget. There is a tendency, understandably, to opt for those projects whose funding may be for a maximum of 3 years rather than 10 years.

Flag days and street collections produce donations from the public. Canvassing of companies may lead to one-off or regular donations, and some companies fund publications by advertising and sponsorship.

All in all the sources of funding are varied and not predictable.

The private agency

In looking at alternative areas of help for

elderly people it is important to consider the role of private agencies offering domestic and nursing help.

As with any business they aim to provide a commodity that the consumer wants, but also the agency must make a profit at the end of the year. For people with financial resources or who chose to spend their money to gain additional help, the private agency offers the client greater opportunity to specify the type of help she receives than would be possible through the local authority or health board services.

All agencies operate their service in different ways. They all must, however, be registered under the Employment Agency Act 1973, and if they are offering a nursing service they have to be registered with the local health board. Annual inspections are made by both the Department of Employment and the health board to ensure that agencies maintain acceptable standards for their employees: customers and licences can be revoked if standards are not satisfactory.

The main areas of help covered by the private agencies are:

1. Nursing service
2. Auxiliary nursing
3. Domestic help
4. Live-in housekeepers.

Nursing services

Qualified registered general nurses and enrolled nurses are the only people who can be employed when the work includes such tasks as applying dressings, or giving medication and injections. If offering such a service an agency must comply with the health board registration procedure which lays down that all assessments for this type of work must be carried out by a registered general nurse. They are also required to offer an emergency on-call service, again manned by a registered general nurse.

Auxiliary nursing service

This is an area of work most in demand. Tasks

cover a wide range of help, from general cleaning and shopping to assistance with personal care. Total care of a client is offered, but as the employee is not a registered nurse no medical procedures can be carried out.

Domestic help

This area overlaps in many ways with the home help service provided by the local authority. The service offers general help at home and a watching eye over an elderly person, ensuring her safety and well-being and providing her with company. Many families request help on behalf of elderly relatives. Family and agency together can persuade a reluctant elderly person to have help, whereas the local authority can only offer a home help if an elderly person fully agrees.

Living-in housekeepers

Housekeepers are very hard to find on a long-term basis, and appear to pose the most difficulties for agencies. Few people want to live 24 hours a day in their place of employment, and sadly those who are interested often have problems of their own not compatible with the task or long-term commitment.

On a short-term basis it is less difficult to find employees. The short-term contract is often used to cover an elderly person's needs when her family goes on holiday or when a carer is ill. This arrangement avoids the disruption of an elderly person's admission to a home or hospital and the understandable distress of a move away from familiar surroundings.

Whatever the task, employees should always have regular contact with the agency to report back concerns and ensure the time available suits the needs of the elderly person.

To operate an agency providing home care requires sound business practice balanced by interest in and care of the employees and clients. Charges must be sufficiently high to cover overheads and produce a profit at the end of the year. Nurses must be paid Whitley Council salaries and domestic helps the equivalent of local authority rates to comply with registration and inspection requirements and trade union rules.

The task of balancing needs with making a profit is not easy, but this is a growing area of service and must be acknowledged as one that the community wants and that people from all walks of life are willing to pay for.

Conclusion

This chapter aims to provide a view of the role of voluntary groups and is very general in its approach.

In preparing it I contacted a variety of organisations and rapidly came to the conclusion that I could not do justice to their role and level of professionalism in brief paragraphs about each.

To gain detailed knowledge of any one voluntary organisation it is necessary to contact them individually. They all produce excellent publicity ranging from pamphlets outlining their role to books giving details of their origins, aims and their future plans: these aim to educate all involved with their particular target group, be it elderly people or those with a specific medical problem. There are also many excellent videos and films for information and training use.

I advise anyone involved in caring for elderly people, either as a professional or carer, to contact the voluntary groups involved with the specific needs of their patient.

Lists of voluntary organisations are available from various sources such as the Scottish Council for Community and Voluntary Organisations and the Scottish Council on Disability whose addresses I have listed in Appendix I. The Scottish Council on Disability publish a most useful list through their information service. This and their other information lists are free to disabled people and regularly updated. It provides the name of the organisation, the address and a brief description of the organisation's role. It is an excellent guide on which group to approach for help for individuals, carers and professionals seeking resources and information.

APPENDIX I

The following list of voluntary organisations is in no way comprehensive but offers a useful starting point to anyone looking for help or information whilst working with elderly people.

I recommend reference is made to the Scottish Council on Disabilities, Information Service and Information Lists, Princes House, 5 Shandwick Place, Edinburgh, EH2 4RG, 031-229-8632.

Age Concern England (National Old People's Welfare Council)
Bernard Sunley House,
60 Pitcairn Road, Mitcham,
Surrey, CR4 3LL
01-640 5431

Alzheimer's Disease Society
Bank Buildings, Fulham Broadway,
London, SW6 IEP
01-387 3177

Arthritis and Rheumatism Council
41 Eagle Street,
London, WC1R 4AR
01-405 8572

The Association of Carers
Lilac House, Medway Homes,
Balfour Road, Rochester, Kent
(0634) 813981

Association of Crossroads Care Attendant Schemes Ltd
Pat Osborne, Chief Executive Officer,
94 Coton Road, Rugby,
Warwickshire, CV21 4LN
Rugby (0788) 61536

British Association of the Hard of Hearing
7-11 Armstrong Road,
London, W3 7JL
01-743 1110/1353 Vistel 01-743 1492

British Heart Foundation
102 Gloucester Place,
London, W1H 4DH
01-935 0185

British Tinnitus Association
c/o The Royal National Institute for the Deaf,
105 Gower Street,
London WC1E 6AH
01-387 8033

Chest, Heart and Stroke Association
Tavistock House (North),
Tavistock Square,
London, WC1H 9JE
01-387 3012

Counsel and Care for the Elderly
John Hobart, General Secretary,
131 Middlesex Street,
London, E1 7JF
01-621 1624

Disablement Income Group (DIG) and Disablement Income Group Charitable Trust
Attlee House, 28 Commercial Street,
London E1 6LR
01-247 2128/6877

Health Education Council
78 New Oxford Street,
London WC1A 1AH
01-637 1881

Help the Aged
32 Dover Street,
London W1A 2AP
01-449 0972

National Council for Carers and their Elderly Dependants
29 Chilworth Mews,
London, W2 3RG
01-262 1451

National Society for Cancer Relief
Michael Sobell House,
30 Dorset Square,
London, NW1 6QL
01-402 8125

Parkinson's Disease Society of the UK Ltd
36 Portland Place,
London, W1N 3DG
01-323 1174

Royal National Institute for the Blind
224 Great Portland Street,
London W1N 6AA
01-388 1266

Women's Royal Voluntary Service
17 Old Park Lane,
London W1Y 4AJ
01-499 6040

APPENDIX II

I am most grateful to the help given to me by the agencies listed below. They all provide a most professional service and their contribution to the care of the elderly and other client groups should never be underestimated.

Age Concern
Alzheimer's Disease Society
Area 5 Action Group
Chest, Stroke and Heart Association
Church of Scotland
Crossroads Care Attendant Scheme
Edinburgh Cripple Aid Society
Edinburgh and Leith Old People Welfare Committee
Helping Hands (Private Agency)
National Society for Cancer Relief
Scottish Council on Disability
Women's Royal Voluntary Service

25

Future trends

M. Helm

In the introduction it was noted that the number of 75-year olds would continue to increase until the turn of this century.

We are aware that the vast majority of elderly people do not live in institutions, nor would it benefit them to do so. To remain independent, motivated, lucid and active it is necessary to maintain a personal daily regime of decision-making and calculated risk-taking to be free to take responsibility for one's own actions. Nevertheless, improved community support and intervention for frail elderly people will have to be increased to avoid medical and social crises and consequent inappropriate hospital referral. Innovation and imagination will be required to provide flexible and varied solutions, as each person's needs will vary.

EXISTING SERVICES AND NEW DEVELOPMENTS

Community-based treatment and care

Improve prophylactic measures

Early detection and treatment of disease/disability prevents the need for institutionalisation later. Health visitors being trained in health education are appropriate members of the primary health care team to identify on the practice age/sex register those elderly people who are vulnerable. They may be recently bereaved, or have an identified medical psychiatric or mood disorder. They may require regular visits, while those who present with few problems will require a bi-annual or annual check. The health visitor can refer to necessary agencies for appropriate services.

— Community nurses are especially helpful to elderly people with psychiatric illness. They monitor drug compliance and administer routine injections. They also advise and support relatives.
— General practitioners could learn from augmented home care schemes (Ch. 12) where elderly patients suffering from infections only have been able to stay at home owing to support from the district nurse, home care services and neighbours. This avoids further confusion from being hospitalised, and has the added benefit of a quicker recovery at home.
— More auxiliary nurses could be employed to supervise/help wash and bath elderly people requiring assistance (identified by the health visitor, hospital nurse or occupational therapist)
— More home chiropody services to keep elderly people mobile.
— More provision of hot or cold meals-on-wheels, the person providing them being an important contact.
— Volunteers who will shop for housebound elderly and who will also accompany them to the shops if necessary.
— Government should provide adequate pensions and augment these pensions for winter months to cover heating costs.

Education — improve amount and accessibility of information

— Information on how to keep fit, warm and nourished should be broadcast, televised and printed regularly in daily and weekly newspapers, with special reference to local facilities and social opportunities.
— General practitioners could have improved liaison with voluntary and statutory agencies so that printed advice for elderly people is available at all health centres.

— More training for volunteers who work with people suffering from dementia.
— All health care workers should be prepared to emphasise that we are all personally responsible for our health — and be prepared to give all small health matters consideration. Reassurance may be all that is required.
— Mobile and permanent exhibitions of aids to independence should be available, advertised and readily accessible to elderly people.
— Pre-retirement courses should be part of training at factories, businesses and hospitals to ensure that people think about future opportunities and positively plan for an active retirement.

Support for carers

— Carers who have given up work to care for an old person should be paid their previous salary.
— Counselling service for carers at health centres from those with professional experience.
— Share care — families or single people could be matched with an old person, taking her into their home periodically to give the carer some respite from continuous care/supervision.
— Sitting services should be extended to allow carers to have time for themselves and the opportunity to maintain social contacts. There are agencies like Crossroads who already provide this excellent support.
— Respite/holiday admission to hospitals and homes for the elderly could be extended if there were fewer old people permanently in residence.
— More night hospitals for dementing patients who tend to wander at night and sleep by day. The wanderers would be free to roam within secure premises, some beds/sofas being available for use when necessary.
— Day hospital hours could be lengthened to include evenings and weekends for attendance, so that carers could enjoy social

activities and days away from home on their own.

— Most day centres are for old people. At present they are only open 5 days a week like day hospitals; 7 days would be useful. Transport is a big problem and if they were open at the weekend people could bring their relatives for the day. At present, except for a few regular disabled pensioners who are brought by mini bus, only fit elderly manage to attend these clubs. More disabled elderly people need to attend.

— Laundry services for people suffering from incontinence could be advertised at health centres so that relatives under strain could avail themselves of this useful service, normally funded jointly by community nursing and social services.

— Different societies financed by charity, for example Chest, Heart & Stroke, Al Anon, Alzheimer Society, CRUSE, offer practical advice and information (see Chs. 21, 24)

Varied accommodation

— There is an urgent need for more conventional sheltered housing with live-in wardens and alarm systems.

— Extra care sheltered housing which offer meals and physical support, are also required.

— Special housing for elderly and disabled elderly people mixed in with regular housing. Ghettos for elderly or disabled people are not what is required.

— Improve insulation, sound proofing, security and heating of existing homes. Government funding should subsidise this. Living in cold damp conditions invites bronchitis and subsequent hospital admission of the old person. Cold homes confine people to one room: this leads to depression and immobility.

— Architects in housing departments should invite community occupational therapist to advise on designing homes for disabled old people with special reference to kitchens, bathrooms, and door furniture.

— Access to public buildings should include ramps and handrails, plus one or two wheelchairs for the use of frail elderly people.

— Safe Homes are required for elderly mentally frail people when day hospitals or night hospitals can no longer provide adequate care.

— Care on a long-term basis is offered by local authorities and voluntary agencies in residential homes. These should be small and homely so that residents maintain individuality and continue to take responsibility, risks and decisions in a modified way.

— Group homes for 3 or 4 elderly people with a variety of disabilities. The mobile mentally frail could live compatibly with alert physically infirm to try to keep them oriented; conversely the active people could help with others' physical problems.

Transport

— Buses could be redesigned for easy access, i.e. low bottom step with bilateral handrails and hydraulic lift to carry the person to deck level.

— Special buses for elderly/disabled/mothers with small children with conductors to help them to get on and off. These buses would stop more often than conventional ones.

— Specially designed taxis for elderly people to take them to doctor/dentist/chiropodist/hairdresser appointments or for day trips, evenings out, should be generally available.

— More forms and sources of transport to bring housebound old people to day centres, lunch clubs, church groups, or clubs run by voluntary groups like Chest, Heart & Stroke or WRVS are urgently required.

CONCLUSION

It will be argued that all these suggested necessities would be a drain on the economy, but if additional forms of support and improvement are not implemented, hospitals will be quite unable to cope with the resultant flood of elderly referrals.

Caring for the older generation must be given the proportional slice of the health budget that their numbers and vulnerability require.

Index